Globalization and Health

Routledge Studies in Health and Social Welfare

Globalization and Health

Pathways, Evidence and Policy

Edited by
Ronald Labonté, Ted Schrecker, Corinne Packer, and Vivien Runnels

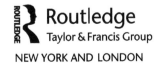

Routledge
Taylor & Francis Group

NEW YORK AND LONDON

First published 2009
by Routledge
605 Third Avenue, New York, NY 10017
4 Park Square, Milton Park, Abingdon, Oxon OX14 4RN

Routledge is an imprint of the Taylor & Francis Group, an informa business

First published in paperback 2012

Library of Congress Cataloging-in-Publication Data

Globalization and health : pathways, evidence, and policy / edited by Ronald Labonté
    . . . [et al.].
      p. ; cm. — (Routledge studies in health and social welfare ; 4)
    Includes bibliographical references and index.
    1. Globalization—Health aspects.   2. World health.   I. Labonte, Ronald N.
II. Series.

[DNLM: 1. Socioeconomic Factors.   2. World Health.   3. Internationality. WA 530.1
G5645 2009]
    RA441.G5853 2009
    362.1—dc22
    2008039911

ISBN13: 978-0-415-99334-0 (hbk)
ISBN13: 978-0-203-88102-6 (ebk)
ISBN13: 978-0-415-64805-9 (pbk)

Contents

Tables

Figures

x *Figures*

Boxes

Abbreviations

ADB	Asian Development Bank
AEC	ASEAN Economic Community
AEI	American Enterprise Institute
AfDF	African Development Fund
AFL-CIO	American Federation of Labor–Congress of Industrial Organizations
AFTA	ASEAN Free Trade Area
ARV	Antiretroviral
ASEAN	Association of Southeast Asian Nations
BI	Bamako Initiative
BMI	body mass index
CAFTA	Central America Free Trade Agreement
CAFTA-DR	Central America-Dominican Republic-United States Free Trade Agreement—also known as DR-CAFTA
CEE	Central and Eastern Europe
CIDSS	Comprehensive and Integrated Delivery of Social Services
CIPIH	Commission on Intellectual Property Rights, Innovation and Public Health
CMH	Commission on Macroeconomics and Health
Codex	Codex Alimentarius Commission

NGO-COD	Nongovernmental Organizations—Coordinating Committee on Development
CPI	Consumer Price Index
CR	Concentration Ratio
CRED	Centre for Research on the Epidemiology of Disasters
CSDH	Commission on Social Determinants of Health
CSIS	Center for Strategic and International Studies
CSO	civil society organization
CTDL	currency transaction development levy
CVD	cardiovascular disease
DAH	development assistance for health
DALYs	disability adjusted life years
DDM	Data for Decision Making
DPT3	Diphtheria, Pertussis, Tetanus vaccine
DRC	Democratic Republic of Congo
DRCD	diet-related chronic diseases
ECLAC	United Nations Economic Commission for Latin America and the Caribbean
EECA	Eastern Europe and Central Asia
EFTA	European Free Trade Association
EIS	Employment Insurance System
EPZs	export processing zones
ERAP	Enhanced Retail Access for the Poor
EU	European Union
FAO	Food and Agriculture Organization of the United Nations
FCTC	Framework Convention on Tobacco Control
FDI	foreign direct investment

FTAs	free trade agreements
G7	Group of Seven
G8	Group of Eight
GAIN	Global Alliance for Improved Nutrition
GATS	General Agreement on Trade in Services
GATT	General Agreement on Tariffs and Trade
GAVI	Global Alliance for Vaccines and Immunization
GBS	general budget support
GDP	gross domestic product
GDP/c	gross domestic product per capita
GDP-PPP	gross domestic product–purchasing power parity
GFATM	Global Fund to Fight AIDS, Tuberculosis and Malaria
GHI	global health initiatives
GHND	Globalization-Health Nexus Database
GKN	Globalization Knowledge Network
GNI	gross national income
GNP	gross national product
GPPN	Global Public Policy Network
GPPPs	Global Public-Private Partnerships
GTZ/GmbH	Gesellschaft für Technische Zusammenarbeit/ German Agency for Technical Cooperation
HHR	health human resources
HIPC	Heavily Indebted Poor Country
HMO	Health Maintenance Organization
IADB	Inter-American Development Bank
IBRD	International Bank for Reconstruction and Development

ICFTU	International Confederation of Free Trade Unions
ICT	Information and Communications Technology
IDA	International Development Association
IDB	International Development Bank
IFAD	International Fund for Agricultural Development
IFC	International Finance Corporation
IFI	international financial institution
IFPMA	International Federation of Pharmaceutical Manufacturers and Associations
IFRC	International Federation of Red Cross and Red Crescent Societies
ILO	International Labour Organization
IMASS	International Mortality and Smoking Statistics
IMF	International Monetary Fund
IMR	infant mortality rate
INGOs	International Non-Governmental Organizations
INPRES	Instruction of the President of the Republic of Indonesia
IOM	International Organization for Migration
IPRs	intellectual property rights
ISO	International Organization for Standardization
ITGA	International Tobacco Growers' Association
IUCN	International Union for the Conservation of Nature
JLI	Joint Learning Initiative (on Human Resources for Health)
KN	knowledge network
LAC	Latin American countries
LEB	life expectancy at birth
LMIC	low- and middle-income countries

Log GDP/c	Log gross domestic product per capita
MDGs	Millennium Development Goals
MDRI	Multilateral Debt Relief Initiative
MEA	Millennium Ecosystem Assessment
MEAs	Multilateral Environmental Agreements
M-EGS	Maharashtra Employment Guarantee Scheme
MENA	Middle East and North Africa
MERCOSUR	Mercado Común Sudamericano/Southern Common Market Agreement
NAFTA	North American Free Trade Agreement
NGO	non-governmental organization
NGO-COD	Non-governmental Organizations—Coordinating Committee on Development
NICs	newly industrialized countries
NPV	net present value
ODA	official development assistance
OECD	Organisation for Economic Co-operation and Development
OLS	ordinary least squares
OOPS	Outside Own Priority Setting
OPEC	Organization of the Petroleum Exporting Countries
ORI	Overall Reform Index
PAHO	Pan American Health Organization
PCT	Patent Cooperation Treaty
PEPFAR	President's Emergency Plan for AIDS Relief
PHC	primary health care
PHR	Partnerships for Health Reform

PRGF	Poverty Reduction Grant Facilities
PRS	Poverty Reduction Strategy
PRSP	Poverty Reduction Strategy Paper
PSP	Private Sector Partnerships
R&D	research and development
RTAs	Regional Trade Agreements
RUDF	Regional Urban Development Fund
SADC	Southern African Development Community
SAP	Structural Adjustment Program
SDH	social determinants of health
SEA-K	self-employment assistance-Kaunlaran
SES	socioeconomic status
SIF	Social Investment Fund
SPLT	Substantive Patent Law Treaty
SPS	Sanitary and Phytosanitary Measures
SSA	sub-Saharan Africa
SWAp	sector-wide approach
TB	Tuberculosis
TBT	Agreement on Technical Barriers to Trade
TFC	transnational food company
TI	Transnational Institute
TLPP	Temporary Livelihood Protection Program
TNC	transnational corporation
TRIPs	Agreement on Trade-Related Aspects of Intellectual Property Rights
TRT	Thai Rak Thai (Thai Love Thai)

U5MR	under-five mortality rate
UHS	Universal Health Scheme
UK DFID	United Kingdom Department for International Development
UK	United Kingdom
UN	United Nations
UNAIDS	Joint United Nations Programme on HIV/AIDS
UNCTAD	United Nations Conference on Trade and Development
UNDP	United National Development Program
UNESCO	United Nations Educational, Scientific and Cultural Organization
UNFPA	United Nations Population Fund
UNICEF	United Nations Children's Fund
UNITAID	International Drug Purchase Facility
UNRISD	United Nations Research Institute for Social Development
UPOV	International Union for the Protection of New Varieties of Plants
U.S.	United States
USA	United States of America
USAID	United States Agency for International Development
USSR	Union of Soviet Socialist Republics
WDR	World Development Report
WFP	World Food Program
WHO	World Health Organization
WHR	World Health Report
WIDER	World Institute for Development Economics Research
WIPO	World Intellectual Property Organization

WSF   World Social Forum

WTO   World Trade Organization

Acknowledgments

The content of this book is largely founded on the many months of work undertaken by the members of the Globalization Knowledge Network established as part of the WHO Commission on Social Determinants of Health. We would like to thank all the members for their impressive commitment and contributions. This work was made possible through funding provided by the International Affairs Directorate of Health Canada (Canada's national ministry of health). However, the views presented here are those of the authors and do not necessarily represent the decisions, policy, or views of Health Canada, WHO, or Commissioners.

We would like to express our deep appreciation to Chloe Davidson, Tanya Andrusieczko, Jodie Karpf, Jessica Melnik-Gauvreau, and (at earlier stages of the research) Elizabeth Venditti and Joëlle Walker at the Institute of Population Health of the University of Ottawa for their assistance in bringing this book to print. Their efforts have been indispensable.

We are grateful to the following for permission to reprint copyrighted material: Bob Sutcliffe, the Food and Agriculture Organization of the United Nations, and the World Health Organization.

1 Introduction

Globalization's Challenges to People's Health

Ronald Labonté and Ted Schrecker

INTRODUCTION: HEALTH EQUITY AND THE SOCIAL DETERMINANTS OF HEALTH

This book describes some of the findings of a research network that examined the relation between contemporary globalization and social determinants of health (SDH), with particular attention to health equity. By social determinants of health, we mean simply those conditions of life and work that make it relatively easy for some people to lead long and healthy lives, and all but impossible for others to do the same. Especially in the global frame of reference, taking SDH seriously means starting from a recognition "that many of the most devastating problems that plague the daily lives of billions of people are problems that emerge from a single, fundamental source: the consequences of poverty and inequality" (Paluzzi & Farmer, 2005, p. 12). We define health equity as "the absence of disparities in health (and in its key social determinants) that are systematically associated with social advantage/disadvantage" (Braveman & Gruskin, 2003, p. 256).

Global commitments to health equity, whether or not stated with reference to that specific phrase, are not new. In 1978, a landmark United Nations conference in Alma-Ata proposed the goal of health for all by the year 2000 (World Health Organization, 1978). Yet in 2007, despite progress toward that goal, millions of people die or are disabled each year from causes that are easily preventable or treatable (World Health Organization, 2004) at a cost that would be regarded as trivial in the high-income countries. For example, more than ten million children under the age of five die each year, 97 percent of them in low- and middle-income countries and from causes of death that are rare or now unheard-of in the industrialized world (Figure 1.1). Undernutrition—an unequivocally economic phenomenon, resulting from inadequate access to the resources for producing food, the income for purchasing it, or simply access to the right food nutrients—is an underlying cause of roughly half these deaths (Bryce, Boschi-Pinto, Shibuya, & Black, 2005), and lack of access to safe water and sanitation contributes to 1.5 million (Black, Morris, & Bryce, 2003). An expanding

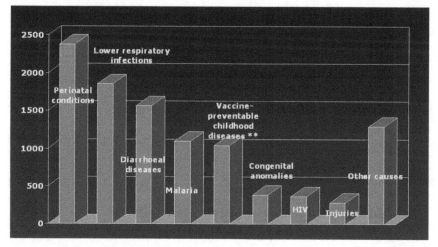

Figure 1.1   Child deaths and diseases of the poor, 2002.
Source: Data from Stein, Inoue, & Fat, 2004.
Notes: *97 percent of which occur in developing countries; ** Measles, pertussis, tetanus.

body of literature describes a similarly unequal distribution of many non-communicable diseases and injuries, with incidence and vulnerability often directly related to poverty, economic insecurity, or economic marginalization (Uauy, Albala, & Kain, 2001; Chopra, Galbraith, & Darnton-Hill, 2002; Peden, McGee, & Sharma, 2002; Nantulya, Sleet, Reich, Rosenberg, Peden, and Waxweiler, 2003; Krug, Dahlberg, Mercy, Zwi, & Lozano, 2003; Monteiro, Moura, Conde, & Popkin, 2004; Monteiro, Conde, & Popkin, 2004; Ezzati et al., 2005).

In 2001, the World Health Organization (WHO) Commission on Macroeconomics and Health turned much conventional wisdom on its head by demonstrating that health is not only a benefit of development but also is indispensable to development (Commission on Macroeconomics and Health, 2001). Illness often leads to "medical poverty traps" (Whitehead, Dahlgren, & Evans, 2001), creating a vicious circle of poor nutrition, forgone education, and still more illness—all of which undermine the economic growth that is necessary, although not sufficient, for widespread improvements in health status. Like the Alma-Ata commitment to health for all, most of the commission's recommendations, which it estimated could have saved millions of lives each year by the end of the current decade, have not been translated into policy. However, the Commission on Macroeconomics and Health did not inquire into how the economic and geopolitical dynamics of a changing international environment ("globalization") support and undermine health, or how these dynamics can be channeled to improve population health.

Knowledge Network Themes

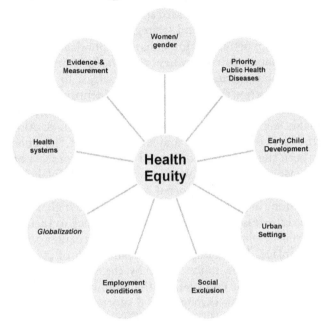

Figure 1.2 The Knowledge Networks of the WHO Commission on Social Determinants of Health.
Source: Commission on Social Determinants of Health.

In 2005, WHO established the Commission on Social Determinants of Health (CSDH), on the premise that action on SDH is the fairest and most effective way to improve and to reduce inequities in health. To inform its work, the commission established nine Knowledge Networks (KNs), charged with critically reviewing research evidence on their respective topics (Figure 1.2). Globalization was the focus of one of the KNs, and most of the chapters in this book are based on research synthesis activities undertaken during the work of the Globalization KN, as background to its final report (Labonté et al., 2007).

GLOBALIZATION AND THE GLOBAL MARKETPLACE

For purposes of its work, the Globalization KN defined globalization as "a process of greater integration within the world economy through movements of goods and services, capital, technology, and (to a lesser extent) labor, which lead increasingly to economic decisions being influenced by global conditions" (Jenkins, 2004, p. 1)—in other words, with reference to the emergence of a *global marketplace*. This definition does not assume away such phenomena as the increased speed with which information about new treatments, technologies, and strategies for health promotion can be diffused, or the opportunities for enhanced political participation and social inclusion that are offered by new, *potentially* widely accessible forms of electronic communication. However, in contrast to simply descriptive accounts of globalization that do not attempt to identify connections among superficially unrelated elements or to assign causal priority to a specific set of mechanisms (e.g., Appadurai, 1990; Pappas, Hyder, & Akhter, 2003), we adopt the view of Woodward and colleagues that "[e]conomic globalization has been the driving force behind the overall process of globalization over the last two decades" (Woodward, Drager, Beaglehole, & Lipson, 2001, p. 876). This view is supported by evidence that many dimensions and manifestations of globalization that are not at first glance economic in nature are nevertheless best explained with reference to their connections to the global marketplace and to the interests of particular powerful actors in that marketplace. For example, the globalization of culture is inseparable from, and in many instances driven by, the emergence of a network of transnational mass media corporations that dominate not only distribution but also content provision through allied sports, cultural, and consumer product industries (McChesney, 2000; Miller, 2002; McChesney & Schiller, 2003). Relatedly, global promotion of brands such as Coca-Cola and McDonald's is a cultural phenomenon but also an economic one (driven by the opportunity to expand profits and markets), even as it contributes to the "global production of diet" (Chopra & Darnton-Hill, 2004) and resultant rapid increases in obesity and its health consequences in much of the developing world, a theme explored in Chapter 10.

We date the emergence of the contemporary global marketplace from approximately 1973: the year in which various events described in Chapter 3 signaled a fundamental change in the nature of the global economic and political order. Choosing a year is less important than recognizing (a) that some time in the early 1970s the world economic and geopolitical environment changed decisively, and (b) that the changes did not "just happen" but rather were a consequence of strategic behavior by economic and political elites (Marchak, 1991; Kozul-Wright & Rayment, 2004). In the mid-1990s, a consortium of social scientists convened to assess the prospects for "sustainable democracy" noted that key Western governments have promoted an "intellectual blueprint . . . based on a belief about the virtues of markets and private ownership" with the consequence that: "For the first time in history, capitalism is being adopted as an application of a doctrine, rather than evolving as a historical process of trial and error" (Przeworski et al., 1995, p. viii). The blueprint has been promoted and implemented by national governments, in particular those of the G7,[1] individually and through multilateral institutions like the World Bank, the International Monetary Fund (IMF), and more recently the World Trade Organization (WTO) (Marchak, 1991; Przeworski et al., 1995; Gershman & Irwin, 2000; Kapur & Webb, 2000). The conditionalities associated with structural adjustment lending by the first two of these organizations, discussed later in this introductory chapter, were a primary channel of influence, establishing the primacy of market-based principles throughout much of the world. Both within and outside the Bank and the fund, networks of academic and professional elites have played an important role in the diffusion of market-oriented ideas about policy design, as shown, for example, by the work of Babb (2002) on academic economists in Mexico, Lee & Goodman (2002) on the World Bank's role in promoting health sector "reform," examined in Chapter 8, and of Brooks (2004, pp. 54–65) and Mesa-Lago & Müller (2002, pp. 709–12) on the Bank's role in promoting privatization of public pension systems, especially in Latin America.

Challenges to the perspectives that emanate from the command centers of the world economy have been many, and in some instances have been facilitated by the technological infrastructure of globalization that, while essential to the needs of its corporate users (Schiller, 1999), have proved amenable to use for quite different purposes. Perhaps the best-known illustration of the political influence of civil society organizations (CSOs) as it relates to health and globalization is their role in challenging the primacy of economic interests as defended by multilateral institutions. In the 1990s, for example, CSO activity contributed to the French government's withdrawal from negotiations on a Multilateral Agreement on Investment, and its subsequent abandonment by the Organization for Economic Cooperation and Development (Birchfield & Freyberg, 2004). In the early 2000s, CSO activism resulted in an interpretation of the Agreement on Trade-Related Aspects of Intellectual Property (TRIPs) that allows health concerns, under some circumstances, to "trump" the harmonized patent protection that was actively promoted by pharmaceutical firms during the negotiations that led to the establishment of the WTO ('t Hoen, 2002; Sell, 2003, 2004; Brysk, 2004). However, concerns remain about the practical effect of this interpretation because of informal pressures from the pharmaceutical industry and industrialized country governments and "TRIPs-plus" provisions in bilateral trade agreements, as discussed in Chapters 5 and 11. Thus, although we insist on the primacy of the economic dimensions of globalization, and on the economic elements of SDH, our view is not narrowly deterministic, and allows for the possibility of effective challenges to the interests that dominate today's global economic and political order.

The outline of the remainder of the chapter is as follows. Immediately following, we summarize some key conceptual and methodological issues in the study of globalization and health. We then address a basic controversy in this field: the extent to which globalization, as defined primarily with reference to trade liberalization, is beneficial to population health because of its contribution to economic growth, poverty reduction, and the availability of resources for public provision of services such as education and health care. Following this discussion, the implications of which are picked up in some subsequent chapters, we address a process that is simultaneously a manifestation of the increasing interconnectedness of national economies and a key "driver" of national commitment to globalization: the debt crises that affected many developing countries, often for reasons outside their control, starting in the 1970s.

We then describe two dimensions of globalization's consequences that are critical areas for future understanding of population health: implications for the form and fabric of the world's cities, and for the natural environment and the life-sustaining ecosystem services that it provides. The brevity of these discussions does not reflect their lesser importance; the lack of attention to them in the course of the operations of the Globalization Knowledge Network (GKN) was simply a manifestation of the prioritization that must be undertaken when time and resources are limited. We conclude with an outline of the book's remaining chapters.

MODELING GLOBALIZATION AND SOCIAL DETERMINANTS OF HEALTH: CONCEPTUAL AND METHODOLOGICAL ISSUES

We begin from the premise that processes comprising globalization affect access to SDH by way of multiple pathways that interact in various ways. Because of our focus on health equity (or reducing health inequities) and given that the effects of globalization on SDH are almost never uniformly distributed across populations, our concern throughout this book is on how globalization affects disparities in access to SDH. This "equity lens" approach also explains our emphasis on what might be described as negative effects of globalization: we presume (based on a large body of international evidence) that disparities in access to SDH lead to deterioration in the health status of those adversely affected, and that when the result is to increase health disparities that deterioration is unacceptable even if offset by positive impacts (e.g., improved health for the well-off) elsewhere in the economy or the society. Stated another way, we regard as prima facie undesirable changes in access to SDH that are likely to steepen the socioeconomic gradients in health that are observable in all countries, rich and poor alike (Marmot, 2006).

In a conceptual framework developed specifically for explaining social disparities in health, Diderichsen and colleagues (Diderichsen, Evans, & Whitehead, 2001, p. 14) identify "four main mechanisms—social stratification, differential exposure, differential susceptibility, and differential consequences—that play a role in generating health inequities." Globalization can affect health outcomes by way of each of these mechanisms, and

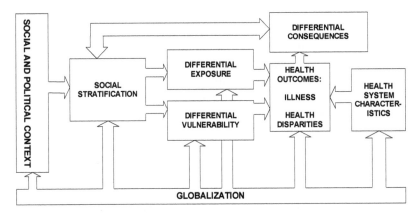

Figure 1.3 Globalization and health: A framework for analysis.
Source: Developed by the authors based on Diderichsen et al. (2001).

the authors' reference to the influence on stratification of "those central engines in society that generate and distribute power, wealth and risks" (Diderichsen et al., 2001, p. 16) is especially apposite in this context. A variant of this model was adopted for purposes of the KN; Figure 1.3 presents this variant in simplified form.

A stylized example shows the model's relevance. Import liberalization may reduce the incomes of some workers in sectors serving the domestic market, or shift workers into the informal economy, thereby affecting social stratification, differential exposure (e.g., as workers are exposed to new hazards), and differential vulnerability (e.g., as income loss means adequate nutrition or essential health care becomes harder to afford, or in the extreme cases in which women are driven to reliance on "survival sex" [Wojcicki & Malala, 2001; Wojcicki, 2002]). Increased vulnerability may also magnify the negative consequences of ill health by reducing the resources available to households to pay for health care or absorb earnings losses, increasing the chance of falling into "poverty traps" (hence the feedback loop to social stratification). Import liberalization may also reduce tariff revenues (and therefore funds available for government to use for public expenditures on income support or health care) in advance of any offsetting increases from income and consumption taxes. In countries with high levels of external debt, the need to conserve funds for repaying external creditors, perhaps by initiating or increasing user fees for health and education, may create a further constraint on social spending. (The rationale for including health systems as a separate element of the diagram now becomes apparent). Conversely, if import liberalization is matched by improved access to export markets, new employment opportunities may be created for specific groups, such as women working in export processing zones, who are thereby empowered to escape patriarchal social structures (social stratification) and reduce their economic vulnerability.

Despite the sense of simplicity created by diagrammatic representations, no single such representation can adequately capture the complexities of globalization and its influences. Globalization comprises multiple, interacting policy dynamics or processes the effects of which may be difficult if not impossible to separate. Pathways from globalization to changes in SDH are not always linear, do not operate in isolation from one another, and may involve multiple stages and feedback loops. Similarities exist with the task of analyzing causal links between environmental change and human health, which "are complex because often they are indirect, displaced in space and time, and dependent on a number of modifying forces," in the words of WHO's synthesis of the health implications of the findings of the Millennium Ecosystem Assessment project (Corvalan et al., 2005, p. 2).

It is therefore necessary to rely on evidence generated by multiple disciplines, research designs, and methodologies—the approach now widely described as transdisciplinary (Somerville & Rapport, 2000)—which comprises both qualitative and quantitative findings. Issues of scale are also relevant: for example, research that situates data from local-scale survey research in the context of structural adjustment in Zimbabwe (Potts & Mutambirwa, 1998; Bassett, Bijlmakers, & Sanders, 2000) and that identifies globalization-related influences on health in South Africa (Gilbert & Gilbert, 2004) demonstrates the need to integrate work using different units of analysis (e.g., the household, the region, the national economy) in order to describe relevant mechanisms of action in sufficient detail, and to reflect intranational disparities (e.g., by region, class, and gender) that are not apparent from national level data (Lozano et al., 2001; Gwatkin, 2002; Henninger & Snel, 2002).

The evidence base for assessing globalization's effects on SDH and identifying opportunities for intervention is therefore different from, and more heterogeneous than, the body of research that is available with respect to clinical and (many) public health interventions. Notably, qualitative research provides information about differential impacts (e.g., by region, gender, kind of employment) that are not revealed by standard indicators, and about such matters as the access problems for the poor created by the imposition of user charges and cost recovery in water and sanitation systems (Lundy, 1996). Within the ethnographic literature, Schoepf (1998, 2002, 2004; Schoepf, Schoepf, & Millen, 2000) demonstrates the value of qualitative evidence in explicating in considerable depth and detail the relations between microlevel outcomes and such macrolevel factors as falling commodity prices, domestic austerity policies that involved cuts in public sector employment and in subsidized access to health care, and migration driven by economic desperation.[2]

Policy-relevant linkages between globalization and SDH are therefore best described, and the strength of evidence evaluated, by way of syntheses that incorporate several elements, including (but not limited to): (a) description of the national and international policy context and its history; (b) country- or region-specific studies that describe changes in determinants of health, such as the level and composition of household income, labor-market changes, access to education and health services; (c) evidence from clinical and epidemiological studies that relates to demonstrated or probable changes in health outcomes arising from those impacts; (d) ethnographic research, field observations, and other firsthand accounts of experience "on the ground." This choice of elements is not random; it recognizes the need for study at the various levels identified in Figure 1.1, and the need not only to connect contextual factors with changes in SDH and their distribution but also to demonstrate where feasible a relation between changes in SDH and changes in health outcomes.

At the same time, the complexity of the evidence base and the relevant causal chains means that rarely will it be possible to state conclusions with the degree of conclusiveness that may be possible in a laboratory situation or even in many epidemiological study designs, where almost all variables can be controlled. In the words of social epidemiologist Michael Marmot, who chaired the CSDH: "The further upstream we go in our search for causes," and globalization is the quintessential upstream variable, the greater the need to rely on "observational evidence and judgment in formulating policies to reduce inequalities in health" (Marmot, 2000, p. 308). The choice and defense of a standard of proof—how much evidence is enough—is also important. As in the context of national public health and regulatory policy (Page, 1978; Schrecker, 2001), the decision must be made with explicit reference to the underlying, potentially competing values. Excessive concern with avoiding false positive findings (Type I errors, or the incorrect rejection of the null hypothesis) can supply, as in other contexts, a credible and convenient rationale for doing nothing. This is the "tobacco industry standard of proof" (Crocker, 1984, pp. 66–67)—so demanding that there is always room to claim that evidence is less than conclusive. In the environmental policy context, Page (1978) has convincingly demonstrated the negative health outcomes that may result when standards of proof are set without explicit reference to the possible consequences of being wrong in different kinds of ways. On this point, it cannot be emphasized too strongly that the choice of a standard of proof is inescapably value-driven, and is not always a choice with respect to which scientific researchers have any special competence.

A choice must also be made about the time frame of concern. In the long run, wealthier societies are healthier, albeit with wide variations in both the health status at a given level of income per capita (World Bank, 1993; Deaton, 2004) and in the distribution of that status within societies. It can be argued that the optimal, or at least most realistic, approach to improving SDH is the one that will maximize economic growth in the countries or regions of concern. However, the empirical uncertainties associated with this position, some of which are described in the next section of the chapter, have led Angus Deaton, one of the leading researchers on the relations between economic growth and health, to warn flatly that "economic growth, by itself, will not be enough to improve population health, at least in any acceptable time" (Deaton, 2006). The issue of acceptable time further raises the ethical question of how long is too long. As suggested by Deaton, diffusion of the benefits of economic growth in ways that lead to widespread improvements in population health is neither automatic nor rapid: it took more than fifty years for such diffusion in the industrial cities of nineteenth-century England, for example (Szreter, 1997, 2003; Szreter & Mooney, 1998). Given the frequency with which globalization has resulted in deterioration in SDH for substantial segments of national populations, despite impressive economic growth as measured by national indicators, this is not just an academic point.

TRADE LIBERALIZATION, GROWTH, AND POVERTY REDUCTION

We accept as given the proposition that poverty (both absolute and relative) is inimical to health equity and undermines access to SDH. Thus, to the extent that trade liberalization (or globalization more generally) could be shown to be positively associated with growth, a presumption would exist in favor of growth-inducing policies *if* growth reliably reduced poverty without other offsetting negative consequences. The argument that globalization is beneficial in terms of population health (Feachem, 2001) often starts from an equation of globalization with trade liberalization: the lowering of tariffs and other barriers to imports that has been a defining characteristic of the post–World War II economic order. As a consequence of such liberalization, the value of world trade doubled from 24 percent of world gross domestic product (GDP) in 1960 to 48 per cent in 2003 (World Bank, 2007).

Widely cited comparative studies of national economies carried out under the auspices of the World Bank (Dollar, 2001, 2002; Dollar & Kraay, 2002, 2004) concluded that during the 1980s and 1990s, the economies of "globalizers" (trade liberalizers) grew faster than "non-globalizers." However, countries held up as model high-performing globalizers (China, India, Malaysia, Thailand, and Viet Nam) actually started out as more closed economies than those nonglobalizers whose economies stalled or declined, mostly in Africa and Latin America (Dollar, 2002). The reason for this seeming anomaly, and the basis for several critiques of the studies, is one of definition. Globalizers in these studies are defined as countries that saw their trade/GDP ratio increase since 1977; nonglobalizers are simply those that saw their ratio drop. Thus, India and China are considered globalizers, even though their trade/GDP ratios at the end of the study period were lower than the average of all countries studied.

Conversely, the nonglobalizers started out more highly integrated into the world economy. The positive globalization to growth relationship becomes an artifact of the studies' design.

Furthermore, the economic problems of the nonglobalizers are at least partly attributable to global factors outside the control of national economic-policy makers: specifically, a decline in most commodity prices (only recently reversed for some) that damaged both export performance and import ability of countries that were heavily reliant on commodity exports, but already highly integrated into the global economy on some measures (Birdsall & Hamoudi, 2002; Milanovic, 2003; Dowrick & Golley, 2004). The decline in commodity prices was partly an effect of other policies that drove countries into intensified export competition with one another in order to pay their debts to external creditors. Further, excluding India and China from the sample—each of which is arguably a special case, albeit for different reasons—actually changes the conclusion: globalizers grew more slowly than nonglobalizers over the period 1980–2000 (Dowrick & Golley, 2004). Added concerns exist about the reliability of data on incomes and household assets and the appropriateness of the World Bank's definitions of poverty with reference to poverty lines or thresholds of United States (US) $1/day and $2/day (Reddy & Pogge, 2005; Woodward & Abdallah, 2008), especially in large metropolitan areas (Satterthwaite, 2003). As just one illustration, Van Doorslaer and colleagues have recently shown, for eleven Asian countries, that the World Bank understates the extent of poverty as measured by the $1/day poverty line because the surveys on which the estimates are based ask questions about the value of household consumption that include out-of-pocket health care costs. Ironically, then, large numbers of households appear to have escaped poverty because of catastrophic medical expenses (van Doorslaer et al., 2006).

Even if for the sake of argument one accepts the World Bank measures of poverty, it is not at all clear that globalization has reliably led to substantial poverty reduction. Between 1981 and 2004, a period during which the value of the world's economic output quadrupled, the number of people in the world living on $1/day or less fell by five hundred million. Although superficially impressive, this net reduction is due entirely to poverty reduction in China, with gains elsewhere in the world being offset by increases in the number of poor people elsewhere, mainly in sub-Saharan Africa. There was almost no change in the number of people worldwide living on $2/day or less: 2.45 billion in 1981, 2.55 billion in 2004. In this case, reductions in China were more than offset by increases in the number of poor people in South Asia (principally India) and sub-Saharan Africa (Chen & Ravallion, 2007). Even globalization's enthusiasts concede that there may be substantial numbers of losers within national economies. This underscores the importance of Chapter 4's focus on labor markets (on which trade policy is just one influence among many) and the global reorganization of production as pathways leading from globalization to changes in access to SDH and in health outcomes; and Chapter 6's discussion of social protection approaches that, with varying degrees of success, buffered some of the Asian financial crises of the late 1990s brought on by liberalization of their capital markets. Thus, the only responsible conclusion is that "the net effects of globalization on the poor can only be judged on the basis of 'context-specific' empirical studies" (Nissanke & Thorbecke, 2006, p. 1340). In other words: Does globalization reduce poverty? It all depends (and some of the factors on which it depends are topics of this book).

A more fundamental critique of growth as a route to poverty reduction, which stands on its own apart from issues of trade policy, arises from calculations by the New Economics Foundation showing that growth is a very ineffective way of reducing poverty. "Of every $100 of growth in income per person in the world as a whole between 1981 and 2001, just $1.30 contributed to reducing poverty as measured by the $1-a-day line, and a further $2.80 to reducing poverty between $1-a-day and $2-a-day lines"; furthermore, the effectiveness of growth in reducing poverty declined in the 1990s relative to the 1980s (Woodward & Simms, 2006, p. 16). This is not just an academic point: recent studies of social policy in Latin America concluded that even a little redistribution of income through progressive taxation and targeted social programs would go farther in terms of poverty reduction than many years of solid economic growth, because of the extremely unequal distribution of income and wealth in most countries in the region (Paes de Barros et al., 2002; de Ferranti, Perry, Ferreira, & Walton, 2004; Jubany & Meltzer, 2004). If global health equity is considered a desirable social goal, then the case for redistribution both within and across national borders is almost incontrovertible—a theme to which we return in the concluding chapter.

DEBT CRISES, STRUCTURAL ADJUSTMENT, AND MARKETIZATION UNDER PRESSURE

A long history of debt crises constrains the ability of many developing countries to meet basic needs in the areas of public health, education, water, sanitation, and nutrition. Recently, debt service payments have contributed to a larger pattern of financial transfers from the South to the North, most importantly to the United States, that contradicts colloquial wisdom about the direction of global financial flows (United Nations Department of Economic and Social Affairs, 2006). The etiology of debt crises varies from country to country and over time (Naylor, 1987; George, 1988; Strange, 1998; Hanlon, 2000) and is discussed in more detail in Chapters 3 and 7, but a stylized list of major causes includes: (a) the oil price shocks of 1973 and 1979–80, which had an especially severe impact on low-income, oil-importing countries; (b) aggressive lending by banks seeking to invest deposits from oil-exporting countries; (c) a rapid increase in real interest rates during the early 1980s generated by the monetary policies of the US Federal Reserve, meaning that debtor countries often had to roll over existing debt at much higher interest rates; (d) falling world prices, that is, deteriorating terms of trade, for the primary commodities that are the key exports of many developing economies; and (e) capital flight, consisting both of outright theft and of the rational, mostly legal shifting of assets abroad by economic elites worried about tax increases and future devaluations. A further precondition is so basic that it is sometimes overlooked. Banks, national governments, and multilateral institutions such as the World Bank have been willing, almost without exception, to accord leaders of developing countries what philosopher Thomas Pogge has called the "borrowing privilege": the right to incur debts on behalf of those they rule without having to defend the legitimacy of their rule. The borrowing privilege is accorded even to leaders who have taken power by force or deceit, maintain it by extreme repression, and are not accountable to citizens in any meaningful way (Pogge, 2002).

The impacts of debt crises cannot be understood without considering structural adjustment. The term entered the international development lexicon in 1980, when the World Bank initiated structural adjustment loans, normally in conjunction with stabilization loans from the IMF, to assist recipient countries to reorganize their economies in order to increase their ability to repay external creditors. The urgency of such lending grew after 1982, when Mexico's announcement that it was prepared to default on billions of dollars in loans, primarily made by major US banks, raised concern about the stability of financial systems in the industrialized world. Conditionalities attached to such loans, and the associated rescheduling of loan payments to the World Bank and IMF, emphasized reduction of subsidies for basic items of consumption such as food; rapid removal of barriers to imports and foreign direct investment (FDI); reductions in state expenditures, particularly on social programs such as health, education, water/sanitation, and housing; and rapid privatization of state-owned enterprises, on the presumption that private service provision was inherently more efficient, and that proceeds from privatization could be used to ensure debt repayment (Milward, 2000; Babb, 2005). In other words, the international financial institutions systematically promoted multiple, more or less coordinated domestic policies of integrating national economies into the global marketplace.

Research on health-related impacts of structural adjustment, however, has had to confront at least three design problems. First, implementation of conditions attached to World Bank and IMF loans was often incomplete (Killick, 2004)—leaving open at least the theoretical possibility that if the reforms in question had been undertaken even more aggressively, outcomes might have been more favorable. However, the recent history of market-oriented development policy in the two regions of the developing world where it has been pursued most aggressively, Latin America and Africa (Eyoh & Sandbrook, 2003; Kaufman, 2003), calls this claim into question. So too does the pattern of magnification of inequality through labor-market outcomes that has resulted from domestic marketization and export orientation (Razavi, Pearson, & Danloy, 2004; van der Hoeven & Saget, 2004). Second, it can be difficult to separate effects of structural adjustment from those of the globalization-related economic crises that preceded and led to engagement with the World Bank and IMF. Third, and relatedly, every assessment of public policy effects relies implicitly or explicitly on a counterfactual: an alternative state of the world against which the state of the world post-introduction of the policy in question is compared (as is the case with the econometric study presented in Chapter 2). If structural adjustment is compared with the continuation of business as usual, which would in many cases have involved (continued) hyperinflation and the isolation of countries from international financial markets, then structural adjustment may appear as the least destructive option. On the other hand, if the comparison is with an alternative set of policy options that would have given priority to meeting basic needs, then conclusions about the necessity and desirability of structural adjustment are likely to be less sanguine. For countries highly exposed to the international economy, this counterfactual requires further assumptions about an alternative international order at least partly driven by solidarity or conceptions of obligations that cross national borders—a point to which we return in the book's final two chapters (13 and 14).

It is also difficult to separate impacts on SDH of domestic policies that were adopted in specific response to lender conditionalities from those adopted in response to the broader diffusion of market-oriented policy ideas. However, the policy changes undertaken as part of structural adjustment programs, which can be generically described as marketization or (re)commodification (Elson & Cagatay, 2000; Bond, 2005), are congruent with the market-oriented policy shifts that are a key element of globalization more generally (Babb, 2002, 2005), succinctly codified by Williamson as the "Washington consensus" on development policy (Williamson, 1990). This "consensus" identified the suite of policies pursued throughout the 1990s to integrate developing countries into the global economy by, inter alia, financial and trade liberalization, domestic deregulation, privatization, fiscal discipline and reduced public expenditure, tax reforms emphasizing consumption rather than income, competitive exchange rates, openness to FDI, and strengthened property rights. It may be interesting to know how much of a country's social and economic policy orientation in years can be attributed to responses to the World Bank and IMF, and how much to national decision makers' interpretation of the available options within an international economic context over which they may have minimal influence. However, even if it were answerable, this question would not alter the fact that if we want to know how globalization affects SDH by way of marketizing domestic social and economic policy and commodifying basic needs, then research on structural adjustment is valuable independent of specific historical connections between lender conditionalities and policy responses. Indeed, it constitutes one of the single most important bodies of evidence available on the effects of globalization—a fact reflected in the discussions of the impacts of structural adjustment on policy space in Chapter 5, on health systems in Chapter 7, and on health worker migration in Chapter 9.

CITIES RESTRUCTURED BY THE GLOBAL MARKETPLACE

Long-distance effects of quite a different kind are evident in changing patterns of urban form and settlement, and assume special importance given the estimate that the world's urban population will have grown by more than two billion people between 2005 and 2030. While not a theme explored by the KN (there was a separate knowledge network devoted to the rapid growth in urban settlements; see Kjellstrom et al., 2007), it has a direct relationship to globalization and potentially profound health-equity effects. Almost all of this population growth will occur in countries with limited resources to provide urban and peri-urban infrastructure that is taken for granted in most of the industrialized world (UN Millennium Project Task Force on Improving the Lives of Slum Dwellers, 2005). A consistent pattern in the transformation of cities and metropolitan areas by transnational economic integration, in countries rich and poor alike, is that gaps between economic winners and losers grow, based on their position within the global economy and the basis of their connection (or lack of connection) to it. Statistics on income disparities capture only part of the picture. Castells's description of the urban impacts of globalization in terms of a "space of flows" (Castells, 1996) is valuable because it reminds us that "connectedness" to the networks of investment and information that characterize the globalized economy may have nothing to do with proximity as viewed on a road map. Castells observes that urban districts whose residents are not part of the "process that connects advanced services, producer centers, and markets in a global network" can become "irrelevant or even dysfunctional: for example, Mexico City's colonias populares (originally squatter settlements) that account for about two thirds of the megapolitan population, without playing any distinctive role in the functioning of Mexico City as an international business centre" (Castells, 1996, pp. 380–81). Thus, large metropolitan areas will contain substantial "local populations that are either functionally unnecessary or socially disruptive" (Castells, 1996, p. 404).

Spatial divisions that reflect or reinforce the pattern of gains and losses from globalization arise in a variety of ways. In parts of the industrialized world, they have been initiated by large-scale job and income losses and economic polarization associated with deindustrialization (Adams, 1997; Reardon, 1997; Storper, 1997; Warf & Holly, 1997). Even in the immensely wealthy United States, some cities with economies built on manufacturing lost half to three-quarters of their manufacturing jobs in the second half of the twentieth century (Abu-Lughod, 1999; Hodos, 2002; Savitch, 2003), with devastating effects on economic opportunities and the social fabric (Kasarda, 1989; Coulton, 2003). Urban "revitalization" may include not only policies that favor more desirable (read: higher-income) residents, but also reconfiguration of urban space in pursuit of profitable commercial development and tourism revenues, similarly leading to displacement of residents and sometimes the literal enclosure of public spaces (see, e.g., Leaf, 1996; Makdisi, 1997; Vasconcellos, 1997; Bunnell & Nah, 2004; Fernandes, 2004; Lakshmi, 2005). Residential segregation deepens through gentrification, suburbanization, and the creation of fortified enclaves with separate private systems of service provision, while those less able to pay are shifted to less desirable locations and rely on inferior services.[3] Policy choices with special significance for the boundaries of inclusion/exclusion involve transportation, specifically the balance between public transit and car-centered development (see, e.g., Leaf, 1996; Alcantara de Vasconcellos, 2005; Pucher, Korattyswaropam, Mittal, & Ittyerah, 2005). In this and other cases, access to essential resources is often determined by individual households' ability to pay or by group/neighborhood attractiveness as a market. Poverty may be criminalized (Wacquant, 2001, 2002). These processes are documented in an indispensable UN Habitat synthesis on *Cities in a Globalizing World* (United Nations Centre for Human Settlements, 2001), hence the lack of more extensive references here.

Bidding contests for urban spaces, which epitomize the interplay of global power relations and local opportunities, are paralleled by contests over locationally valuable nonurban resources, notably those associated with the expanding business of tourism. These contests can exclude current, low-value, or low-productivity users of a resource either by degradation, for example, by using surface or groundwater as a sink for the disposal of toxic wastes (Stonich, 1998), or by enclosure, for example, by pricing the use of specific locations and resources out of reach of all but the wealthy (Griffith, 2000; Richter, 2001; Leatherman & Goodman, 2005). The common analytical denominators in these conflicts are: (a) in the global marketplace, some resources simply command too high a price to be used for the basic needs of people with limited purchasing power, and (b) domestically, the polarization of income and wealth that accompanies economic integration shifts the political allegiances of decisive political pluralities in the direction of private service provision rather than collective action.

GLOBALIZATION, NATURAL RESOURCES, AND ENVIRONMENTAL EXPOSURES

The unprecedented scale of recent human impacts on the natural environment (Turner, Clark, Kates, Richards, Matthews, & Meyer, 1993), exemplified by global climate change, is in itself an important health-related dimension of globalization. On a smaller scale, exposures to environmental hazards that arise from the operation of the global marketplace comprise an important and complex set of influences on SDH. At least two mechanisms can be identified: (a) urbanization and intraurban disparities in exposure to such hazards as vehicle traffic and air and water pollution, and (b) global migration of hazardous industries, production processes, and waste. Some authors argue that "agroindustrialization," as production is reorganized into global, input-intensive commodity chains, constitutes yet another mechanism (Barrett, Barbier, & Reardon, 2001). To some extent these pathways overlap or interact with other elements of globalization, as when agroindustrialization and associated environmental damage are driven by the imperative of increasing revenues from exports destined for foreign consumers. For example, Stonich and Bailey (2000, pp. 23–24) argue that pressure to increase export earnings leads governments to promote "export-oriented aquacultural development regardless of the social and environmental consequences," creating situations in which "the increasing use of low-value fish species in the production of fishmeal for aquacultural feeds in effect puts the poor in competition with shrimp," and with the rich consumers who can afford to buy them (see also Stonich & Vandergeest, 2001).

This is one instance of a pattern noted by the health synthesis of findings from the Millennium Ecosystem Assessment (MEA) project,[4] which explicitly recognized economic globalization as one of the drivers of change in ecosystems and human well-being: "Historically, poor people disproportionately have lost access to ecosystem services as demand from wealthier populations has grown" (Corvalan et al., 2005, p. 28). The ecosystem services in question (such as safe drinking water or waste decomposition) may themselves be essential to health, or else may be essential sources of livelihood the loss of which leads to economic insecurity and deprivation. The difference globalization makes is that winning bidders may be half a world away, as in Stonich's aquaculture example and in the case of markets for tropical timber, oil in Nigeria (where abundant resource revenues have failed to improve the grinding poverty and poor health status of much of the country's population), and coltan and other minerals in the Democratic Republic of the Congo (Sizer & Plouvier, 2000; Montague, 2002; United Nations Security Council, 2002, 2003; Ferguson, 2005; Gellert, 2005; Watts, 2005).

In many cases, as globalization increases aggregate demand for marketable resources and ecological services, it simultaneously fosters policies and institutions that facilitate control over gains and losses across entire regional economies by local elites and the dominant actors in global commodity chains (see, e.g., United Nations Security Council, 2002, 2003). One analysis of investment in developing countries by transnational logging companies in response to increasing global demand for tropical timber was strongly critical of the sustainability of forest management practices, and further noted that:

Where analysis is available . . . the economic benefit is minor, even in the short-term, and certainly far less than it could be if contracts were structured and negotiated differently. While large amounts of capital are involved, the revenue to national treasuries can be small because most of the profits leave the country or accrue in the hands of very few, often already wealthy and powerful local people. (Sizer & Plouvier, 2000, p. 29, citations omitted)

Transnational mineral firms are often the beneficiaries of large-scale financial support from export credit and insurance agencies in their home countries (Rich, Horta, & Goldzimer, 2000; Moody et al., 2005)—an element of global influence that appears to have received little research attention outside a rather specialized community of CSOs. In such cases, global asymmetries of economic power are reflected in extreme inequalities in the distribution of benefits domestically.

The MEA health synthesis noted another set of differential exposures and vulnerabilities: "Poor populations are more vulnerable to adverse health effects from both local and global environmental changes" (Corvalan et al., 2005, p. 27), because they are more likely to be exposed to hazards from which the rich can remove themselves. Disasters in Bhopal and New Orleans provide dramatic evidence of this point, as do the routine conditions of urban life for hundreds of millions of people worldwide (Stephens, 1996). It is estimated that more than 850 million people now live in slums, with the number projected to rise to 1.4 billion in 2020 in the absence of effective policy interventions (UN Millennium Project Task Force on Improving the Lives of Slum Dwellers, 2005). Slum residence is an imperfect but nevertheless useful proxy for exposure to urban environmental hazards including infectious disease related to inadequate sanitation and industrial pollution, as well as other quotidian risks exemplified by the collapse of a rain-soaked open rubbish dump that killed some of the residents of Manila's informal settlements in 2000 (Aglionby, 2000; Mydans, 2000).

Some studies find a clear pattern of migration of hazardous industries to lower-income countries, notably to export processing zones (EPZs) (Kopinak & Barajas, 2002; Frey, 2003). Other, quantitative studies that do not focus on particular regions suggest that evidence for the emergence of industrial "pollution havens" is equivocal or absent (Wheeler, 2001; Cole & Elliott, 2005). An impressionistic assessment of such "negative" findings is that many are compromised by (a) failure to focus on the global restructuring of production within specific industries or sectors; (b) concentration on foreign direct investment (FDI), without considering contractual arrangements such as outsourcing that are not recorded in FDI statistics but are extensively described in the literature on commodity or value chains; (c) inability to distinguish causal effects of lax environmental regulation on relocation of production (what the pollution-haven hypothesis is all about) from those of other variables, such as low wages and flexible working conditions, that tend to operate in parallel; and (d) failure to distinguish between changes in pollution exposures attributable to industrial processes and to such factors as increased vehicle traffic. Substantial evidence also exists of the emergence of a global trade in hazardous wastes, with disposal in low-income countries becoming increasingly attractive and met with policy responses that are at best only partially effective (Clapp, 2001, 2002; Puckett et al., 2002; Iles, 2004).

In the background is the question of whether such environmental changes and their health impacts should be regarded as normal, in the sense that they are comparable to those undergone by the industrialized countries at comparable stages of their own economic development. Evidence of the extent to which contemporary technology allows for "technological leap-frogging" (Goldemberg, Johansson, Reddy, & Williams, 2001) and "dematerialization" (Ayres & Ayres, 2002), which avoid many environmentally destructive forms of industrial production and consumption, suggests that this conclusion should be rejected. However, environmental and resource impacts can alternatively be considered with reference to a green counterfactual that assumes transfer of clean technologies on favorable terms, along with serious efforts by the industrialized economies to reduce their consumption of natural resources and ecological services, and to adopt policies that minimize negative environmental and resource impacts outside their borders. Thus, globalization's negative effects on SDH that operate by way of the environment, like those that operate in other ways, must be regarded primarily as consequences of political choices and avoidable failures of governance.

OVERVIEW OF THE BOOK

The GKN commissioned thirteen monograph-length research synthesis papers, each of which undertook substantial evidence reviews related to their themes. The reviews drew on studies that crossed disciplines and methodologies; incorporated research, testimony, and analyses from civil society organizations; and attended carefully to issues of geography, scale, and (particularly) gender. Each paper was subject to extensive critique and review within the network, before being externally blind-reviewed. The review process focused on three key questions: Was important evidence related to the theme missed? Was the analysis derived from the evidence based solidly on the evidence reported? Were the policy inferences (either known or implied) linked logically and coherently to the evidence? The reviews were important to the final knowledge products of the KN, since the potential evidence base for each theme explored was almost endlessly vast.

The chapters in this book are derived (with some updating) from these background papers, many of which have been Web published for readers wishing to examine each issue in greater depth. New evidence and argument surrounding globalization (generally) and how it affects health (generally or via the themes explored in these chapters) are continually being generated. What we present in this book is the most rigorous assessment of "state-of-the-art" knowledge as of late 2007. While certain facts and trends could change rapidly, especially given the current prospect of global recession, the underlying dynamics of globalization that pose particular health risks explored in the following chapters are unlikely to alter substantially without the types of policy changes addressed throughout the book, and particularly in our final two chapters.

We begin, in Chapter 2, with a study of how globalization-related policies have affected health outcomes. Cornia, Rosignoli, and Tiberti first summarize existing evidence of change along a number of pathways by which globalization influences morbidity and mortality, notably: material deprivation; acute psychosocial stress; unhealthy lifestyles; high levels of social stratification and lack of social cohesion; and positive and negative "shocks." Although 1980–2005 was characterized by a series of favorable political and economic "dividends" that should have led to faster improvements in health status and declines in health inequality within and across countries and regions, the period recorded a slowdown in health improvements and an increase in health inequality worldwide. The chapter explores the reasons for this phenomenon using an econometric regression model comparing global and regional trends in life expectancy at birth since 1980 attributable to globalization-related policies, against a counterfactual continuation of trends in the preglobalizing decades of 1960–80.

In Chapter 3, Bond adds depth to understanding how these globalization-related policies reflected major shifts in global political economy and geopolitics since the 1970s. These shifts brought together processes of governance and liberalization in often uncomfortable ways and with profound implications for health and SDH policies. Geopolitical realignments and neoliberal policy ascendancy are observed in a series of "moments" in which key events reflected important power shifts. The broader global context has been a series of durable economic problems: stagnation, financial volatility, and uneven development. One reaction to these persisting problems has been the turn to what the chapter describes as "extra-economic" relationships between markets and nonmarket social and ecological values; an unhealthy development when global political discourses are dominated by neoliberal and neoconservative forces.

Chapter 4 focuses on one of globalization's main health-determining pathways: the substantial and dramatic changes that have occurred in global labor markets. Schrecker examines the relation between labor-market outcomes and poverty; the global reorganization of production and the associated emergence of a genuinely global labor market; the tendency of globalization to increase economic inequality and demands for labor-market "flexibility"; and the impact of financial crises on employment and labor income. He argues that among the key objectives of economic policy should be creation of an economic environment that generates adequate and secure livelihoods for all, which requires "bringing employment back in" as a central concern of economic and development policy—a direct challenge to the neoliberal economic nostrums described in Chapter 3.

Chapter 5 discusses a more subtle and complex way by which globalization is affecting health and SDH: the contraction of policy space available to national governments for purposes of regulation. One of the means of doing so (trade agreements) is already well known, since the purpose of such treaties is precisely to reduce the policy flexibilities governments can use with respect to international economic transactions in order to maximize the free movement of goods, services, and capital. Koivusalo, Schrecker, and Labonté examine the many ways in which trade treaties affect policy space, extending beyond the agreements themselves to the processes by which they are negotiated. A second force reducing policy space is financial-market liberalization, which imposes an "implicit conditionality" on the range of options from which governments might select. While noting that not all international constraints on policy space are potentially health-negative (human rights treaties and multilateral environmental agreements are cited as health-positive constraints), the authors argue the importance of protecting policy flexibilities for health and SDH.

Chapter 6 focuses on one set of policies that governments can use to buffer the inherently "disequalizing" outcomes of global market liberalization: the use (and expansion) of social protection policies. Globalization generally and trade liberalization specifically create winners and losers in domestic economies as well as among countries. The negative impacts are not limited to one-time adjustments to trade reforms but more generally to the greater frequency and scope of economic restructuring in an open economy. Using the experience of East Asian country responses to the financial crisis of the late 1990s, Bhusan and Blouin assess the impact of differing national policies aimed at reducing economic vulnerability arising from trade or financial-market liberalization. The evidence underscores the importance of improving (broadening, deepening) general social safety nets prior to or alongside ongoing global market integration—a conclusion reached recently, and explicated forcefully, in the 2008–2009 *Chronic Poverty Report* by a university/CSO partnership organization known as the Chronic Poverty Research Centre (Addison et al., 2008).

Social protection policies, such as publicly financed health care, education, active labor market programs, employment insurance, and direct income transfers, have costs associated with them; many lower-income countries will be unable to self-finance effective social protection programs for some decades into the future. Chapter 7 examines two critical and enjoined issues related to improving their financing capacities: aid and debt relief. After reviewing trends in aid disbursements, Taylor and Rowson confront the heated debate regarding aid effectiveness, suggesting that new evidence shows that aid is not only essential for the health and welfare of poorer countries, but that, despite its many well-documented problems associated in the first instance with donor country practices and condition-alities, it has been effective in promoting economic development and in improving health outcomes. Aid effectiveness, however, has been hampered by countries' continued servicing of foreign (and to lesser extent, domestic) debt. Debt relief or cancellation for a group of nations known as the Heav-ily Indebted Poor Countries has been compromised by a lack of speed and creditor dominance. There is also an urgent need to reframe the process of debt cancellation from one which focuses on the detail of countries' economic vulnerability to debt to one which focuses on the idea of "debt responsibility," involving greater public scrutiny of lending, the establish-ment of international mediation processes between debtors and creditors, and placing social needs ahead of debt repayments.

Chapter 8 narrows the examination of globalization's health impacts by focusing on one critical sector: health systems. Lister and Labonté argue that, since the 1980s, and particularly after the move by the World Bank into health-system financing in the 1990s, health-system reform globally has followed a "marketization" model emphasizing cost recovery (user fees), privatization, competition, technical/disease-specific interventions, and other policy approaches that undermined the earlier Alma-Ata Dec-laration on Primary Health Care's call for universal, comprehensive public systems. The results of the imposition of these reforms, through structural adjustment, aid, or debt-relief initiatives, has been largely health-negative, leading to recent calls for a return to broader and more integrated mod-els of health care delivery. Even as these public interventionist policies are reemerging in global policy discourse, however, ongoing trade negotiations continue to emphasize the economic value of opening up international trade in health services. More developing than developed countries have already committed to do so, while private health providers and insurers from devel-oped countries are most likely to benefit. Some believe that opening health services to foreign investment and providers can improve access by bring-ing new capital and expertise to national systems. Others worry that it will only mean better access for a very small portion of the population with higher incomes. The recent trade-related boom in "medical tourism," in which patients from high-income countries receive hospital care in low-income nations, provides a cautionary tale in this respect.

Chapter 9 highlights another facet of globalization's effect on health systems: the "crisis" in global health workforce migration. Deteriorating economic and broader social and environmental conditions at least partly attributable to liberalization or other forms of global market integration are "pushing" out health workers in many developing (and especially low-income) countries. At the same time, the main destination countries of health worker migrants suffer their own health worker shortages and increasingly rely on the immigration of foreign-trained health workers to relieve them. These countries are able to offer higher pay, better working conditions, and greater opportunities to save money, effectively pulling in foreign health workers. Whether this flow of health workers globally constitutes a "brain drain," as critics contend, or a "brain circulation," as others argue, the short-term impact is a dramatic shortage of health workers in countries facing the greatest need. Packer, Labonté, and Runnels conclude by examining the feasibility and desirability of various policy options that have been proposed to manage global health workforce migration more ethically and equitably.

Chapter 10 introduces the concept of "nutrition transition," a term referring to the globalization of poor quality energy-dense diets leading to obesity and diet-related chronic diseases. Hawkes, Chopra, and Friel explore how globalization is affecting the development of "overnutrition" in a world still plagued by undernutrition. They identify the supply-side globalization processes to the increase of poor quality diets, focusing on three particular processes: the growth of transnational food companies, international food trade, and global food advertising and promotion. The evidence finds that these processes are affecting the availability, price, accessibility, and desirability of different foods, driving uneven dietary development between different socioeconomic groups. The chapter ends by discussing the policy implications of the evidence presented.

Chapter 11 explores inequalities in health outcomes emerging from the existing intellectual property-rights regime, one of the most visible and contentious of globalization's policies having direct health-related effects. Correa examines the impact of the internationalization of the IPR system and, in particular, the adoption of minimum standards of protection in the WTO Agreement on Trade-Related Intellectual Property Rights. The chapter highlights some of the features of innovation in the pharmaceutical field and the changes under way in the predominant business model for research and development. It notes that, in this shifting context, patents fail to encourage research and development in diseases prevailing in developing countries, while creating barriers to drug access, particularly affecting the poor. The chapter concludes by assessing how policy interventions can improve such access through strengthened flexibilities in trade treaties (e.g., for compulsory licenses) and various models for financing drug research outside of patent regimes.

Chapter 12 extends the discussion of alternatives to the current system of globalization's various trade and investment rules to the broader terrain of global governance for health. Lee and her contributing authors document the transition taking place towards global governance related to SDH in terms of institutional actors and their relative roles, power, and authority. The chapter then assesses how emerging forms of global governance may be influencing the SDH, posing the question: How might various institutions, and the distribution and use of power and authority among them, affect the SDH? The authors answer this question, in part, by assessing the quality of emerging forms of global governance against recognized "good governance" criteria. The chapter finally identifies how global governance can play a transformational role in addressing the SDH.

Chapter 13 summarizes and distils the arguments from the previous chapters. It brings forward some of the key policy recommendations emanating from the book's chapters, and identifies a global policy agenda that responds to globalization's present asymmetries structured around the "three Rs" of redistribution, regulation, and rights. The international human rights framework is discussed for the opportunities it presents for limiting commodification and the spread of the global marketplace in ways that undermine health equity. More generally, Chapter 13 describes the new forms of coordinated action on an international scale by national governments and multilateral institutions that the "three Rs" demand, highlighting a number of productive areas for policy innovation while warning that their potential is unlikely to be realized in the absence of decisive leadership and political action.

Chapter 14 offers an invited, reflective commentary by David Sanders, one of the founders of the People's Health Movement and a long-time, African-based activist public health physician. The chapter focuses on the evidence for how power inequalities lie at the heart of both the health inequities associated with contemporary globalization, and on the historically rooted necessity of civil society struggles to challenge and alter these toxic inequalities.

NOTES

1. The Group of 7 leading industrialized nations includes Canada, Italy, France, Japan, Germany, the United Kingdom (UK), and the United States of America (USA). Formed in 1976 to manage potentially damaging issues arising from global economic activities, the G7 became the G8 in 1997 with the addition of Russia.
2. For further illustrations of the value of qualitative research, see, e.g., the World Bank's Voices of the Poor study (Narayan, Patel, Schafft, Rademacher, & Koch-Schulte, 1999; Narayan, Chambers, Shah, & Petesch, 2000); the report of the Structural Adjustment Participatory Review International Network (Bhattacharya et al., 2002); and a summary of studies of sources of livelihood in KwaZulu-Natal, South Africa by Lund (2004). For description of a similar approach adopted by another of the commission's KNs, see Employment Conditions Knowledge Network (2007, pp. 25–29).
3. A telling example of this, and of the global reach of marketization: a commission meeting in Nairobi included a presentation where an official explained why it made sense to sell to private developers the land where the city's largest slum had grown over past decades, since the slum now abutted the growing downtown and had become valuable property. Profits from the sale, it was argued, would be used to relocate the millions of slumdwellers to the city's periphery, a location devoid of any services, shops, schools, or transportation.
4. The final report is downloadable, on a chapter-by-chapter basis, from http://www.millenniumecosystemassessment.org. For a description of the MEA's findings at a level of detail that will suffice even for many sophisticated users, see Alcamo et al., 2005; Butler & Oluoch-Kosura, 2005; Carpenter, Bennett, & Peterson, 2005; Cork, Peterson, Bennett, Petschel-Held, & Zurek, 2005; Nelson et al., 2005; Rodriguez et al., 2005.

REFERENCES

Abu-Lughod, J. (1999). *New York, Chicago, Los Angeles: America's global cities.* Minneapolis: University of Minnesota Press.
Adams, C. T. (1997). The Philadelphia experience. *Annals of the American Academy of Political and Social Science,* 551, 222–34.
Addison, T., Harper, C., Prowse, M., Shepherd, M., Barrientos, A., Braunholtz-Speight, T., et al. (2008). *The Chronic Poverty Report 2008–09.* Manchester, UK: Chronic Poverty Research Centre. Retrieved from: http://www.chronicpoverty.org/pubfiles/CPR2_whole_report.pdf.
Aglionby, J. (2000). Life and death on a rubbish dump. *Guardian* [online] July 14.
Alcamo, J., van Vuuren, D., Ringler, C., Cramer, W., Masui, T., Alder, J., et al. (2005). Changes in nature's balance sheet: Model-based estimates of future worldwide ecosystem services. *Ecology and Society,* 10.
Alcantara de Vasconcellos, E. (2005). Urban change, mobility and transport in São Paulo: Three decades, three cities. *Transport Policy,* 12, 91–104.
Appadurai, A. (1990). Disjuncture and difference in the global cultural economy. *Theory, Culture, and Society,* 7, 295–310.
Ayres, R. U., & Ayres, L. W., eds. (2002). *A handbook of industrial ecology.* Cheltenham, UK: Edward Elgar. Retrieved from:http://books.google.com/books?ie=UTF-8&hl=en&id=g1Kb-xizc1wC&dq=Ayres+dematerialization&prev=http://scholar.google.com/olar%3Fq%3DAyres%2Bdematerialization%26num%3D100%26hl%3Den%26lr%3D%26sa%3DG&pg=PR4&printsec=3&lpg=PR4&sig=uIFZhpFsoTg96uO0T6ykidla6lU.
Babb, S. (2002). *Managing Mexico: Economists from nationalism to neoliberalism.* Princeton, NJ: Princeton University Press.
———. (2005). The social consequences of structural adjustment: Recent evidence and current debates. *Annual Review of Sociology,* 31, 199–222.
Barrett, C. B., Barbier, E. B., & Reardon, T. (2001). Agroindustrialization, globalization, and international development: The environmental implications. *Environment and Development Economics,* 6, 419–33.
Bassett, M. T., Bijlmakers, L. A., & Sanders, D. (2000). Experiencing structural adjustment in urban and rural households of Zimbabwe. In M. Turshen (ed.), *African women's health* (pp. 167–91). Trenton, NJ: Africa World Press.
Bhattacharya, D., Moyo, T., Terán, J. F., Morales, L. I. R., Lóránt, K., Graham, Y., et al. (2002). *The policy roots of economic crisis and poverty: A multi-country participatory assessment of structural adjustment* (1st ed.). Washington, DC: Structural Adjustment Participatory Review International Network (SAPRIN) Secretariat. Retrieved from: http://www.saprin.org.
Birchfield, V., & Freyberg, A. (2004). Constructing opposition in the age of globalization: The potential of ATTAC. *Globalizations,* V1, 278–304.
Birdsall, N., & Hamoudi, A. (2002). *Commodity dependence, trade, and growth: When "openness" is not enough.* CGD Working Papers No. 7. Washington, DC: Center for Global Development.
Black, R., Morris, S., & Bryce, J. (2003). Where and why are 10 million children dying every year? *Lancet,* 362, 2226–34.
Bond, P. (2005). Globalisation/commodification or deglobalisation/decommodification in urban South Africa. *Policy Studies,* 26, 337–58.
Braveman, P., & Gruskin, S. (2003). Defining equity in health. *Journal of Epidemiology and Community Health,* 57, 254–58.
Brooks, S. M. (2004). International financial institutions and the diffusion of foreign models for social security reform in Latin America. In K. Weyland (ed.), *Learning from foreign models in Latin American policy reform* (pp. 53–80). Washington, DC: Woodrow Wilson Center Press.

Bryce, J., Boschi-Pinto, C., Shibuya, K., & Black, R. E. (2005). WHO estimates of the causes of death in children. *Lancet, 365,* 1147–52.

Brysk, Alison (2004). *Human rights and private wrongs: Constructing norms in global civil society.* Paper presented at the International Studies Association annual conference, Montreal. Retrieved from: http://archive.allacademic.com/publication/index.php?PHPSESSID=691c5c9a256aaa8d53eba3a0f45373fd.

Bunnell, T., & Nah, A. M. (2004). Counter-global cases for place: Contesting displacement in globalising Kuala Lumpur metropolitan area. *Urban Studies, 41,* 2447–67.

Butler, C. D. & Oluoch-Kosura, W. (2005). Linking future ecosystem services and future human well-being. *Ecology and Society,* 11.

Carpenter, S. R., Bennett, E. M., & Peterson, G. D. (2005). Scenarios for ecosystem services: An overview. *Ecology and Society,* 11.

Castells, M. (1996). *The rise of the network society.* Oxford, UK: Blackwell.

Chen, S., & Ravallion, M. (2007). *Absolute poverty measures for the developing world, 1981–2004.* World Bank Policy Research Working Paper WPS4211. Washington, DC: World Bank. Retrieved from: http://d.repec.org/n?u=RePEc:wbk:wbrwps:4211&r=ltv.

Chopra, M., & Darnton-Hill, I. (2004). Tobacco and obesity epidemics: Not so different after all? *British Medical Journal, 328,* 1558–1560.

Chopra, M., Galbraith, S., & Darnton-Hill, I. (2002). A global response to a global problem: The epidemic of overnutrition. *Bulletin of the World Health Organization, 80,* 952–58.

Clapp, J. (2001). *Toxic exports: The transfer of hazardous wastes from rich to poor countries.* Ithaca, NY: Cornell University Press.

———. (2002). Seeping through the regulatory cracks. *SAIS Review, 22,* 141–55.

Cole, M. A., & Elliott, R. J. R. (2005). FDI and the capital intensity of "dirty" sectors: A missing piece of the pollution haven puzzle. *Review of Development Economics, 9,* 530–48.

Commission on Macroeconomics and Health. (2001). *Macroeconomics and health: Investing in health for economic development.* Geneva: World Health Organization. Retrieved from: http://www.cid.harvard.edu/cidcmh/CMHReport.pdf.

Cork, S. J., Peterson, G. D., Bennett, E. M., Petschel-Held, G., & Zurek, M. (2005). Synthesis of the storylines. *Ecology and Society,* 11.

Corvalan, C., Hales, S., McMichael, A., Butler, C., Campbell-Lendrum, D., Confalonieri, U., et al. (2005). *Ecosystems and human well-being: Health synthesis.* Geneva: World Health Organization. Retrieved from: http://www.millenniumassessment.org.

Coulton, C. J. (2003). Metropolitan inequities and the ecology of work: Implications for welfare reform. *Social Service Review, 77,* 159–89.

Crocker, T. (1984). Scientific truths and policy truths in acid deposition research. In T. Crocker (ed.), *Economic perspectives on acid deposition control.* Boston: Butterworth.

Deaton, A. (2004). Health in an age of globalization. *Brookings Trade Forum,* 83–130.

———. (2006). Global patterns of income and health. *WIDER Angle, 2,* 1–3.

de Ferranti, D., Perry, G., Ferreira, F. H., & Walton, M. (2004). *Inequality in Latin America & the Caribbean: Breaking with history?* Washington, DC: World Bank. Retrieved from: http://wbln0018.worldbank.org/LAC/LAC.nsf/0/4112F1114F594B4B85256DB3005DB262?Opendocument.

Diderichsen, F., Evans, T., & Whitehead, M. (2001). The social basis of disparities in health. In M. Whitehead, T. Evans, F. Diderichsen, A. Bhuiya, & M. Wirth (eds.), *Challenging inequities in health: From ethics to action* (pp. 13–23). New York: Oxford University Press.

Dollar, D. (2001). *Globalization, inequality, and poverty since 1980.* Washington, DC: World Bank. Retrieved from: http://www.sfu.ca/~akaraiva/e455/dollar-glob.pdf.

———. (2002). Global economic integration and global inequality. In D. Gruen, T. O'Brien, & J. Lawson (eds.), *Globalisation, living standards and inequality: Recent progress and continuing challenges.* Proceedings of a conference held in Sydney, 27–28 May, 2002 (pp. 9–36). Canberra: Reserve Bank of Australia. Retrieved from: http://www.rba.gov.au/PublicationsAndResearch/Conferences/2002/.

Dollar, D., & Kraay, A. (2002). *Growth is good for the poor.* Washington, DC: World Bank. Retrieved from: www.worldbank.org/research.

———. (2004). Trade, growth, and poverty. *The Economic Journal,* 114, F22–F49.

Dowrick, S., & Golley, J. (2004). Trade openness and growth: Who benefits? *Oxford Review of Economic Policy,* 20, 38–56.

Elson, D., & Cagatay, N. (2000). The social content of macroeconomic policies. *World Development,* 28, 1347–64.

Employment Conditions Knowledge Network. (2007). *Employment conditions and health inequalities: Final report to the WHO Commission on Social Determinants of Health (CSDH).* Barcelona, Spain: Health Inequalities Research Group, Occupational Health Research Unit, Department of Experimental Sciences and Health, Universitat Pompeu Fabra. Retrieved from: http://www.who.int/social_determinants/resources/articles/emconet_who_report.pdf .

Eyoh, D., & Sandbrook, R. (2003). Pragmatic neo-liberalism and just development in Africa. In A. Kohli, C. Moon, & G. Sørensen (eds.), *States, markets, and just growth: Development in the twenty-first century* (pp. 227–57). Tokyo: United Nations University Press.

Ezzati, M., Vander Hoorn, S., Lawes, C. M., Leach, R., James, W. P., Lopez, A. D., et al. (2005). Rethinking the "diseases of affluence" paradigm: Global patterns of nutritional risks in relation to economic development. *Public Library of Science Medicine,* 2, 1–9.

Feachem, R. G. A. (2001). Globalisation is good for your health, mostly. *British Medical Journal,* 323, 504–06.

Ferguson, J. (2005). Seeing like an oil company: Space, security, and global capital in neoliberal Africa. *American Anthropologist,* 107, 377–82.

Fernandes, L. (2004). The politics of forgetting: Class politics, state power and the restructuring of urban space in India. *Urban Studies,* 41, 2415–30.

Frey, R. S. (2003). The transfer of core-based hazardous production processes to the export processing zones of the periphery: The maquiladora centers of northern Mexico. *Journal of World-Systems Research,* 9, 317–54.

Gellert, P. K. (2005). The shifting natures of "development": Growth, crisis, and recovery in Indonesia's forests. *World Development,* 33, 1345–64.

George, S. (1988). *A fate worse than debt.* London: Penguin.

Gershman, J., & Irwin, A. (2000). Getting a grip on the global economy. In J. Y. Kim, J. V. Millen, A. Irwin, & J. Gershman (eds.), *Dying for growth: Global inequality and the health of the poor* (pp. 11–43). Monroe, ME: Common Courage Press.

Gilbert, T., & Gilbert, L. (2004). Globalization and local power: Influences on health matters in South Africa. *Health Policy,* 671, 245–55.

Goldemberg, J., Johansson, T. B., Reddy, A. K., & Williams, R. H. (2001). Energy for the new millennium. *Ambio: A Journal of the Human Environment,* 30, 330–37.

Griffith, D. (2000). Social capital and economic apartheid along the coasts of the Americas. *Urban Anthropology,* 29, 255–84.

Gwatkin, D. (2002). *Who would gain most from efforts to reach the millennium development goals for health?* Washington, DC: World Bank.

Hanlon, J. (2000). How much debt must be cancelled? *Journal of International Development,* 12, 877–901.

28   *Ronald Labonté and Ted Schrecker*

Henninger, N., & Snel, M. (2002). *Where are the poor? Experiences with the development and use of poverty maps.* Washington, DC: World Resources Institute. Retrieved from: http://www.povertymap.net/pub.htm.

Hodos, J. (2002). Globalization, regionalism, and urban restructuring: The case of Philadelphia. *Urban Affairs Review, 37,* 358–79.

Iles, A. (2004). Mapping environmental justice in technology flows: Computer waste impacts in Asia . *Global Environmental Politics, 4,* 76–107.

Jenkins, R. (2004). Globalization, production, employment and poverty: debates and evidence. *Journal of International Development, 16,* 1–12.

Jubany, F., & Meltzer, J. (2004). *The Achilles' heel of Latin America. The state of the debate on inequality,* FPP-04-5. Ottawa: Canadian Foundation for the Americas (FOCAL).

Kapur, D., & Webb, R. (2000). *Governance-related conditionalities of the international financial institutions.* G-24 Discussion Paper Series, No.6. Cambridge, MA: United Nations/Center for International Development, Harvard University.

Kasarda, J. D. (1989). Urban industrial transition and the underclass. *Annals of the American Academy of Political and Social Science, 501,* 26–47.

Kaufman, R. R. (2003). Latin America in the global economy: Macroeconomic policy, social welfare, and political democracy. In A. Kohli, C. Moon, & G. Sørensen (eds.), *States, markets, and just growth: Development in the twenty-first century* (pp. 97–126). Tokyo: United Nations University Press.

Killick, T. (2004). Politics, evidence and the new aid agenda. *Development Policy Review, 22,* 5–29.

Kjellstrom, T., Mercado, S., Satterthwaite, D., McGranahan, G., Friel, S., & Havemann, K. (2007). *Our cities, our health, our future: Acting on social determinants for health equity in urban settings—Report to the WHO Commission on Social Determinants of Health from the Knowledge Network on Urban Settings.* Kobe, Japan: WHO Centre for Health Development. Retrieved from: http://www.who.int/social_determinants/resources/knus_report_16jul07.pdf.

Kopinak, K., & Barajas, R. (2002). Too close for comfort? The proximity of industrial hazardous wastes to local populations in Tijuana, Baja California. *Journal of Environment and Development, 11,* 215–46.

Kozul-Wright, R., & Rayment, P. (2004). *Globalization reloaded: An UNCTAD perspective.* UNCTAD Discussion Paper No. 167. New York: United Nations Conference on Trade and Development.

Krug, E. G., Dahlberg, L. L., Mercy, J. A., Zwi, A. B., & Lozano, R., eds. (2003). *World report on violence and health.* Geneva: World Health Organization.

Labonté, R., Blouin, C., Chopra, M., Lee, K., Packer, C., Rowson, M., et al. (2007). *Towards health-equitable globalization: Rights, regulation and redistribution, Globalization Knowledge Network Final Report to the Commission on Social Determinants of Health.* Ottawa: Institute of Population Health, University of Ottawa. Retrieved from: http://www.who.int/social_determinants/resources/gkn_final_report_042008.pdf.

Lakshmi, Rama. (2005, August 5). Bombay moves to push out the poor: Slums are razed as plans envisage reinvented city. *Washington Post.*

Leaf, M. (1996). Building the road for the BMW: Culture, vision, and the extended metropolitan region of Jakarta. *Environment and Planning A, 28,* 1617–35.

Leatherman, T. L., & Goodman, A. (2005). Coca-colonization of diets in the Yucatan. *Social Science and Medicine, 61,* 833–46.

Lee, K., & Goodman, H. (2002). Global policy networks: The propagation of health care financing reform since the 1980's. In K. Lee, K. Buse, & S. Fustukian (eds.), *Health policy in a globalising world* (pp. 97–119). Cambridge: Cambridge University Press.

Lozano, R., Zurita, B., Franco, F., Ramirez, T., Hernandez, P., & Torres, J. (2001). Mexico: Marginality, need, and resource allocation at the county level. In M. Whitehead, T. Evans, F. Diderichsen, A. Bhuiya, & M. Wirth (eds.), *Challenging inequities in health: From ethics to action* (pp. 276–95). New York: Oxford University Press.

Lund, F. (2004). *Livelihoods (un)employment and social safety nets: Reflections from recent studies in KwaZulu-Natal.* Hatfield, South Africa: Southern African Regional Poverty Network. Retrieved from: http://www.sarpn.org.za/documents/d0000925/index.php.

Lundy, P. (1996). Limitations of quantitative research in the study of structural adjustment. *Social Science and Medicine,* 42, 313–24.

Makdisi, S. (1997). Laying claim to Beirut: Urban narrative and spatial identity in the age of solidere. *Critical Inquiry,* 23, 660–705.

Marchak, P. (1991). *The integrated circus: The new right and the restructuring of global markets.* Montreal: McGill-Queen's University Press.

Marmot, M. (2000). Inequalities in health: Causes and policy implications. In A. Tarlov & R. St. Peter (eds.), *The society and population health reader, vol. 2: A state and community perspective* (pp. 293–309). New York: New Press.

———. (2006). Health in an unequal world. *The Lancet,* 368, 2081–94.

McChesney, R. (2000). *Rich media, poor democracy: Communications politics in dubious times.* New York: New Press.

McChesney, R., & Schiller, D. (2003). *The political economy of international communications:* Foundations for the emerging global debate about media ownership and regulation. Technology, Business and Society Programme Paper No. 11. Geneva: UNRISD.

Mesa-Lago, C., & Müller, K. (2002). The politics of pension reform in Latin America. *Journal of Latin American Studies,* 34, 687–715.

Milanovic, B. (2003). The two faces of globalization: Against globalization as we know it. *World Development,* 31, 667–83.

Miller, M. C. (2002). What's wrong with this picture? *The Nation* [online]. Retrieved from: http://www.thenation.com/doc.mhtml?i=20020107&s=miller.

Milward, B. (2000). What is structural adjustment? In G. Mohan, E. Brown, B. Milward, & A. B. Zack-Williams (eds.), *Structural adjustment: Theory, practice and impacts* (pp. 24–38). London: Routledge.

Montague, D. (2002). Stolen goods: Coltan and conflict in the Democratic Republic of Congo. *SAIS Review,* XXII, 103–18.

Monteiro, C., Conde, W., & Popkin, B. (2004). Obesity and inequities in health in the developing world. *International Journal of Obesity,* 28, 1181–86.

Monteiro, C., Moura, E., Conde, W., & Popkin, B. (2004). Socioeconomic status and obesity in adult populations of developing countries: A review. *Bulletin of the World Health Organization,* 82, 940–46.

Moody, R., Gedicks, A., Smith, S. D., Bank Information Center, Bosshard, P., Membup, J., et al. (2005). *The risks we run: Mining, communities, and political risk insurance.* Utrecht, Netherlands: International Books.

Mydans, Seth. (2000, July 18). Before Manila's garbage hill collapsed: Living off scavenging. *New York Times.*

Nantulya, Vivand M., et al., eds. (2003). Road traffic injuries and health equity. *Injury Control and Safety Promotion,* (special issue)10, 1–2.

Narayan, D., Chambers, R., Shah, M. K., & Petesch, P. (2000). *Voices of the poor: Crying out for change.* Oxford: Oxford University Press for the World Bank.

Narayan, D., Patel, R., Schafft, K., Rademacher, A., & Koch-Schulte, S. (1999). *Can anyone hear us? Voices from 47 countries.* Washington, DC: Poverty Group, PREM, World Bank.

Naylor, R. T. (1987). *Hot money: Peekaboo finance and the politics of debt.* Toronto: McClelland & Stewart.

Nelson, G. C., Bennett, E., Berhe, A. A., Cassman, K., DeFries, R., Dietz, T., et al. (2005). Anthropogenic drivers of ecosystem change: An overview. *Ecology and Society,* 11.

Nissanke, M., & Thorbecke, E. (2006). Channels and policy debate in the globalization-inequality-poverty nexus. *World Development,* 34, 1338–60.

Paes de Barros, R., Contreras, D., Feres, J. C., Ferreira, F. H. G., Ganuza, E., Hansen, E., et al. (2002). *Meeting the millennium poverty reduction targets in Latin America and the Caribbean.* Santiago: United Nations Economic Commission for Latin America and the Caribbean.

Page, T. (1978). A generic view of toxic chemicals and similar risks. *Ecology Law Quarterly,* 7, 207–44.

Paluzzi, J. E., & Farmer, P. E. (2005). The wrong question. *Development,* 48, 12–18.

Pappas, G., Hyder, A. A., & Akhter, M. (2003). Globalization: Toward a new framework for public health. *Social Theory and Health,* 1, 91–107.

Peden, M., McGee, K., & Sharma, G. (2002). *The injury chart book: A graphical overview of the global burden of injuries.* Geneva: WHO.

Pogge, T. (2002). *World poverty and human rights.* Cambridge: Polity.

Potts, D., & Mutambirwa, C. (1998). "Basics are now a luxury": Perceptions of structural adjustment's impact on rural and urban areas in Zimbabwe. *Environment and Urbanization,* 10, 55–76.

Przeworski, A., Bardhan, P., Bresser Pereira, L. C., Bruszt, L., Choi, J. J., Comisso, E. T., et al. (1995). *Sustainable democracy.* Cambridge: Cambridge University Press.

Pucher, J., Korattyswaropam, N., Mittal, N., & Ittyerah, N. (2005). Urban transport crisis in India. *Transport Policy,* 12, 185–98.

Puckett, J., Byster, L., Westervelt, S., Gutierrez, R., Davis, S., Hussain, A., et al. (2002). *Exporting harm: The high-tech trashing of Asia.* Seattle, WA: The Basel Action Network.

Razavi, S., Pearson, R., & Danloy, C., eds. (2004). *Globalization, export-oriented employment and social policy: Gendered connections.* Houndmills, UK: Palgrave Macmillan.

Reardon, K. M. (1997). State and local revitalization efforts in East St. Louis, Illinois. *Annals of the American Academy of Political and Social Science,* 551, 235–47.

Reddy, S. G., & Pogge, T. W. (2005). *How not to count the poor, Version 6.2.* New York: Columbia University. Retrieved from: http://www.undp-povertycentre.org/publications/poverty/HowNOTtocountthepoor-SANJAYREDDY.pdf.

Rich, B., Horta, K., & Goldzimer, A. (2000). *Export credit agencies in sub-Saharan Africa indebtedness for extractive industries, corruption and conflict.* Washington, DC: Environmental Defense. Retrieved from: http://www.environmentaldefense.org/documents/638_ACF666.pdf.

Richter, L. (2001). Tourism challenges in less developed nations: Continuity and change at the millennium. In D. Harrison (ed.), *Tourism and the less developed world: Issues and case studies* (pp. 47–59). Oxford: CABI Publishing.

Rodriguez, J. P., Beard, T. D., Bennett, E. M., Cumming, G. S., Cork, S. J., Agard, J., et al. (2005). Trade-offs across space, time, and ecosystem services. *Ecology and Society,* 11.

Satterthwaite, D. (2003). The Millennium Development Goals and urban poverty reduction: Great expectations and nonsense statistics. *Environment and Urbanization,* 15, 181–90.

Savitch, H. (2003). How suburban sprawl shapes human well-being. *Journal of Urban Health, 80, 590–607.*

Schiller, D. (1999). *Digital capitalism: Networking the global market system.* Cambridge, MA: MIT Press.

Schoepf, B. G. (1998). Inscribing the body politic: AIDS in Africa. In M. Lock & P. Kaufert (eds.), *Pragmatic women and body politics* (pp. 98–126). Cambridge: Cambridge University Press.

———. (2002). "Mobutu's disease": A social history of AIDS in Kinshasa. *Review of African Political Economy, 29, 561–73.*

———. (2004). AIDS in Africa: Structure, agency, and risk. In E. Kalipeni, S. Craddock, J. R. Oppong, & J. Ghosh (eds.), *HIV & AIDS in Africa: Beyond epidemiology* (pp. 121–32). Oxford: Blackwell.

Schoepf, B. G., Schoepf, C., & Millen, J. V. (2000). Theoretical therapies, remote remedies: SAPs and the political ecology of poverty and health in Africa. In J. Y. Kim, J. V. Millen, A. Irwin, & J. Gershman (eds.), *Dying for growth: Global inequality and the health of the poor* (pp. 91–126). Monroe, ME: Common Courage Press.

Schrecker, T. (2001). Using science in environmental policy: Can Canada do better? In E. Parson (ed.), *Governing the environment: Persistent challenges, uncertain innovations* (pp. 31–72). Toronto: University of Toronto Press.

Sell, S. K. (2003). *Private power, public law: The globalization of intellectual property rights.* Cambridge: Cambridge University Press.

———. (2004). The quest for global governance in intellectual property and public health: Structural, discursive and institutional dimensions. *Temple Law Review, 77, 363–99.*

Sizer, N., & Plouvier, D. (2000). *Increased investment and trade by transnational logging companies in Africa, the Caribbean and the Pacific: Implications for the sustainable management and conservation of tropical forests.* Brussels: World Wide Fund for Nature-Belgium and World Wide Fund for Nature-International.

Somerville, M. A., & Rapport, D., eds. (2000). *Transdisciplinarity: (Re)creating integrated knowledge.* London: UNESCO/EOLSS Publishers.

Stein, C. E., Inoue, M., & Fat, D. M. (2004). The global mortality of infectious and parasitic diseases in children. *Seminars in Pediatric Infectious Diseases, 15, 125–29.*

Stephens, C. (1996). Healthy cities or unhealthy islands? The health and social implications of urban inequality. *Environment and Urbanization, 8, 9–30.*

Stonich, S. (1998). Political ecology of tourism. *Annals of Tourism Research, 25, 25–54.*

Stonich, S. C., & Bailey, C. (2000). Resisting the blue revolution: Contending coalitions surrounding industrial shrimp farming. *Human Organization, 59, 23–36.*

Stonich, S. C., & Vandergeest, P. (2001). Violence, environment, and industrial shrimp farming. In N. Peluso & M. Watts (eds.), *Violent environments* (pp. 261–86). Ithaca, NY: Cornell University Press.

Storper, M. (1997). *The Regional World: Territorial development in a global economy.* New York: Guilford Press.

Strange, S. (1998). The new world of debt. *New Left Review, 230, 91–114.*

Szreter, S. (1997). Economic growth, disruption, deprivation, disease, and death: On the importance of the politics of public health for development. *Population and Development Review, 23, 693–728.*

Szreter, S. (2003). Health and security in historical perspective. In L. Chen, J. Leaning, & V. Narasimhan (eds.), *Global health challenges for human security* (pp. 31–52). Cambridge, MA: Global Equity Initiative, Asia Center, Harvard University.

Szreter, S., & Mooney, G. (1998). Urbanization, mortality, and the standard of living debate: New estimates of the expectation of life at birth in nineteenth-century British cities. *Economic History Review, 51*, 84–112.

't Hoen, E. (2002). TRIPS, Pharmaceutical patents and access to essential medicines: A long way from Seattle to Doha. *Chicago Journal of International Law, 3*, 27–46.

Turner, B. L., Clark, W. C., Kates, R. W., Richards, J. F, Matthews, J. T. , & Meyer, W. B., eds. (1993). *The Earth as transformed by human action: Global and regional changes in the biosphere over the past 300 years.* Cambridge: Cambridge University Press.

Uauy, R., Albala, C., & Kain, J. (2001). Obesity trends in Latin America: Transiting from under- to overweight. *The Journal of Nutrition, 131*, 893S–899S.

UN Millennium Project Task Force on Improving the Lives of Slum Dwellers. (2005). *A home in the city.* London: Earthscan. Retrieved from: http://www.millenniumproject.org.

United Nations Centre for Human Settlements. (2001). *Cities in a globalizing world: Global report on human settlements 2001.* London: Earthscan. Retrieved from: http://www.unhabitat.org/pmss/getPage.asp?page=bookView&book=1618.

United Nations Department of Economic and Social Affairs. (2006). *World economic situation and prospects 2006.* New York: United Nations. Retrieved from: http://www.un.org/esa/policy/wess/wesp2006files/wesp2006.pdf.

United Nations Security Council. (2002). *Final report of the panel of experts on the illegal exploitation of natural resources and other forms of wealth of the Democratic Republic of the Congo* No. S/2002/1146. New York: United Nations. Retrieved from: http://www.tcf.org/Publications/InternationalAffairs/report1.pdf.

United Nations Security Council. (2003). *Final report of the panel of experts on the illegal exploitation of natural resources and other forms of wealth of the Democratic Republic of the Congo* No. S/2003/1027. Retrieved from: http://www.tcf.org/Publications/InternationalAffairs/report2.pdf.

van der Hoeven, R., & Saget, C. (2004). Labour market institutions and income inequality: What are the new insights after the Washington consensus? In G. A. Cornia (ed.), *Inequality, growth, and poverty in an era of liberalization and globalization* (pp. 197–220). Oxford: Oxford University Press.

van Doorslaer, E., O'Donnell, O., Rannan-Eliya, R. P., Somanathan, A., Adhikari, S. R., Garg, C. C., et al. (2006). Effect of payments for health care on poverty estimates in 11 countries in Asia: An analysis of household survey data. *The Lancet, 368*, 1357–64.

Vasconcellos, E. (1997). The making of the middle-class city: Transportation policy in São Paulo. *Environment and Planning A, 29*, 293–310.

Wacquant, L. (2001). The penalisation of poverty and the rise of neo-liberalism. *European Journal on Criminal Policy and Research, 9*, 401–12.

———. (2002). Toward a dictatorship over the poor? Notes on the penalization of poverty in Brazil. *Punishment Society, 5*, 197–205.

Warf, B., & Holly, B. (1997). The rise and fall and rise of Cleveland. *Annals of the American Academy of Political and Social Science, 551*, 208–21.

Watts, M. J. (2005). Righteous oil? Human rights, the oil complex, and corporate social responsibility. *Annual Review of Environment and Resources, 30*, 373–407.

Wheeler, D. (2001). Racing to the bottom? Foreign investment and air pollution in developing countries. *Journal of Environment and Development, 10*, 225–45.

Whitehead, M., Dahlgren, G., & Evans, T. (2001). Equity and health sector reforms: Can low-income countries escape the medical poverty trap? *The Lancet*, 358, 833–36.

Williamson, J. (1990). What Washington means by policy reform. In J. Williamson (ed.), *Latin American adjustment: How much has happened?* (pp. 7–38). Washington, DC: Institute for International Economics.

Wojcicki, J. M. (2002). "She Drank His Money": Survival sex and the problem of violence in taverns in Gauteng Province, South Africa. *Medical Anthropology Quarterly*, 16, 267–93.

Wojcicki, J. M., & Malala, J. (2001). Condom use, power and HIV/AIDS risk: Sexworkers bargain for survival in Hillbrow/Joubert Park/Berea, Johannesburg. *Social Science and Medicine*, 53, 99–121.

Woodward, D., Drager, N., Beaglehole, R., & Lipson, D. (2001). Globalization and health: A framework for analysis and action. *Bulletin of the World Health Organization*, 79, 875–81.

Woodward, D., & Abdallah, S. (2008). *How poor is "poor"? Towards a rights-based poverty line (technical version)*. London: New Economics Foundation.

Woodward, D., & Simms, A. (2006). *Growth isn't working: The unbalanced distribution of benefits and costs from economic growth*. London: New Economics Foundation. Retrieved from: http://www.neweconomics.org/NEF070625/NEF_Registration070625add.aspx?returnurl=/gen/uploads/hrfu5w555mzd3-f55m2vqwty502022006112929.pdf.

World Bank. (1993). *World development report 1993: Investing in health*. New York: Oxford University Press.

———. (2007). World development indicators [online]. World Bank [online]. Retrieved from: http://devdata.worldbank.org/wdi2006/contents/index2.htm

World Health Organization. (1978). Declaration of Alma-Ata, International Conference on Primary Health Care, Alma-Ata, USSR, 6–12 September. World Health Organization [online]. Retrieved from: http://www1.umn.edu/humanrts/instree/alma-ata.html

———. (2004). *World health report 2004: Changing history*. Geneva: World Health Organization.

2 An Empirical Investigation of the Relation between Globalization and Health[1]

Giovanni Andrea Cornia, Stefano Rosignoli, and Luca Tiberti

INTRODUCTION

During the last quarter century, economic trends were favorably affected by five major changes: the end of the Cold War, the collapse of communism and spread of democratic institutions, the introduction of market reforms in dirigiste economies, a sharp deceleration in birth rates and a parallel growth of the labor force, the spread of information and communications technologies (ICT), and the biomedical revolution. The last quarter century also witnessed the spread of an economic paradigm that emphasizes domestic liberalization, privatization, and trade and financial liberalization. Its proponents claim that these measures reduce rent-seeking, increase competition, improve export opportunities, and promote the convergence of the income per capita and health status of poor countries towards those of the advanced ones (Dollar, 2001). However, such claims have seldom been validated, and economic and health performance in countries following such an approach has often been disappointing (see Chapter 9, this volume).

This chapter tries to shed some light on this apparent contradiction by discussing the relation between globalization policies,[2] socioeconomic determinants of health, and mortality. This task faces huge methodological and data challenges, and the establishment of a causal nexus between globalization policies and health status can only be tentative. Nevertheless, the literature reviewed and econometric analyses presented in this chapter suggest that, in spite of the five changes mentioned earlier witnessed during the last quarter century, the social determinants of health and indicators of population health themselves improved at a slower pace than during the previous two decades. The blame for this slowdown cannot necessarily be placed on globalization, as it could have been caused by random shocks and endogenous changes. Yet, it is possible that economic policy changes implemented under conditions of structural rigidities, incomplete markets and institutions, persistent protectionism, and a high cost of technology transfer may have delayed progress in health status.

MORTALITY TRENDS DURING THE
CURRENT ERA OF GLOBALIZATION

Between 1980 and 2000, the rate of improvement of the main health indicators slowed down in most regions (Deaton, 2004). Cornia and Menchini (2006) confirm that during the 1980s and 1990s there was a statistically significant slowdown in the global rate of improvement of (100-LEB),[3] a result that is robust to the removal from the sample of countries analyzed of the

Table 2.1 Average Annual Population-Weighted[a] Rates of Change[b] of (100-LEB) and Infant Mortality Rate, 1960–2004

	(100-LEB)				IMR			
	60–80	80–90	90–00	00–04	60–80	80–90	90–00	00–04
High-income countries	−0.84	−0.93	−0.97	−0.35***	−4.8	−3.9***	−3.6	−1.3***
China	−3.21[a]	−0.63***	−0.45***	−1.01***	−5.5[a]	−2.5***	−1.4***	−5.8***
East Asia & Pacific excl. China	−1.27	−1.28	−1.03**	−1.00	−2.5	−2.1	−3.3***	−2.6*
Eastern Europe & Central Asia (EECA)	−0.53	−0.70	−0.32***	−0.70***	−2.1	−2.1	−1.9	−3.3***
Latin America & Caribbean	−1.07	−1.04	−1.02	−0.93	−2.5	−3.5***	−3.6	−2.7***
Middle East & North Africa	−1.17	−1.58***	−1.33***	−1.06***	−2.7	−4.4***	−1.9***	−2.9**
India	−0.97	−1.14***	−0.97***	−0.36***	−1.3	−3.4***	−1.6***	−2.4***
South Asia excl. India	−0.94	−1.07	−1.25	−1.26	−1.2	−1.6	−2.1	−1.8
Sub-Saharan Africa	−0.68	−0.22***	0.64***	−0.05***	−1.7	−0.7 ***	−0.7	−0.7
World	−1.42[a]	−0.88***	−0.65***	−0.74*	−2.2[a]	−2.2	−1.0***	−1.6***
World without SSA	−1.48[a]	−0.94***	−0.79***	−0.83	−2.4[a]	−2.9***	−1.6***	−2.5***
World without SSA and EECA	−1.84[a]	−1.16***	−0.95***	−0.98	−2.6[a]	−3.2***	−2.1***	−2.8***

Source: Authors' elaboration based on World Bank (2007) and United Nations (2004).
Notes: East Asia does not include Japan; the unweighted rates of change in IMR and (100-LEB) confirm the trends revealed using the weighted data; the asterisk indicates that the rate of change is different from that of the prior period at the following probability level: ***< 0.01, **between 0.01 and 0.05, *between 0.05 and 0; the variance of the "universe" used to carry out the test is the population-weighted variance of the decennial rates of change for the countries of each region for the years 1960–2000. [a]These values are influenced by the Chinese famine of 1958–62 and would be smaller if their long-term trend value were used. Regional averages are obtained by weighting country data with the data on live births in the case of IMR and the population in that of (100-LEB).

HIV-affected sub-Saharan Africa (SSA) and the hard-hit transitional economies of Eastern Europe (Table 2.1). This slowdown was most widespread
in the 1990s, suggesting the presence of systemic problems possibly related
to policy changes recorded during that decade (Table 2.1). The infant mortality rate (IMR) trends are similar, except that in most regions the fastest
decline was recorded in the 1980s, rather than in the 1970s. This was due
to the rapid increase in child immunization rates and the coverage of other
primary health care (PHC) measures. In contrast, as confirmed by Ahmad
et al. (2000), the rate of reduction of IMR and under-five mortality rates
(U5MRs) diminished sharply in the 1990s in almost all regions. This global
slowdown was probably caused by the decline or premature leveling off of
vaccination and other key health programs, in turn caused by a decline in
their international financing (Cutler, Deaton, & Lleras-Muney, 2006); the
difficulties encountered in regions with IMRs below 30–40 per thousand
in tackling complex and costly to remove perinatal and neonatal problems;
and the rise in AIDS-related deaths among young children in sub-Saharan
Africa (Cornia & Zagonari, 2002). Yet, while all relevant, these factors do
not fully explain the IMR trends recorded in other regions. Factors including a slower growth of household incomes, greater income volatility, shifts
in health financing, and others probably contributed to this outcome.

MORTALITY MODELS AND PATHWAYS
OF HEALTH IMPACT

Five main mortality models can help to explain the slowdown in the rate
of health improvement discussed previously: material deprivation, progress
in health technology, acute psychosocial stress, unhealthy lifestyles, and
income inequality, hierarchy, and social disintegration.

Material deprivation. In this model, an increase in material resources or a
reduction in environmental contamination reduces mortality due to infectious,
parasitic, airborne, waterborne, and nutritional-related diseases. The first of
such resources is real household income. Income stability is also important for
health as households may be exposed to life-threatening income fluctuations.
Thirdly, given an average gross domestic product (GDP) per capita, an egalitarian distribution improves health status by ensuring that most households
control enough income to satisfy their basic needs, while high inequality limits
the access of the poor to basic resources. In addition, increases in the relative
price of essential goods (e.g., food and drugs) reduce household real consumption and worsen health status. The level of education of family members, and
of mothers in particular, is also a major determinant of the health status of
family members, notably children: better-educated parents have been shown
to make more rational consumption decisions and better use of public health
services, and to absorb new health knowledge more readily. Next, access to
public or private health services and their quality are closely associated with

health outcomes (World Health Organization, 2006). However, for any given amount of health resources, allocations to different levels of care and methods of financing are equally important (see Chapter 8, this volume). Public provision of free basic health services is the least discriminatory approach. This advantage persists when nominal user fees are introduced to reduce service overuse but disappears when substantial user fees are adopted. Private health financing is the most exclusionary; the impact of health insurance is regressive in economies with a large informal sector. Health outcomes also depend on demographic factors, as families with high dependency ratios tend to have worse health outcomes. Finally, environmental contamination affects life expectancy, particularly among the poor who are exposed to air-, water-, and vector-borne diseases, pollutants, industrial wastes, and pesticides.

Progress in health technology. During the post–World War II period, progress in health technology sharply reduced mortality due to infectious, parasitic, and communicable diseases in low-income countries (Preston, 1976), while medical advances in controlling cardiovascular problems explain 70 percent of the seven-year gains in LEB recorded in the United States between 1960 and 2000 (Cutler et al., 2006). The health impact of such discoveries depends on their accessibility, which in turn depends on the existence of nonexclusionary delivery channels. In developing countries, progress in health technology can be proxied by the coverage rate of immunization, oral rehydration, clinic-based delivery, and access to fresh water, while in countries with an elderly population it can be proxied by the rate of screening for chronic and degenerative diseases.

Acute psychosocial stress. Stress is a key factor in deaths due to heart problems, hypertension, alcohol psychosis, suicide, accidental deaths, and cirrhosis. In countries hit by social upheavals, death due to acute stress results from increased pressures to adapt to new situations, the absence of coping strategies, and weak public policy responses. Epidemiological research has shown that stress leads to physiological and psychological arousal, which provokes sudden changes in heart rate, blood pressure and viscosity, loss of emotional balance, sense of powerlessness, and loss of personal control and purpose in life (Marmot & Bobak, 2000). Acute stress has been shown to lead to increased consumption of health-damaging stress relievers such as alcohol and drugs, which further affects mental balance and social behavior.

As suggested by the Social Readjustment Rating Scale, stress may also arise from loss of employment, especially if this is unanticipated and unaddressed by public policy. Marmot and Bobak (2000) estimate that jobless workers face on average a 20 percent greater risk of death than the employed. In addition to a loss of income, unemployment causes a loss of skills, cognitive abilities, motivation, and sense of control, while giving rise to feelings of being unwanted, unproductive, dependent, and without a role. Unemployment may also erode social norms and cause an increase in crime rate and family violence. Stress may also arise from the sense of frustration caused by failure to fulfill one's own obligations, rapid changes in social hierarchies, and changes in personal living arrangements such as widowhood, divorce, and distress migration.

Unhealthy lifestyles. According to this model, the promotion of health information and changes in personal behavior are the most important determinants of health status. Smoking is a main factor in premature deaths due to cancer, emphysema, cardiovascular diseases, cirrhosis, and nonmedical fatalities. Smoking kills one in every ten people, with 85 percent of them in developing countries where quit rates are very low (Ezzati et al., 2005). Excessive consumption of salt and saturated fats raises the incidence of cardiovascular problems, especially if associated to lack of physical exercise, while a low intake of antioxidants is associated with a high risk of myocardial infarction. In addition, excessive alcohol consumption is related to deaths due to cirrhosis of the liver, psychosis, accidents, and injury. For years, the unhealthy-lifestyles model has guided mortality analyses in developed countries but recent literature on "nutritional transition" and "communicability of smoking to developing countries" suggests it applies also to the urban population of middle- and low-income countries (see Chapter 10, this volume).

Income inequality, hierarchy, and social disintegration. High income inequality affects health by increasing social stratification and eroding social cohesion (Wilkinson, 1996). Highly stratified societies feature a high degree of heterogeneity, divergent social objectives, limited capacity to undertake collective action, low taxation and provision of public health services, residential segregation, and restricted political participation. Such phenomena are not the prerogative of advanced countries but have been observed also in poor rural settings, as shown by the study of Godoy et al (2006) on thirteen Bolivian villages. According to this model, high inequality erodes social cohesion and control, which are essential factors in the diffusion of health information, control over deviant health behavior and criminal activity, and promotion of interpersonal help among community members (Kawachi, Kennedy, & Wilkinson, 1999). One particular source of such stress is a hierarchical organization of work in which decisions are concentrated in the hands of a few people, while the rest have little control over work decisions. One suggested explanation is the "learned helplessness" model, a concept first developed from animal studies to describe an apparent resignation to harmful noxious events beyond control even when barriers to control were removed.

CHANGES IN THE DETERMINANTS
OF HEALTH FROM 1980–2005

Changes that occurred from 1980–2005 in the economic and social determinants of health discussed in the context of the five mortality models discussed previously are reviewed in the text that follows.

Growth of GDP per capita. Trends in this area are well known (Table 2.2). To begin, world growth slowed down from 1980–2000 (the present era of globalization) compared to the previous twenty years, 1960–1980. Growth was particularly weak in the 1990s owing to stagnation in Europe, Japan, Latin America, Middle East, and North Africa (MENA), the effect of the 1997 financial crisis on the Asian economies, and to recession in the transition economies and sub-Saharan Africa. Second, negative or zero growth was recorded in 32 percent of the countries analyzed, and growth of less than 1 percent was recorded in another eighteen countries where, *ceteris paribus*, health status deteriorated or improved only slowly. In contrast, growth improved in East and Southeast Asia, India, and China. Third, the engine of world growth shifted from the Organisation for Economic Co-operation and Development (OECD) to the Asian countries. However, given their low initial weight, their surge in growth was overshadowed by the slowdown in the OECD countries, thus leading to a global growth deceleration. Finally, during the period 2000–2005, the growth rate of GDP per capita showed a mild recovery due to continued growth in the Asian economies, a moderate recovery in sub-Saharan Africa and Japan, and strong growth in transitional Europe.

Table 2.2   Period GDP per Capita Growth Rates[a] by Main Regions

	1960–1970	1970–1980	1980–1990	1990–2000	1960–1980	1980–2000	2000–2005
High-income countries	4.11	2.60	2.39	1.88	3.35	2.13	1.45
China	1.49	4.31	7.71	9.26	2.89	8.48	8.77
East Asia & Pacific (excl. China)	2.87	4.51	3.47	3.18	3.69	3.32	3.60
Eastern Europe & Central Asia	5.0*	2.3*	2.1*	−1.03	n.a.	n.a.	5.07
Latin America & Caribbean	2.54	3.15	−0.89	1.68	2.85	0.39	0.94
Middle East & North Africa	n.a.	n.a.	0.14	1.88	n.a.	1.01	2.15
India	1.69	0.68	3.58	3.62	1.19	3.60	5.25
South Asia (excl. India)	2.60	0.40	2.82	1.93	1.50	2.38	2.52
Sub-Saharan Africa	2.31	0.76	−1.04	−0.32	1.53	−0.68	1.96
World	3.25	1.83	1.38	1.41	2.54	1.39	1.53

Source: Authors' calculation based on World Bank (2007).
Notes: The regional aggregates refer only to the developing countries (e.g., East Asia does not include Japan); the data in the columns refer to the periods 1960–70, 1970–80, 1980–90 and are from Cornia & Danziger (1997); [a]average yearly compounded and population weighted growth rates computed on a point-to-point decennial basis.

Economic instability. In most low- and high-income countries, macro instability remained broadly unchanged during the last quarter century (Table 2.3), though micro instability rose in several of them. For instance, in Japan the unemployment rate rose from zero in the late 1980s to 5.4 per cent in 2002 following the scrapping of the old lifetime employment system. While mortality due to most causes declined, the number of suicides grew by 80 percent between 1990 and 2000, affecting mainly unemployed workers and bankrupt managers (Lamar, 2000). In contrast, macro and micro instability rose in most middle-income countries. Indeed, globalization appears to have heightened the instability of GDP per capita (Table 2.3) due to an epidemic of banking, financial, and currency crises which followed the financial deregulation of the mid-1980s and the capital account liberalization of the 1990s.

The health impact of growing instability is increasingly documented. A study of sixty-eight developing countries by Guillaumont et al. (2006) found that growing volatility of GDP per capita growth rate negatively correlated with the survival rate of children of under five years of age. The most shocking case of increased mortality caused by macro instability is that observed during the transition in the former Soviet Union. Micro studies on the health impact of instability are less common but point in the same direction. One example is the sharp rise of suicides among cotton farmers in Andra Pradesh (Cornia, 2004) following the abolition in July 1991 of state subsidies to agriculture, rising input costs, the liberalization of cotton imports, rising volatility in world cotton prices, and the absence of price stabilization mechanisms.

Income inequality. From the early 1980s income inequality began to rise in the majority of OECD countries, Latin America, transitional Europe, and China (Table 2.4). An increase of income inequality was observed also in the egalitarian economies of East Asia and, after the liberalization of 1991, in India. Jäntti and Sandstrom (2005) show that inequality rose in most of the 115 countries they analyzed, while Table 2.4 suggests that it increased in sixty of the eighty-five countries for which it was possible to construct a long-term trend. However, in eleven of those sixty countries, inequality stabilized in the 1990s or 2000s after the shift from Keynesian to liberal policies was completed (as in the United Kingdom) or following a return to GDP growth in the early 2000s (as in some transitional economies).

Table 2.3   Average Standard Deviation of GDP per Capita Growth Rate by Country Groups, 1960–2005

	1960–1970	1970–1981	1982–1990	1990–2005
Low-income	4.69	6.32	4.95	4.58
Middle-income	2.77	3.48	4.44	5.62
High-income	1.93	2.69	1.91	2.58

Source: Authors' elaboration on World Bank (2007).

Notes: The above values are obtained by computing the decadal standard deviation of each country, which were then averaged for each of the three areas.

Table 2.4   Trends in the Gini Coefficients of the Distribution of Income from the 1950s
to the 2000s in 85 Developed, Developing, and Transitional Economies

Inequality Trend	OECD Countries	Transition Countries	Developing Countries	World	% of Countries	% of Populations	% of GDP-PPP[a]
Rising	13	24	23	60	70	76	71
Constant	1	1	14	16	19	19	18
Declining	6	0	3	9	11	5	12
Total	20	25	40	85	100	100	100

Source: Authors' calculation based on World Income Inequality Database (United Nations University & World Institute for Development Economics Research, 2008).

Notes: The higher a Gini coefficient, the more unequal the distribution of income in a jurisdiction; [a]/gross domestic product–purchasing power parity.

Inflation and prices of basic goods. Inflation rates declined almost everywhere for most of the 1980s and 1990s due to the emphasis placed by many governments on the achievement of low inflation. Yet, the reforms of the last quarter century emphasized measures, such as price liberalization and the removal of subsidies to essential goods and devaluation, that could have led to faster rises in food prices than in the consumer price index (CPI). The trend of the food price index per CPI ratio, however, does not provide evidence of such an effect except for the transition economies.

Taxation, public health expenditure, and health financing. In advanced countries, health expenditure rose because of aging and the high income elasticity of the demand for health care. Developing countries behaved in a heterogeneous way. With the reduction of budget deficits following the introduction of stabilization policies, the spending capacity of governments was increasingly determined by the tax revenue collected. In this regard, reduction of tariffs following trade liberalization diminished, *ceteris paribus*, government spending capacity. Furthermore, developing countries reduced corporate income tax and introduced tax holidays for foreign investors. As a result of these and other changes, the average tax/GDP ratio of a number of developing countries dropped by 1 percentage point over the 1980s and 1990s, as opposed to a rise of 1.6 points between the 1970s and 1980s (Chu, Davoodi, & Gupta, 2000). These trends may be behind the drop in public health expenditure observed in several countries, such as in China between 1978 and 1990, and in India after 1991. However, in other countries, public health expenditure remained the same or even increased.

Health status and access to health care were also influenced by changes in health financing. These changes were often instituted in the wake of the budget crises of the early to mid-1980s and basically introduced user fees in state clinics, opened up health care provision to private providers, privatized government hospitals, and introduced private health insurance. These health sector reforms reduced service utilization in sub-Saharan Africa (Reddy &

Vandermoortele, 1996) while a survey-based review of eleven Asian countries (van Doorslaer et al., 2006) shows that out-of-pocket payments for charges at public hospitals, drug purchases, and insurance copayments rose markedly, with the exception of Malaysia and Indonesia. In turn, following the introduction of private health insurance in 1994 in Vietnam, there was an 11.6 percent rise between 1993 and 1998 in the share of sick people not seeking care (Tiberti, 2006). In China, as a result of the health reforms of the 1980s and 1990s, out-of-pocket payments rose from 20 to 56 percent of total health expenditure from 1978 to 2003 and became the only way to secure medical care, while a sizable part of the population was left with no coverage (Aiguo, 2006).

Migration and family arrangements. In 2005, the world stock of migrants reached 190 million. Migration may have helped to improve the health of people in countries of destination (OECD and Gulf States) through better staffing of health services and care of the elderly by migrants. Second, migrants generally work in low-skilled jobs no longer filled by locals, contributing in this way to overall growth. Migration also moderates growth in wages, thus preserving economic competitiveness. In the countries of origin, the outflow of medical practitioners caused "brain drain," but migrant remittances raised the consumption of food and drugs and as a result may have contributed to better health outcomes. A declining density of health workers in low-income countries with high burdens of disease, however, is associated with higher rates of maternal, infant, and U5MR, indicating at best an ambiguous health outcome for several so-called source countries (see Chapter 9, this volume).

Technical progress in health. Assessing the impact of medical progress on health worldwide requires answering three questions: Has globalization enhanced incentives to produce new drugs addressing the health problems of advanced and developing countries? Have trade and technology transfer policies facilitated the shift of health knowledge to less advanced countries? And have domestic policies enhanced access to transferred technologies?

First, it is difficult to prove whether liberalization has led to an acceleration in health discoveries. What is clear, however, is that research continued to focus on health conditions typical of advanced countries. Only 10 percent of research expenditure is currently allocated to diseases which are common in developing countries and which account for 90 percent of the global burden of disease.

Second, trade liberalization favorably affected the transfer of health knowledge by reducing tariffs. Likewise, cheaper and faster transmission of data via the Internet sped up the diffusion of health information. The last twenty years also recorded the diffusion in poor countries of vaccines, oral rehydration salts, nutritional supplements, antibiotics, aspirin, and drugs following patent expiration. The spread of these low-cost health technologies played a key role in reducing infant and overall mortality. Combined diphtheria, polio, and tetanus (DPT) immunization rates, for instance, rose sharply between 1980 and 1990, though after 1990 they

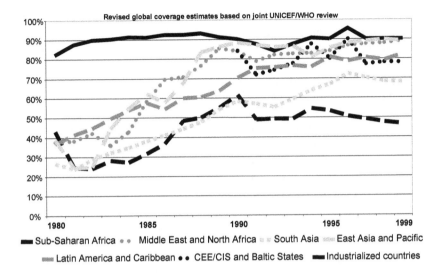

Figure 2.1 DPT percentage immunization rate, 1980–99.
Source: Authors' elaboration on United Nations Children's Fund (UNICEF) data.

stagnated or fell (Figure 2.1). The transfer of sophisticated drugs and technologies including beta-blockers, screening equipment, cardiac units, and
antiretroviral drugs was more limited, as the Agreement on Trade-Related
Aspects of Intellectual Property Rights (TRIPS) raised the cost of newly
patented drugs and medical technologies (see Chapter 11, this volume). As
put by Deaton (2004, p. 30), "There is clearly a long way to go before the
[health] habits and technology of the rich countries are fully adopted even
in middle-income countries."

Third, the free-market policies adopted in the health sector emphasized
the introduction of user fees in state facilities and privatization of health:
measures that tend to exclude the poor from health care.

Smoking, drinking, and obesity. During the last quarter century, these
risk factors became relevant for a growing share of the population of
developing countries. The International Mortality and Smoking Statistics (IMASS) database shows that, after rising from 1960 to 1980, smoking incidence among men fell steadily in OECD countries as a result of
awareness campaigns, a variety of prohibitions (including pricing policies,
tobacco advertising, and promotional campaigns), and class actions against
tobacco companies. In contrast, smoking prevalence continues to rise for
both men and women in Eastern Europe and developing countries, partly
because the liberalization of foreign direct investment (FDI) made possible the relocation of tobacco transnational corporations (TNCs) to these
countries. In developing countries, purchases of highly processed foods and
drinks rich in salt, sugar, and fat from supermarkets have risen steadily,

and now account for a quarter of total food purchases (Hawkes, 2005). The result of this nutritional transition to calorie-dense inexpensive food has been a rapid increase in obesity, cholesterol, blood pressure, cardiovascular diseases, and diabetes among the urban poor in both developing and developed countries. Finally, with the exception of low-income nations, there has been an increase over the last twenty years in the consumption of alcohol, particularly in the transition economies.

Random shocks. The last quarter century also witnessed a sharp rise in the number of internal wars, ethnic struggles, and complex humanitarian emergencies, which climbed from twenty-five per year in the early 1980s to almost sixty in the mid-to-late 1990s. Conflicts have raised the number of deaths due to violence, starvation, and infectious diseases. While in some cases the related mortality spikes quickly returned to precrisis levels at the end of the shock, this has not been the case in parts of sub-Saharan Africa where conflicts have become endemic. The Centre for Research on the Epidemiology of Disasters (CRED)[4] database shows that the number of casualties involved in such conflicts was 200,000 to 500,000 in Rwanda, 100,000 in Angola in 1994, 100,000 in Burundi in 1993, and 100,000 in Mozambique in 1992, about 50,000 in Liberia in 1993, and smaller but not negligible numbers in Sudan and South Africa in 1993. Increases in mortality were also due to the spread of HIV-AIDS that currently kills 2.3 million people a year worldwide. Its incidence is highest in Eastern and Southern Africa, where in the late 1990s, adult prevalence rates ranged from 12 percent in Tanzania to 35 percent in Botswana.

ECONOMETRIC MODELS OF LIFE EXPECTANCY AT BIRTH, INFANT MORTALITY RATE, AND UNDER-FIVE MORTALITY RATE

Globalization-Health Nexus Database (GHND). The estimation of an econometric model linking mortality indicators to the health determinants described earlier required the development of a GHND database[5] which includes LEB, IMR, and U5MR, their determinants, indexes of policies for Latin America and Eastern Europe that may influence the determinants of health, and random shocks. Information for these variables was compiled for the 1960–2005 period for 136 countries and ten quinquennia (1960, and every five years thereafter) and, in the case of the European economies in transition, for the years 1985–2005. If data for all countries and years were available, the "quinquennial GHND" would count 1,360 (136 × 10) data points for each variable. Missing data at the beginning and end of the period reduce the number of country-years for which all data are available. When missing data for one or two years concerning a qualitatively well-known phenomenon threatened to reduce the number of complete data strings, the missing data were interpolated on the basis of information taken from the literature. The data points added in this way represent 6 percent of the total number of observations, except for DPT vaccination for which estimated data account for 18 percent of the data[6] used in regression analysis. The 136 countries included in GHND were grouped into eight regions (sub-Saharan Africa, South Asia, Southeast and East Asia, MENA, Latin America, OECD, Eastern Europe, and the former USSR), which were further grouped into "low-income developing countries" (sub-Saharan Africa, South Asia, and China), "middle-income developing countries" (Southeast and East Asia excluding China, Latin America, and MENA), a third group which includes the European transitional economies, and a fourth containing the OECD countries.

Model specification and regression plan. GHND is organized as a tridimensional matrix, with 136 countries on one axis, ten quinquennia on the second, and the dependent and explanatory variables on the third. This kind of dataset requires that the procedure chosen for the estimation of the mortality model takes into account that each country is observed over several periods. The model takes therefore the following form: where y is the dependent variable, x is a vector of explanatory variables, the subscripts i and t represent respectively the countries and the quinquennia of the panel, u_i the error term for each country, ε_{it} a joint error term for countries and time periods, and α and β the parameters to be estimated. Given the nature of GHND, the Ordinary Least Squares (OLS) procedure yields inefficient estimates and distorts the values of α and β, as information on the countries' fixed effects would be neglected (Baltagi, 2005). The estimation procedure best suited to situations in which u_i varies from country to country is the fixed effects model[7] in which u_i is not treated as a random variable. The Hausman test confirmed that such a model is the most appropriate under these circumstances. To improve the goodness of fit and the robustness of the estimates, and to avoid multicollinearity problems, a few explanatory variables were either dropped or normalized. For instance, to remove its inverse correlation with GDP per capita, the Gini coefficient was in some cases standardized for the time trend (proxied by "year-1959"). In turn, the variable "log doctors per 1,000 people" was divided by the Gini coefficient or by the log of GDP per capita, obtaining an index of availability of distribution of health personnel relative to the GDP per capita norm. Output volatility was proxied by the maximum value in any five-year period of the five-year rolling standard deviation of GDP per capita. The health impact of technical progress was proxied with DPT immunization coverage and regional time dummies for 1985–2005 in relation to 1960–80. All other variables were included without changes. The age dependency ratio was used only for transition economies, where it changed markedly in recent years, while it was dropped in other regions as it correlates too closely with GDP per capita.

Estimation results: the global mortality model. Table 2.5 presents the results of the estimation of the global relation between health status measured by LEB, IMR, and U5MR. The parameters in Table 2.5 capture the average global impact of the explanatory variables included in the five mortality pathways analyzed, and of the random shocks discussed in the "Mortality models and pathways of health impact" sections of the chapter. Given the large number of different countries and long time span considered, the estimates of this "multipathway model" are quite stable. The regression results on LEB are presented separately for the entire 1960–2005 period and for the periods of 1960–80 (the so-called Second Golden Age of globalization) and 1985–2005 (the current era of globalization).

Models (1), (4), and (5) present the results of the estimation of a multipathway mortality model over the 1960–2005 period. Though based on 556 observations (553 for U5MR) out of a theoretical maximum of 1,360 for ninety-seven countries (out of 136), the estimates in Table 2.5 are satisfactory. Practically all variables have the expected sign as well as plausible and statistically significant coefficients.[8] These models suggest that an important part of the gains in LEB, IMR, and U5MR (ranging between 0.74 years in the OECD to 3.4 LEB years in South Asia and MENA) was due to technical progress in health realized over the 1985–2000 period. The negative value recorded by this variable in the transition economies is correct and reflects the collapse of the socialist health care model during the 1990s. However, "technical progress in health" is proxied by a time dummy that could capture unexplained effects such as, in the case of the economies in transition, the institutional shock experienced after 1990. The impact of technical progress in health is captured also by the highly significant value of the coefficient of DPT vaccination.

Log GDP/capita is also highly significant for the 1960–2005 period as well as for its two subperiods. The same is true for the volatility of GDP per capita that negatively affects LEB, IMR, and U5MR. In turn, income inequality affects strongly and significantly all three health indicators. Quinquennial increases in income inequality greater than 4 Gini points were also found to be significant in the LEB models, though they are, as expected, weakly significant in the case of IMR and U5MR. For instance, rises in the Gini coefficient of ten points from one quinquennium to the next reduce LEB by one year, thus supporting the conclusions of prior studies. Female illiteracy is strongly significant in all five models, and a reduction of ten points reduces U5MR by 8.2 points. The availability of health services (measured by log physicians per 1,000/Gini) is significant in all five models but weakly so for the 1960–80 period. In turn, adopting health-damaging health behaviors, such as excessive alcohol consumption, affects LEB and, surprisingly, IMR. Finally, the model confirms a positive, if small, impact of migrant stocks greater than 3.5 percent of the resident population on the LEB of the countries of destination.

As for random shocks, HIV-AIDS appears to have a large and significant health effect. Raising the HIV prevalence rate by thirty points reduces LEB by a staggering twenty-five years (as observed in Botswana) and raises child mortality by fifty-two points. In contrast, disasters, wars, and humanitarian emergencies are nonsignificant and often have the wrong sign (i.e., not

Table 2.5 Results of Worldwide Regression Analysis for 1960–2005 on LEB[a], IMR, and U5MR

	LEB			IMR	U5MR
	1960–2005	1960–1980	1980–2005	1960–2005	1960–2005
	(1)	(2)	(3)	(4)	(5)
Constant term	38.966***	52.707***	39.673***	165.088***	254.926***
Dummy tech progr. 1980–05 OECD	0.792*	....	....	3.818	8.297** ws
Dummy tech progr. 1980–05 E.Asia	1.362**	....	....	1.192	1.051
Dummy tech progr. 1980–05 Trans	−2.461***	....	....	−3.064	1.2714
Dummy tech progr. 1980–05 Latin American Countries (LAC)	3.311***	....	....	−21.126***	−31.583***
Dummy tech progr. 1980–05 MENA	3.432***	....	....	−44.478***	−56.951***
Dummy tech progr. 1980–05 S.Asia	3.397***	....	....	−8.411**	−25.279***
Dummy tech progr 1980–05 SSA	2.438**	....	....	−12.971***	−18.3312***
Log GDP/capita	3.203***	2.307***	3.148***	−14.19***	−21.75***
GDP/capita volatility	−.0009**	−.0007	−.0008*	.0042*	.0093***
Gini income distribution	−0.057**	−.1058**	−.0498***	.3215***	.4424**
Δ Gini coeff . > 4 points	−.0423*–	−.0645	−.0398	.0861	.2821
Female illiteracy (%)	−.098***	−.2763***	−.0427*	.5779***	.9464***
Log physicians per 1,000 people/Gini	36.89***	7.305	55.392*–	−90.98*–	−158.69*
DPT Immunization rate (%)	.0861***	.1425***	.0828***	−.3631***	−.6155***
Immigrants stock/ Total population	.0026***	.0040***	.0042*–	−.0007	−.0042
Alcohol consumption/capita	−.2536***	−.4074***	−.2702***	.4841*	.3820
War and humanitarian emergencies	14.95**ws	−24.420	13.56*–		
ws	−15.63	−4.332			
Disasters	.2864	.4415	.2106	2.6132*	3.2774*–
HIV/AIDS	−.8495***	−2.099***	−.7737***	1.1505***	1.8334***
F statistic	126.89***	56.45***	77.02***	113.39***	113.64***
R square	.897	.847	.890	.820	.845
Number of observations	556	234	385	556	553
Number of countries	97	65	97	97	97

Source: Authors' calculations based on GHND.

Notes: ***significant at the 1% level; **between 1 and 5% level; *between 5 and 10% level; *–significant at 10–15%; ws = wrong sign; [a]/the use of LEB (instead of 100-LEB, as in Table 2.1) does not change the results of the model, as every linear transformation of the dependent variable in a regression model does not change the value of the parameters which, however, change their sign.

the sign expected). This may be due to their low frequency or poor approximation of the variable in the GHND.

REGIONAL RESULTS

The mortality models described in Table 2.5 were validated separately on high-, middle-, and low-income countries, and transition economies. The variables that do not influence mortality in specific regions were omitted (e.g., the relative price of food, wars, and disasters in the advanced countries), while it is expected that the sign of some variables (e.g., migrant stock) might change from region to region, and that of parameters of log GDP/capita may become small or insignificant in high-income groups. In turn, female education was proxied by the percentage of women who completed primary education in low-income countries, postsecondary education in high-income countries and transition countries, and female illiteracy in middle-income countries. When available, regional variables were added, as was smoking for the high-income group, while variables with no or only a few regional observations were omitted. Finally, the estimation of regional models entails dividing the sample of 556 observations into four subsamples causing, by definition, a loss of significance of the parameters, particularly in regions with fewer data. This was the case for transition countries, where the lack of a sufficient number of quinquennial data required testing the model on annual data for 1980–2005.

The results for the high-income countries (130 observations) are satisfactory (Table 2.6). Of the ten variables explaining LEB, all but one (log of physicians per 1,000/log GDP/capita) have the right sign and are significant. Smoking and drinking depress LEB in a significant way, while immigration has a positive (if modest) effect on LEB. As predicted by the Preston curve, GDP per capita is not significant if considered alone but is significant if interacted with its volatility. Likewise, increases in Gini coefficients > 4 are not significant as this phenomenon was seldom observed in the region. All other variables have correct signs and plausible parameters. In the case of IMR and U5MR, half of the variables have the right sign and are statistically significant, though the economic variables measuring stress and resources (log GDP/volatility, income inequality, and sudden changes in inequality) have, as expected, nonsignificant signs. As expected, smoking and migrant stock are also not significant, suggesting that they do not significantly affect the survival of children.

The mortality model is validated in an equally satisfactory way for the middle-income countries (218 observations), as all twelve variables (including war and disasters) have the expected sign and are highly significant, with the exception of Δ Gini > 4, GDP volatility, disasters, wars, and medical progress in East Asia. Similar results are obtained for IMR and U5MR. Interestingly, both IMR and U5MR rise when the "migrant stock" increases, possibly signaling a kind of brain-drain effect, though the related parameters are weak or nonsignificant.

Table 2.6 Results of the Regression Analysis on LEB, IMR, U5MR for the High- and Middle-Income Countries (Quinquennial Data, 1960–2005)

	High-income countries			Middle-income countries		
	LEB 1960–2005	IMR 1960–2005	U5MR 1960–05	LEB 1960–05	IMR 1960–05	U5MR 1960–05
Constant term	94.43***	2.5942*-	-5.4486	38.56***	158.22***	208.53***
Dummy med progr 80–05 OECD	1.06***	-3.9686***	-5.1890***	0.6603	9.19**ws	12.49*–ws
Dummy med progr 80–05 E.Asia				1.8315***	-13.40***	-19.07***
Dummy med progr 80–05 LAC				1.2796*	-22.96***	-34.55***
Dummy med progr 80–05 MENA				2.5239***	-13.31***	-18.37***
Log GDP/capita	⋯⋯	⋯⋯	⋯⋯	.0071	.0169*	
Log GDPcapital/ volatility	74.78***	-30.22	-102.16			
GDP/capita volatility	-.0482*	.3415***	-.00003			
Gini income distribution	⋯⋯	⋯⋯	⋯⋯	-.0679***	.2534***	.4695***
Gini income distribution/t	.1002	-.5582	.5013***	-.0456	.1780	.6743–
Δ Gini coeff. > 4 points	.2888***	-.7689***	-.7957			
% women > 25 with post2ary educ	⋯⋯	⋯⋯	-.9792***	-.1918***	1.1433***	1.7979***
Female illiteracy	-28.9***ws	20.80	36.57	11.2796***	-14.75	-31.33
Log phys. per 1000/ Log GDP/capita	.0775***	-.1969***	-.2514***	.0701***	-.3296***	-.5999***
DPT Immunization rate (%)	.0017***	.0029*	.0027	.0035*–	-.0099	.0128
Immigrants stock/ Population	-.2582***	.4301**	.5003***			
Alcohol consumption/capita	-.0544***	-0.0210	-.0306	-.4350***	1.4932***	1.7121*-
Smoking				No data	No data	No data
War and human emergencies	Unobserved	Unobserved	Unobserved	-10.3808	94.22	136.06
Disasters	Unobserved	Unobserved	Unobserved	-.2075	1.6205	1.3079
HIV/AIDS	Unobserved	Unobserved	Unobserved	Unobserved	Unobserved	Unobserved
F statistic	69.81***	40.97***	40.85***	185.63***	115.03***	127.17***
R square	.287	.509	.513	.837	.684	.721
Number of observations	130	130	130	212	212	212
Number of countries	22	22	22	34	34	34

Source: Authors' calculations.
Notes: ws = wrong sign.

Table 2.7   Results of the Regression Analysis on LEB, IMR, U5MR for Low-Income (Quinquennial Data for 1960–2005) and Transitional Economies (Yearly Data for 1980–2005)

	Low-income countries			Transitional countries		
	LEB	IMR	U5MR	LEB	IMR	U5MR
Constant term	22.10**	158.73***	291.25***	54.37***	80.29***	67.92***
Dummy tech progr 80–05	3.041***	−19.06***	−33.58***			
Dummy trans 90–05	……	……	……	−.15139	−1.128**	−.9778*–
Log GDP/capita	3.6640***	−7.8231*	−18.91**	1.6664**	−2.9997**	−2.2838
GDP/capita volatility	−.0064*	.0065	.0396*–	−.0012***	0.0007*–	.0009*–
Gini income distribution	−.2032***	.8179***	1.5343***	−.0062	−.2843*** ws	−.3061*** ws
Δ Gini income > 4 pts	.0641	−.2959	−.7060	−.1421**	.3840***	.7762***
% enrolment in secondary education	……	……	……	.0346***	−.0761***	−.0504***
% women with completed primary education	.1913**	−.6223*	−1.0926*	……	……	……
Log physicians × 1,000 people/ Log GDP/capita	14.2350**	−14.48	−24.7722	8.6528**	−36.66***	−32.9712***
DPT immunization rate (%)	.1147***	−.5339***	−.8950***			
Immigrants stock/ population	−.0276**	.0030	.0818	……	……	……
Age dependency ratio	……	……	……	−15.2211***	45.395***	59.2501***
Alcohol consumption/capita	−.0240	−.2135	−1.4582	No data	No data	No data
War	26.66	−198.94	−291.25	No data	No data	No data
Disasters	.0246	4.7663**	7.353*	No data	No data	No data
HIV/AIDS	−.7208***	.6006***	.9750***	Unobserved	Unobserved	Unobserved
F statistic	32.21***	32.60***	27.49***	28.95***	43.66***	45.36***
R square	.743	.661	.613	.170	.586	.605
Number of observations	123	123	114	325	316	316
Number of countries	23	23	22	24	24	24

Source: Authors' calculations.

Notes: The years 1960 and 2005 have a low coverage; ws = wrong sign.

For the low-income countries (125 observations), the LEB model shows very satisfactory results (Table 2.7) as all variables have the expected sign (except for alcohol consumption, disasters, and wars, which are also non-significant), and are statistically significant (but for Δ Gini > 4), thus confirming the conclusions arrived at on the basis of the global model. It must be noted that the value of the parameters of log GDP/capita, Gini, DPT, and others is generally greater than in the global or middle-income-countries model, confirming the theoretical expectations that changes in such variables have a greater health impact in poor than in rich countries.

Finally, the estimates for the transition countries are less comprehensive than those of the other three regions, as the estimation was carried out on yearly data for 1980–2005 and no data are available for DPT immunization, migration, alcohol consumption, war, and disasters. Several of the key effects are, however, also correctly estimated in this case: the LEB model (Table 2.7) captures most effects related to negative gain in medical progress, volatility, GDP per capita, large Gini increments, female education, availability of doctors, and dependency ratio (which captures the region's demographic collapse of the 1990s). The Gini of income distribution is nonsignificant, but its larger than four-points increment is significant. Similar results were obtained for IMR and U5MR, though in these two models the Gini of income distribution had the wrong sign, and log GDP was nonsignificant.

A confirmation of the good results of the estimations presented in Tables 2.7 and 2.8 is given by Figure 2.2, which describes the good fit of the LEB

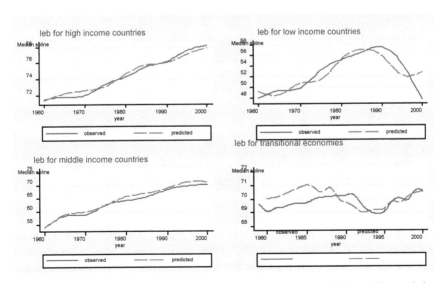

Figure 2.2 Trend in the observed (solid line) and estimated (dotted line) of the median spline of the life expectancy at birth in the four subregions.
Source: Authors' calculations.

estimates (dotted lines) in relation to the observed values (solid line) for the respective reference periods and regional groups.

SIMULATION OF LEB CHANGES DUE TO GLOBALIZATION AND SHOCKS

The preceding models can be used to assess whether the changes observed recently in the policy-driven determinants of health (growth of GDP per capita, inequality, instability, and health provision), random shocks (HIV-AIDS, wars, and disasters), and endogenous medical progress led in 2000 to LEB values higher than, equal to, or lower than those which would have been achieved under a "counterfactual scenario" in which all the LEB determinants followed the trend observed over 1960–80. In practice, this means first fixing for each variable a 2000 value obtained by prolonging the 1960–80 trend or keeping constant its 1980 value and, secondly, simulating on the basis of these counterfactual values and of the regional LEB models in Tables 2.7 and 2.8 the values that LEB would have taken by 2000. The specific hypotheses in the counterfactual scenario are:

1. The log of GDP/capita*Gini, log of physicians per 1,000/log GDP/capita, and migration stock rise between 1985 and 2005 according to their 1960–80 trend.
2. DPT immunization rates, female illiteracy (or primary or secondary education), and alcohol consumption rise according to their 1960–90 trend.
3. GDP volatility, the Gini index of the distribution of income, age dependency ratio, and smoking incidence remain at their 1980 or 1985 level. As a result, the change in Gini is equal to zero.
4. There is no progress in health technologies between 1985 and 2005.
5. HIV-AIDS incidence remains at its 1980 level and there are no disasters and wars.

Thus, for each region the *simulated* LEB values in 2000 (LEB^s_i) are equal to the sum of the products of the simulated 2000 values of explanatory variables by the parameters of equations (1) in Tables 2.7 and 2.8.[9]

The observed values of LEB in 2000 (LEB^o_i) are the sum of the products of the observed 2000 values of the explanatory variables by the parameters of equations (1) in Tables 2.7 and 2.8.[10]

It is now possible to compute, region by region, the difference between LEB^o_i and LEB^s_i as the sum of the differences between the observed and simulated values of each explanatory variable multiplied by the parameters α_1, α_2, etc. of equation (1) in Tables 2.7 and 2.8.[11]

In this way, for each country or region in Table 2.8, it is possible to derive, variable by variable, the LEB gains (+) and losses (−) in 2000 due to the impact of globalization on the determinants of health, endogenous changes, and random shocks in relation to a "business as usual" counterfactual. World changes in LEB are obtained by weighting regional LEB changes by their populations. At the global level, changes in variables depending on globalization policies appear to have reduced LEB by 1.52 years as a result of several offsetting effects. Higher income inequality than in the counterfactual scenario depressed LEB by 0.77 years. This loss is counterbalanced by LEB gains (0.73 years) due to growth in GDP per capita faster than in the counterfactual scenario in China, India, and the rest of South Asia (in most regions, however, a GDP growth slower than between 1960 and 1980 contributed to a decline in LEB). LEB losses of 0.08 years were due to large intraperiod rises of income inequality, while rising GDP per capita volatility appears to have reduced LEB in most regions. A rise during the 1980s and 1990s in the number of physicians per 1,000 people, slower than in the counterfactual scenario, led to a global LEB loss of 0.51 years. Smaller effects were observed for female illiteracy, while improvements in health behavior (alcohol consumption and cigarette smoking in the OECD) and a rise in the migrant stock faster than in the past generated small but telling improvements in world LEB. To these policy-driven LEB changes, one has to add the LEB changes due to endogenous progress in medical technology and, for the economies in transition, in dependency ratios, and subtract those due to AIDS, wars, and disasters. Interestingly, at the global level, the gains due to medical progress cancel out the LEB losses due to policy changes and shocks. One thus wonders how large these gains could have been had policies towards the transfer of health technology been more favorable. A disturbing message of this simulation is that a perceptible LEB loss (0.47 years) was due to the stagnation or decline in DPT vaccination since 1990, a result in line with the findings of Cutler et al. (2006). Finally, wars and disasters did not affect health perceptibly, though this result may be due to data and specification problems.

As expected, the biggest losers from the policy-driven changes are sub-Saharan Africa and the two regions in transition, but less obvious findings emerge from this simulation. Among the winners, one finds the OECD and East Asia, excluding China. The latter experienced LEB losses due to growing inequality, sudden and large inequality rises, and a GDP per capita slowdown that were offset by gains in medical staffing, reduced alcohol consumption, and eradication of female illiteracy. Surprisingly, MENA experienced large policy-driven LEB gains due to a growth in doctors, migrants, and especially female education at a faster rate than in the past. Interestingly, the two "growth superstars," China and India, suffered a policy-driven loss of LEB, as the effect of a GDP per capita growth at a faster rate than in the counterfactual was offset by losses due to a rise in inequality and volatility, a poor performance in reducing female illiteracy, increased alcohol consumption, less availability of physicians, and stagnant DPT vaccination. In both China and India, LEB gains due to technical

Table 2.8   Gains (Nonitalic) and Losses (Italic) in LEB Years by 2000 Due to 1980s/1990s Changes in Policies, Endogenous Changes, and Random Shocks

Region	OECD	TRANS	USSR	E. Asia	China	L. Amer.	MENA	India	S. Asia	SSA	WORLD
Policy-driven LEB changes	2.02	*–1.78*	*–3.92*	0.49	*–3.61*	*–1.54*	2.19	*–1.07*	*–1.59*	*–5.63*	*–1.52*
Log GDP/c	0.00	*–0.43*	*–1.91*	*–1.22*	3.98	*–0.80*	*–2.07*	1.71	0.69	*–0.99*	0.73
Log GDP/c on volatility	*–0.46*	0.00	0.00	0.00	0.00	0.00	0.00	0.00	0.00	0.00	*–0.07*
Gini of income inequality	*–0.03*	*–0.07*	*–0.12*	0.00	*–2.14*	0.00	0.00	*–1.15*	*–0.61*	*–0.45*	*–0.77*
Gini of income inequality/ (year 1959)	0.00	0.00	0.00	0.00	0.00	*–0.01*	*–0.01*	0.00	0.00	0.00	0.00
GDP/c Volatility	0.00	*–0.72*	*–0.49*	*–0.05*	*–1.26*	0.01	0.04	*–0.63*	*–0.32*	*–0.09*	*–0.44*
Intra-period D Gini > 4 points	0.02	*–0.58*	*–1.60*	*–0.08*	0.00	*–0.03*	0.00	0.00	0.00	0.14	*–0.08*
Log physicians per 1,000/Log GDP/c	*–0.44*	0.02	0.37	1.10	*–1.67*	0.25	0.73	*–0.97*	*–0.44*	*–0.60*	*–0.51*
Migrant stock/ population	0.07	0.00	0.00	0.41	0.00	0.01	0.39	0.00	*–0.12*	0.06	0.07
DPT immunization coverage	0.31	0.00	0.00	0.70	*–0.73*	*–0.05*	*–0.29*	*–0.18*	*–0.58*	*–3.37*	*–0.47*
Female education	0.52	0.00	*–0.16*	*–0.57*	*–1.78*	*–1.14*	3.41	0.15	*–0.21*	*–0.32*	*–0.31*
Cigarette smoking/c	0.82	0.00	0.00	0.00	0.00	0.00	0.00	0.00	0.00	0.00	0.12
Alcohol consumption/c	1.21	0.00	0.00	0.20	0.00	0.22	*–0.01*	0.00	0.00	0.00	0.22
Endogenous-driven LEB changes	1.07	0.36	0.35	0.66	3.04	1.83	1.28	3.04	3.04	3.04	2.15
Age dependency ratio	0.00	0.66	0.66	0.00	0.00	0.00	0.00	0.00	0.00	0.00	0.05
Technical progress in health field	1.07	*–0.31*	*–0.31*	0.66	3.04	1.83	1.28	3.04	3.04	3.04	2.10
Shocks-driven LEB changes	0.00	0.00	0.00	0.00	*–0.02*	*–0.04*	*–0.05*	*–0.57*	*–0.34*	*–6.36*	*–0.76*
War and humanitarian conflicts	0.00	0.00	0.00	0.00	0.00	0.00	0.00	0.00	*–0.01*	0.18	0.02
Disasters	0.00	0.00	0.00	0.00	*–0.02*	*–0.04*	*–0.05*	*–0.02*	*–0.02*	*–0.01*	*–0.02*
HIV-AIDS	0.00	0.00	0.00	0.00	0.00	0.00	0.00	*–0.54*	*–0.31*	*–6.54*	*–0.76*
Total LEB changes	3.08	*–1.42*	*–3.57*	1.15	*–0.59*	0.25	3.42	1.41	1.11	*–8.95*	*–0.13*

Source: Authors' calculations based on the parameters of the regional models (Tables 2.6 and 2.7).

Notes: The results of the above simulation based on the parameters of the global model (Table 2.6) are similar for the world as a whole. As for the ten regions, the signs of the variations are similar, but the size of the variations are different, as the parameters of the explanatory variables vary substantially between the global model (that measures an "average" effect) and the regional models (which reflect different regional circumstances).

progress in health offset the LEB losses due to economic changes, with the result that the actual outcome was—on balance—more favorable than in the counterfactual scenario.

Though plausible, these conclusions are weakened by a few methodological problems. First of all, except for AIDS, wars, disasters, and changes in health technologies and dependency ratios, all LEB changes are attributed to the impact of globalization policies on growth, inequality, volatility, vaccination, and so on, while other factors (e.g., institutions and external financing) may be in part responsible for the changes recorded in these variables. This problem is addressed in part in the next section. Second, lack of data prevented the inclusion in the model of important health determinants such as diet and smoking. Third, technical change in health is proxied by a period dummy that captures also the part of LEB explained by variables omitted in the model. Yet, as the number of variables included in the analysis is fairly high, this argument may not be too relevant.

IMPACT OF POLICY CHANGES ON HEALTH DETERMINANTS

This section tests to what extent the negative changes observed during the last two decades in GDP per capita, its volatility, and income inequality can be attributed to a premature adoption of globalization policies that neglected the specific economic and social characteristics of the countries in question. In this type of analysis, most researchers rely on sectoral and overall reform indexes developed by Lora (2001) for Latin America and by Campos for the European economies in transition. Each sectoral policy index varies between zero (no reform) and one (complete reform). The overall reform index is the average of the five sectoral indexes.

Reasons of space allow only a cursory allusion to prior research in this field. Dollar & Kraay (2003) analyzed the effect of openness on growth and conclude that trade openness is a key growth determinant. However, these results were often criticized by noting that growth is determined mainly by the quality of institutions, which "trumps" everything else, including economic openness. Other studies analyzed the impact of liberalization and globalization on income inequality. An analysis of the impact of economic liberalization in eighteen Latin American countries from 1980 to 1998 (Behrman, Birdsall, & Székely, 2000) found that these policies had a significant disequalizing effect over the short and medium term. Trade liberalization did not affect inequality significantly, but capital account liberalization, followed by domestic financial liberalization and tax reform, had strong disequalizing effects. Likewise, a review of the effects of liberalization and globalization policies during twenty-one reform episodes over the last two decades (Taylor, 2005) found that inequality rose in thirteen cases, remained constant in six, and improved in two. Other analyses (Cornia, 2004) emphasize that the standard theory is unable to predict the growth, inequality, and volatility impact of liberalization and globalization policies, as it is based on models relying on highly restrictive assumptions that ignore the impact of institutional weaknesses, structural rigidities, incomplete markets, asymmetric information, and persistent protectionism.

Conscious of these limitations, this section tests the impact of liberalization-globalization policies proxied by Lora's Overall Reform Index (ORI) on three determinants of health—GDP per capita, income inequality, and income volatility—that explain about half of the LEB changes simulated in Table 2.8. To avoid distortions in the parameters (due to the fact that ORI covers only the 1980–2000 period), GDP per capita was proxied as a GDP index (1980 = 100) or as a deviation from its 1960–80 trend. The volatility of GDP per capita was also expressed as deviation from its 1960–80 trend.

In models (1) and (4) in Table 2.9 on income inequality, the ORI lagged by five years, as reforms take time to affect income inequality, while the reform increments over the subsequent five years were introduced to assess the time profile of the reforms' impact (Behrman et al., 2000). In addition, ORI was interacted with the initial value of the Gini coefficient (G_0) to test whether the impact of the reform varied with the initial inequality level. A GDP per capita index and its square were also included among the regressors to test if the impact of the reforms varies with the countries' income levels. Instead, in models (2) and (5) on the impact of reforms on GDP per capita, ORI was expressed in quadratic form as, in the economies in transition, the reform impact followed a concave pattern. The same approach was followed in models (3) and (6) on the impact of reforms on the deviation of GDP per capita volatility from its 1960–80 trend. Finally, to remove the confounding effects of other nonpolicy factors, several control variables were included among the regressors.

Table 2.9 presents the econometric estimates of a fixed-effects model for the two regions and periods indicated following. In both Eastern Europe and Latin America, the Reform Index t-5 has a significant positive effect on income inequality, as do the subsequent reform increments. The interaction between ORI and initial inequality is negative, indicating that globalization reforms especially affect countries with a low initial inequality. Finally, the parameters of the GDP index and its square suggest that the impact of the reforms are more pronounced in low-income countries.

Regressions (2) and (4) confirm that growth is affected by reforms in a concave way in Eastern Europe and in an increasingly concave way in Latin America. Similar conclusions apply to GDP per capita volatility. Also, in this case the negative effect is particularly strong in the initial phase of reforms. Finally, among the control variables only the real interest rate, inflation, and money supply are significant. These results would seem to provide some initial support to the hypothesis that, in the two regions considered, the policy reforms of the last twenty years negatively affected three key health

Table 2.9 Results of the Regression of Lora's ORI on Income Inequality, GDP per Capita, and Volatility of GDP per Capita

	European transition economies (1989–01)			Latin America (1980–1999)		
	Income Inequality	GDP/c index (1989 = 100)	GDP volatility (deviation from 60–80 trend)[a]	Income Inequality	GDP/c (deviation from 1960–80 trend)[a]	GDP volatility (deviation from 60–80 trend)[a]
	(1)	(2)	(3)	(4)	(5)	(6)
Constant	18.70***	1.09***	12.61***	37.37***	−.5285***	8.43***
Reform Index	....	−1.71***	31.29***	....	−.2328***	8.62**
Reform Index²	....	1.74***	−36.68***	....	−.2090***	−10.57***
Reform Index* Gini 0	....	....	....	−.1851***	....	....
Reform Index t–5	15.19***	....	....	13.53***	....	....
Reform increment t 4–5	12.58***	....	....	14.27***	....	....
Reform increment t 3–4	12.42***	....	....	11.28***	....	....
Reform increment t 2–3	10.64***	....	....	14.73***	....	....
Reform increment t 1–2	9.47***	....	....	13.58***	....	....
Reform increment t 0–1	6.40***	....	....	12.01***	....	....
Money supply (M2/GDP)	−.0672***	.0019***	....	.0179 ws	.0004	....
Total external debt	....	1.66*–	....	2.36***	−1.08***	....
Real interest rate	−.0020***	−.00004	−.0273*–	....	−.0003	.0152**
External terms of trade	no data	no data	no data	−.0047	−.0003*–	.0122ws
Inflation	−.0025**ws	....	.0100***	.00008	.000001***	.0006**
GDP index	29.08***	....	....	14.99***	.6133***	....
GDP index²	−14.79***	....	....	−4.01**	....	....
F statistic	22.41***	29.81***	18.60***	10.08***	80.12***	2.39**
R square	.018	.280	.047	.005	.680	.009
Number of observations	120	127	306	183	191	191
Number of countries	17	17	24	12	17	17

Source: Authors' calculations.
Notes: [a]/Computed as the difference between the observed values of the variable and the value obtained by a prolongation of the 1960–80 trend, divided by the value extrapolated on the basis of the 1960–80 trend; ***significant at the 1% level; **between 1 and 5% level; *between 5 and 10% level; *–significant at 10–15%; ws = wrong sign.

determinants examined. In the case of inequality, the impact appears to be somewhat delayed and to most affect countries with low initial inequality and GDP per capita. With all the necessary precaution, one can tentatively conclude that there is some initial evidence of the potentially adverse effect of recent globalization policies on the determinants of health.

However, as noted by Rodrik, this kind of growth-policy regression can be misleading. In particular, Rodrik notes that:

> as long as policy interventions are not random and their presence responds to unobservables, regressing an economic performance variable on policy is uninformative about the degree to which market failures exist, the extent to which policy interventions are targeted on them,

the effectiveness with which government policies are deployed, or the extent to which policy interventions are used to create and divert rents for political purposes. (Rodrik, 2005, p. 11)

For these reasons, it is impossible conclusively to attribute the negative effect of the reforms to a premature implementation of liberal reforms, rather than to other factors. Yet, while one can only speculate about what lies behind the negative association found between liberalization-globalization policies, poor economic performance, and unsatisfactory health trends, it is also evident that—for whatever reason—this association seems to be robust.

IN LIEU OF CONCLUSIONS

This chapter is not meant to provide policy recommendations, as these would require considerable space and make sense only in country-specific contexts. Yet, some observations on the direction of policymaking and future research can be tentatively advanced.

First, the chapter confirms prior findings about the slow growth, instability, inequality, and reduced access to health care observed in many countries over the last quarter century, and on the link between such trends and globalization policies introduced in the 1980s and 1990s. Contrary to expectations, such policies caused a systemic increase in instability and inequality, and a weakening of the role of the state in providing basic services. In turn, the TRIPS Agreement reduced the potential impact of the transfer of medical technologies. In addition, while greater awareness of good health behaviors appears to have spread in OECD countries, external liberalization contributed to an increase in smoking, drinking, and poor nutritional habits in developing countries. For these reasons, there is some merit in the view that sees unsatisfactory health trends of the recent era of globalization to be related to a premature and acritical application of liberal policies.

Confirmation of the negative effects of premature liberalization and globalization on key determinants of health (GDP per capita, inequality, volatility, and health provision) provided in this chapter requires reconsidering the present approach to policy reform. It is quite possible that if properly managed, some (if not all) globalization policies could lead to health gains. Under ideal conditions, liberalization would reward effort and entrepreneurship, increase employment opportunities, and improve health by raising family earnings and reducing consumer prices. In turn, declining trade protection in developed countries could incorporate developing nations with narrow domestic markets into the global economy, while less restrictive policies in the field of property rights would facilitate a North-South transfer of drugs, medical equipment, and health knowledge. But the conditions for the success of such policies are, at the moment, met only in some countries, and it is doubtful whether, under the rules of access prevalent in international markets, any further textbook liberalization and globalization would help developing countries improve their market position, economic efficiency, or health status. For these countries, a selective integration into the world economy, linked to the reduction of major global asymmetries, is preferable to destabilizing big-bang globalization policies.

NOTES TO CHAPTER 2

1. The authors would like to acknowledge the comments provided on earlier versions of this chapter by Ben Crow, Patrick and Silvyane Guillaumont, Roberto De Vogli, Corinna Hawkes, Ronald Labonté, Ted Schrecker, participants in seminars held at the University of Clermont Ferrand in December 2006, and the University of California at Santa Cruz in December 2007.
2. In keeping with the approach of the Globalization Knowledge Network, economic globalization is defined here as a process of integration of countries in the world economy through the liberalization of their markets for goods, services, investments, finance, technology, information, and labor.
3. Conclusions about changes in health status based on life expectancy at birth (LEB) are biased by the fact that this variable is upper bounded at around 100 years of age, a fact which forces smaller absolute and relative gains in countries with an already high life expectancy. For this reason, this chapter relies on (100-LEB), a variable that measures the life years lost in relation to the maximum life years attainable. Such a measure has the advantage of being scale invariant, that is, its rate of change is independent from its level at the beginning of each period.
4. Available at http://www.cred.be.
5. Available at http://www.dse.unifi.it/sviluppo/database_eng.html.
6. The vaccination data imputed in the database are 44 percent of all DPT data, but only 18 percent was used in the regression analysis. Not using this 18 percent of imputed data would have prevented the use of all information for the years 1960–75. In any case, the descriptive statistics before and after imputation change little.
7. The estimates of the fixed effects model include an intercept for each of the 136 countries in the GHND panel. Such intercepts capture specific country effects due to geography, institutions, and unobservables.
8. This does not exclude, however, the possibility of reverse causation which is tested by means of the Granger test. However, such a test is not suitable for the GHND quinquennial dataset in which each variable has at best ten observations (Hurlin & Venet, 2001). It is therefore more appropriate to deal with this problem in theoretical terms. In this regard, it must be noted that reverse causality makes no sense in the majority of the relations in Table 2.5. For instance, it is not plausible that an increase in IMR can raise economic volatility, or that a fall in LEB will raise the interperiodal Gini variations more than four points. The only relation in which reverse causation may be plausible is that between LEB and GDP per capita. In this case, however, the relation between rising LEB (due, for instance, to a fall in U5MR) and higher GDP per capita would be characterized by time lags, thus excluding the possibility of reverse causation on synchronous data. The parameters are also affected by estimation bias caused by the omission in the regression analyses of a few

variables discussed in the "Mortality models and pathways of health impact" section, such as out-of pocket health costs and health insurance coverage, which were dropped because of insufficient data. In addition, the parameters may be further distorted by the possible endogeneity of some explanatory variables, which are simultaneously determined by the dependent and policy variables. Solving formally this endogeneity problem by means of a simultaneous equations system, however, is a difficult task in a panel with 136 countries. In addition, such a problem is less severe if one considers that economic theory does not suggest, with the possible exception mentioned earlier, that LEB is currently a main determinant of the explanatory variables.

9. That is: $LEB^s_i = \alpha_0 + \alpha_1$ Dummy Health Progr^s (= 0) + α_2 Log GDP/c^{s*} Gini—α_3 GDPvolatility ^{s}—α_4 Gini ^{s}—α_5 ΔGini>4^s—α_6 Female Illiteracy ^{s} + α_7 Log Phys per 1000/Log GDP/c^s + α_8 DPT^s + α_9 Migrant stock^s—α_{10} Alcohol/c ^{s}—α_{11}AIDS^s.

10. That is: $LEB^o_i = \alpha_0 + \alpha_1$ Dummy Health Progr^o (= 1) + α_2 Log GDP/c^{o*} Gini—α_3 GDPvolatility^o—α_4 Gini^o—α_5 ΔGini>5°—α_6 Female Illit^o + α_7 Log Phys per 1000/Log GDP/c^o + α_8 DPT^o + α_9 Migrant stock^o—α_{10} Alcohol/c ^{o}—α_{11} AIDS^o.

11. That is: LEB^o_$LEB^s = \alpha_1$ [Dummy Health Progr^o (= 1)—Dummy Health Progr^s (= 0)] + α_2 [Log GDP/c^{o*} Gini—Log GDP/c^{s*} Gini]—α_3 [GDPvolatility^o—GDPvolatility^s]—α_4 [Gini^o—Gini^s]—α_5 [ΔGini>5°—ΔGini>5^s]—α_6 [Female Illit^o—Female Illit^s] + α_7 [Log Phys per 1000/Log GDP/c^o—Log Phys per 1000/Log GDP/c^s] + α_8 [DPT^o—DPT^s] + α_9 [Migrant stock^o_Migrant stock^s]—α_{10}[Alcohol/c ^{o}—Alcohol/c ^{s}]—α_{11} [AIDS^o–AIDS^s].

REFERENCES

Ahmad, O. B., Lopez, A. D., & Inoue, M. (2000). The decline in child mortality: A reappraisal. *Bulletin of the World Health Organization, 78*, 1175–91.

Aiguo, L. (2006). *Transition, inequality, stress and health status in China.* Paper prepared for the project "Health and Social Upheavals" sponsored by the John D. and Catherine T. MacArthur Foundation, Institute of World Economics and Politics, Chinese Academy of Social Sciences, Beijing.

Baltagi, B. H. (2005). *Econometric analysis of panel data.* Chichester, UK: John Wiley and Sons.

Behrman, J., Birdsall, N., & Székely, M. (2000). *Economic reform and wage differentials in Latin America*, Research Department Working Papers No. 435. Washington, DC: Inter-American Development Bank.

Chu, K., Davoodi, H., & Gupta, S. (2000). *Income distribution and tax and government social spending policies in developing countries*, UNU/WIDER No. 214. Helsinki: World Institute for Development Economics Research.

Cornia, G. A., ed. (2004). *Inequality, growth, and poverty in an era of liberalization and globalization.* Oxford: Oxford University Press.

Cornia, G. A. (2004). Sudden change and mortality crises. In *Popolazione e Storia.*

Cornia, G. A., & Zagonari, F. (2002). *An econometric investigation of changes in IMR and U5MR in AIDS affected countries during the last twenty years.* Florence, Italy: UNICEF-IRC.

Cornia, G. A., & Danziger, S., eds. (1997). *Child poverty and deprivation in industrialized countries, 1945–1995.* Oxford: Clarendon Press.

Cornia, G. A., & Menchini, L. (2006). *Health improvements and health inequality during the last 40 years*, Research Papers 2006/10. Helsinki: World Institute for Development Economics Research. Retrieved from: http://www.wider.unu.

edu/publications/working-papers/research-papers/2006/en_GB/rp2006–10/_files/78091769993299557/default/rp2006–10.pdf.

Cutler, D., Deaton, A., & Lleras-Muney, A. (2006). The determinants of mortality. *Journal of Economic Perspectives, 20.*

Deaton, A. (2004). Health in an age of globalization. *Brookings Trade Forum,* 83–130.

Dollar, D. (2001). Is globalization good for your health? *Bulletin of the World Health Organization, 79,* 827–33.

Dollar, D., & Kraay, A. (2003). *Institutions, trade, and growth: Revisiting the evidence.* World Bank Policy Research Working Paper.

Ezzati, M., Vander Hoorn, S., Lawes, C. M., Leach, R., James, W. P., Lopez, A. D., et al. (2005). Rethinking the "diseases of affluence" paradigm: Global patterns of nutritional risks in relation to economic development. *Public Library of Science Medicine, 2,* 404–12.

Godoy, R. A., Reyes-García, V., McDade, T., Huanca, T., Leonard, W. R., Tanner, S., et al. (2006). Does village inequality in modern income harm the psyche? Anger, fear, sadness, and alcohol consumption in a pre-industrial society. *Social Science and Medicine, 63,* 359–72.

Guillaumont, P., Korachais, C., & Subervie, J. (2006). *How macroeconomic instability lowers child survival,* WIDER Research Papers. Helsinki: World Institute for Development Economics Research. Retrieved from: http://www.wider.unu.edu/publications/working-papers/research-papers/2008/en_GB/rp2008–51/.

Hawkes, C. (2005). The role of foreign direct investment in the nutrition transition. *Public Health Nutrition, 8,* 357–65.

Hurlin, C., & Venet, B. (2001). *Granger causality test in panel data models with fixed coefficients.* Paris: EURIsCO Université de Paris.

Jäntti, M., & Sandstrom, S. (2005). Trends in income inequality: A critical examination of the evidence in WIID2. In *The future of development economics.* Helsinki.

Kawachi, I., Kennedy, B. P., & Wilkinson, R. (1999). *Inequality and health: A reader.* New York: New York Press.

Lamar, J. (2000). Suicides in Japan reach a record high. *British Medical Journal, 321,* 528.

Lora, E. (2001). *El crecimiento económico en América Latina después de una década de reformas estructurales.* Washington, DC: Banco Interamericano de Desarrollo, Departamento de Investigación.

Marmot, M., & Bobak, M. (2000). Psychological and biological mechanisms behind the recent mortality crisis in Central and Eastern Europe. In G. A. Cornia & R. Paniccia (eds.), *The mortality crisis of transitional economies.* Oxford: Oxford University Press.

Preston, S. H. (1976). *Mortality patterns in national populations.* New York: Academic Press.

Reddy, S., & Vandermoortele, J. (1996). *User financing of basic social services: A review of theoretical arguments and empirical evidence.* New York: UNICEF.

Rodrik, D. (2005). *Why we learn nothing from regressing economic growth on policies.* Harvard University.

Taylor, L. (2005). External liberalisation, economic performance and distribution in Latin America and elsewhere. In G. A. Cornia (ed.), *Inequality, growth and poverty in an era of liberalization and globalization.* Oxford: Oxford University Press.

Tiberti, L. (2006). *Changes in health financing and health status: The case of Vietnam.* In UNU-WIDER Conference on Advancing Health Equity, Helsinki.

United Nations. (2004). *World population prospects: The 2002 revision* (vol. III: Analytical Report). New York: United Nations Publications. Retrieved from: http://www.un.org/esa/population/publications/wpp2002/WPP2002_VOL_3.pdf.

United Nations University & World Institute for Development Economics Research (2008). UNU-WIDER World Income Inequality Database. World Institute for Development Economics Research [online]. Retrieved from: http://www.wider.unu.edu/research/Database/en_GB/database/.

van Doorslaer, E., O'Donnell, O., Rannan-Eliya, R. P., Somanathan, A., Adhikari, S. R., Garg, C. C., et al. (2006). Effect of payments for health care on poverty estimates in 11 countries in Asia: An analysis of household survey data. *The Lancet, 368*, 1357–64.

Wilkinson, R. G. (1996). *Unhealthy societies: The afflictions of inequality.* New York: Routledge.

World Bank. (2007). *World development indicators* [online] 2006. World Bank. Retrieved from: http://devdata.worldbank.org/wdi2006/contents/index2.htm.

World Health Organization. (2006). *The world health report 2006: Working together for health.* Geneva: WHO.

3 Global Political-Economic and Geopolitical Processes, Structures, and Trends

Patrick Bond

INTRODUCTION

This chapter provides a commentary on major shifts in global political economy and geopolitics since the 1970s which have brought together processes of governance and liberalization in often uncomfortable ways. These processes have important manifestations in society, including the generation of structural constraints on policies that would improve health. Geopolitical realignments and neoliberal policy ascendancy can be observed in a series of several dozen moments in which key events reflect important power shifts. The context has been a series of durable economic problems: stagnation, financial volatility, and uneven development. Political alignments have followed and remain in an adverse balance of power from the standpoint of redistributive socioeconomic reforms essential to improving global health equity. Any expectation that global governance offers solutions, at least within prevailing political-economic and geopolitical processes, structures, and trends, requires careful and critical evaluation.

Such an evaluation begins by locating public health challenges related to globalization within a broader context combining *political economy* and *geopolitics*. Political economy is an analysis concerned with the interaction of economic processes and power relations. Geopolitics involves considerations of relations between territorially based actors—not just national states—which have interests in defending or expanding their spatial power. Globalization is an explicitly geographical phenomenon, and hence we must seek an analytical framework capable of considering not only macropolitical and global economic forces but also microfoundational aspects of markets and political actors' interests. That is the challenge for this chapter, which provides a compressed account of four subjects: (1) major defining events since the early 1970s, (2) ideological development, (3) explanatory theory, and (4) empirical tendencies that will shape the immediate future.

The gyrations and stumbles are documented in the next section. While the neoliberal project may have failed to meet its sponsors' promises, a replacement strong enough to reshape the world has yet to emerge. The forces in Washington that support economic neoliberalism (the World

Bank, International Monetary Fund [IMF], United States Treasury, United States [US] Federal Reserve and associated think tanks) and political neo-conservatism (the White House, Pentagon, US Department of State and think tanks) are both suffering major legitimacy problems. But their fusion in many multilateral agencies—notwithstanding some reform rhetorics—suggests a difficult period ahead for those desiring either global post-Washington Consensus reforms (see Table 3.1), or more national sovereignty for low/middle-income states, or global/local justice. Before addressing prospects for changing the power balance, as well as competing agendas, it is important to set out the three-decade-long geopolitical process, as well as deeper political economic dynamics, and then provide some theoretically informed explanation for these.

GEOPOLITICAL REALIGNMENT, NEOLIBERAL ASCENDANCY, AND ECONOMIC VOLATILITY

A catalog of geopolitical changes since the 1970s would emphasize at least four major developments. First, the 1975 defeat of the United States by the Vietnamese guerrilla army reduced the US public's willingness to use its own troops to maintain overseas interests. Second, the Soviet bloc collapsed in the early 1990s, as a result of economic paralysis, foreign debt, bureaucratic illegitimacy, and burgeoning democracy movements. Third, several Middle East wars occurred during the period, with Israel generally dominant as a regional power since the 1973 war with Egypt, notwithstanding its 2006 defeat in Lebanon. Fourth, China emerged as a potent competitor to the West in political as well as economic terms during the 1990s and 2000s.

These were merely the highest-profile of crucial political developments, leaving a sole superpower in their wake. Yet this superpower is one with much lower levels of legitimacy, dubious military and cultural dominance, slower economic growth, higher poverty and inequality, and vastly reduced financial stability over the past third of a century. One critical aspect of the struggle between classes associated with these developments was the waning of the Third World nationalist project and a dramatic shift in class power, away from working-class movements that had peaked during the late 1960s, towards capital and the upper classes.

Chronologically, several other crucial moments helped define the splintered, polarized political sphere since the 1970s. Formal democratization arrived in large parts of the world—Southern Europe during the mid-1970s, the Cone of Latin America during the 1980s and the rest of Latin America during the 1990s, and many areas of Eastern Europe, East Asia, and Africa during the early 1990s—partly through human/civil rights and mass democratic struggles and partly through top-down reform. Yet, because democratization occurred against a backdrop of economic crisis in

Latin America, Africa, Eastern Europe, the Philippines, and Indonesia, the subsequent period was often characterized by instability, in which "dictators passed debt to democrats"[1] who were compelled to impose austerity on their subjects, leading to persistent unrest.

In the wake of transformations in Nicaragua, Iran, and Zimbabwe in 1979–80, the ebbing of Third World revolutionary movements was hastened by the US government's attacks during the 1980s on Granada, Nicaragua, Angola, and Mozambique, sometimes carried out directly but often by proxy. It was also a period of attacks on liberation movements in El Salvador, Palestine (via Israel), and Colombia, as well as on former Central Intelligence Agency client regimes in Panama and Iraq. During this period, low/middle-income governments and their citizenries were thus warned not to stray from Washington's mandates, a message amplified by the 1989–90 demise of the Soviet Union. Indeed, after the Cold War ended, Western aid payments to Africa, for example, quickly dropped by 40 per cent with the evaporation of formerly Cold-War patronage competition, until its resurgence subsequent to Chinese interest in Latin America and Africa during the 2000s (Greenhill & Watt, 2005, p. 36).

The consolidation of European political unity followed corporate centralization within the European Economic Community, as the 1992 Maastricht Treaty ensured a common currency (excepting the British pound, which was battered by speculators just prior to its attempt to join the Euro zone), and as subsequent agreements established stronger political interrelationships. This occurred at a time when most European social democratic parties turned neoliberal in orientation and voters swung between conservative and center-right rule, in the context of slow growth, high unemployment, and rising reflections of citizen dissatisfaction. Meanwhile, persistent 1990s conflicts in "failed states" gave rise to Western humanitarian interventions with varying degrees of success, in Somalia (early 1990s), the Balkans (1990s), Haiti (1994), Sierra Leone (2000), Côte d'Ivoire (2002), and Liberia (2003). However, other sites in Central Africa—Rwanda in 1994 and since then Burundi, northern Uganda, the eastern part of the Democratic Republic of the Congo, Somalia, and Sudan's Darfur region—have witnessed several million deaths, with only rather ineffectual regional interventions that involved Western powers, if at all, only peripherally.

The 2001 attack on the World Trade Center and the Pentagon (followed by attacks in Indonesia, Madrid, and London) signaled an increase in conflict between Western powers and Islamic extremists. These followed earlier bombings of US targets in Kenya, Tanzania, and Yemen, which in turn prompted US reprisals against Islamic targets in Sudan (actually, a medicine factory) and Afghanistan in 1998 and Yemen in 2002. This shift in global militarism was accompanied, in the early-mid 2000s, by a rise of left political parties in Latin America including major swings in Venezuela (1999), Bolivia (2004), and Ecuador (2006), as well as turns away from pure neoliberal economic policies in Brazil, Argentina, Uruguay, and Chile.

These were joined during the mid-2000s in Europe by left coalitions in Norway and Italy.

This list of political moments should not obscure other important trends that seem to have accompanied them: social and cultural change, including postmodernism, the "network society," demographic polarizations and family restructurings; new technologies brought about by the transport, communication, and computing revolutions; major environmental stresses including climate change, natural disasters, depletion of fisheries, and worsening water scarcity; and health epidemics, such as AIDS, drug-resistant tuberculosis and malaria, severe acute respiratory syndrome, and the human health risks of bovine spongiform encephalopathy and avian flu. Although these are topics beyond the scope of the current chapter, their importance in the realm of ideology must not be neglected. Moreover, given the rise of neoliberal and neoconservative philosophies (formerly "modernization" and colonialism), there have been sometimes spectacular counter-reactions ranging from Islamic fundamentalism and resurgent Third World nationalism, to post-Washington Consensus and global governance reform proposals (see Chapter 12, this volume), to global justice movement protests, as discussed later.

Meanwhile, in the sphere of economics, a variety of key moments marked the rise and then decline of neoliberal policy influences across the world. In 1973 the Bretton Woods agreement on fixed exchange rates disintegrated when the United States unilaterally ended the convertibility of the US dollar to gold, representing a default of approximately US$80 billion. The agreement, by which one ounce of gold was valued at US$35 between 1944 and 1971, had served to anchor other major currencies. As a result of the US move, the price of gold rose to US$850 per ounce within a decade. Also in 1973, several Arab countries led a reduction in oil supply by the Organization of the Petroleum Exporting Countries (OPEC) cartel that raised the price of petroleum dramatically and resulted in a similarly dramatic transfer of resources from the world's oil consumers to the coffers of the OPEC countries. In the same year, Augusto Pinochet staged a coup against the elected government of Salvador Allende in Chile. The coup opened up the opportunity for *los Chicago Boys*, a term referring to Chilean bureaucrats trained at the University of Chicago in Milton Friedman's neoliberal economic orthodoxy, to reshape radically the Chilean economy.

In 1976 the IMF signaled its growing power by forcing austerity on Britain at a point where the ruling Labour Party was desperate for a loan, even before Margaret Thatcher's ascent to power in 1979. In 1979, the US Federal Reserve addressed its country's currency decline and inflation problem by dramatically raising interest rates. In turn this catalyzed a severe recession and the Third World debt crisis, especially in Mexico and Poland in 1982, Argentina in 1984, South Africa in 1985, and Brazil in 1987 (in the latter case leading to a default that lasted only six months due to intense pressure on the Sarnoy government to repay). At the same time, the World

Bank shifted from project funding to the imposition of structural and sectoral adjustment (supported by the IMF and the Paris Club cartel of donor nations), in order to assure surpluses would be drawn for the purpose of debt repayment (see Chapter 7, this volume), and in the name of making countries more competitive and efficient.

During the late 1980s and early 1990s Washington adopted a series of financial crisis-management techniques, such as the US Treasury's Baker and Brady plans, to enable banks in New York, London, Frankfurt, Zurich, and Tokyo to write off (with tax breaks) part of the US$1.3 trillion in potentially dangerous debt they were owed by creditors in Latin America, Asia, Africa, and Eastern Europe. Notwithstanding this socialization of the banks' losses, debt relief was denied to the borrowers.

In late 1987 crashes on a scale unprecedented since 1929 occurred on the New York and Chicago financial markets. Further damage was narrowly averted with a promise of unlimited liquidity by US Federal Reserve Chairman Alan Greenspan. The promise was based on a philosophy which in turn allowed the bailout of the savings and loan industry and various large commercial banks (including Citibank) in the late 1980s notwithstanding a recession and serious real estate crash during the early 1990s. Similarly in 1998, when a New York hedge fund, Long Term Capital Management, lost billions on bad investments in Russia and in the process threatened the integrity of the world financial system, the New York Federal Reserve Bank arranged a bailout. The US Treasury's management of the "emerging markets" offered further bailouts for investment bankers exposed in various regions and countries—Eastern Europe (1996), Thailand (1997), Indonesia (1997), Malaysia (1997), Korea (1998), Russia (1998), South Africa (1998, 2001), Brazil (1999), Turkey (2001), and Argentina (2001)—whose hard currency reserves were suddenly emptied by runs.[2]

Finally, while the various excesses of an overinflated US economy, the various excesses of which have occasionally unraveled, as with the bursting of dot.com stock market (2000–2001) and real estate (2007–2008) bubbles, China and India picked up the slack in global materials and consumer demand during the 2000s. However, this development is not without stresses and contradictions that in coming years may threaten world finances, geopolitical arrangements, and environmental sustainability.

These major events reflect tensions and occasional eruptions, but never genuine resolutions, to the growing overall problems of volatility that have wracked world politics and economics since roughly the start of the 1970s. These events were also critical from the standpoint of public health, given how many were associated with drastic increases in mortality and morbidity (see Chapters 1 and 5, this volume). The overall sense of chaos in global political economy and geopolitics contrasts to a more stable, predictable, prosperous, and evenly distributed set of political-economic relations during the immediate post–Second World War quarter century (1945–70).

What explanations can be generated to help come to grips with volatile global political economy and geopolitics?

DURABLE ECONOMIC PROBLEMS

The merits of classical political-economic theory include the identification of durable economic problems—also termed *crisis tendencies*—at the core of the market's laws of motion. But these tendencies are typically met by countervailing management techniques that stabilize the market. Crisis displacement techniques have become much more sophisticated since the Great Depression of the 1930s, which had compelled John Maynard Keynes (1936) to write his *General Theory of Employment, Interest, and Money,* which advocated much greater state intervention so as to boost purchasing power.

The difference today is that such drastic problems have been averted, largely through *shifting and stalling* the devaluation of exposed, uncompetitive capitals—that is, what Joseph Schumpeter (1942) called "creative destruction" necessary to recover from a depression and restore momentum to a new round of accumulation. The stalling entails moving devaluation across time (via the credit system) and the shifting entails its movement across space by powerful actors (the Bretton Woods Institutions, World Trade Organization [WTO], donor agencies) to areas that are less able to withstand the adjustment. Moreover, in the search for temporary fixes to its problems, capital also draws on nonmarket spheres (environmental commons, women's unpaid labor, indigenous economies) for new surpluses by way of extraeconomic coercions ranging from biopiracy and privatization to deepened reliance on unpaid women's labor for household reproduction.

As a result, the global economy's vast financial expansion and the use of geographical power have devalued large parts of the low-income countries and various emerging market sites, as well as some vulnerable markets in the North that have suffered substantial "corrections" in past years. Extraeconomic coercion, including gendered and environmental stress, has intensified in the process. The result is an economy that concentrates wealth and poverty in more intense ways geographically and brings markets and the nonmarket spheres of society and nature together in ways adverse to the latter. This phenomenon is sometimes termed *uneven and combined development,* to which we return next.

Consider three central components to this political-economic argument about global economic problems:

1. The persistent late twentieth-century condition of overaccumulation of capital witnessed huge gluts in many markets, declining rates of

growth in per capita GDP, and falling corporate profit rates (Brenner, 2002; Harvey, 2003; Gérard & Lévy, 2004). The consequences were displaced and mitigated (shifted and stalled geographically and temporally), at the cost of much more severe tensions and potential market volatility in months and years ahead, particularly when, from 2007, the financial bubbling of real estate markets in the United States and many other settings burst.

2. The temporary dampening of crisis conditions through increased credit and financial market activity has resulted in the expansion of "fictitious capital." This is especially so in real estate but other speculative markets based on trading paper representations of capital (derivatives), far beyond the ability of production to meet the paper values.

3. Geographical shifts in production and finance continue to generate economic volatility and regional geopolitical tensions, contributing to unevenness in currencies and markets as well as pressure to combine market and nonmarket spheres of society and nature in search of restored profitability.

As noted following, the interlinked problems of overaccumulation, financialization, and globalization brought pressures for war, as witnessed by battles for resources especially in the Middle East, Central Asia, and Central Africa. Circumstances mainly associated with hyperexpansion of commerce in a context of technological/transport changes also generated threats of catastrophic climate change and new pandemics.

The world macroeconomic context since about 2000 includes some incongruent experiences, especially in the United States, the Euro Area, and Japan (Bank for International Settlements, 2005, pp. 12–32). These experiences include a recovery in trade, foreign investment flows (especially mergers and acquisitions), and stock market values after early 2000 downturns; rising US and Japanese fiscal deficits; and an unprecedented US trade deficit (especially due to increased Chinese imports), while nearly all emerging market economies—aside from Turkey, Mexico, South Africa, the Czech Republic, and Poland—ran large current account surpluses. As well, there has been an upturn in raw material prices from early 2002 (especially in energy and minerals/metals); an uptick in corporate profits as a share of gross domestic product (GDP) accompanied by sluggish private fixed investments; and real interest rates below 1 percent since 2001, in spite of seventeen small rate increases by the US Federal Reserve since 2004, prior to reversals from 2007. But these trends have been companioned with a fast-rising household debt/income ratio in the United States; uncertainty in global property markets—especially US housing—after apparent mortgage-driven peaks in 2005 and a potential real estate devaluation of US $6 trillion in the United States; a 25 per cent fall in the value of the US dollar from its early 2002 high until year-end 2007; and the ongoing role of emerging Asian economies as the engine of world growth.

Recent orthodox analysis of economic disequilibria, especially US trade/budget deficits, often relies upon four key variables by way of an explanation for the tensions that have emerged:

1. Extremely low US national (especially household) savings rates.
2. The positive implications of the "new economy" for US investments (which have been stable at just lower than 20 per cent of GDP during the 1990s–2000s, roughly equal to Europe and Latin America but lower than Japan's 25 per cent and other East Asian countries' 33 per cent).
3. The argument that a global savings glut (roughly 2 per cent higher than 1990s levels) permits relatively low interest rates in the United States in addition to capital inflows.
4. A Sino-American codependency situation due to risk avoidance by Asian investors in the wake of the 1997–98 crisis (Bank for International Settlements, 2005, p. 24).

For Barry Eichengreen, "the four sets of factors supporting the global imbalance and the US deficit will not last forever. There will have to be adjustment, the question being whether it will come sooner or later and whether it will be orderly or disorderly" (2006, p. 14). In 2007 that adjustment began, but repeated vast financial bailouts of major banks and institutional investors (and even US mortgage guarantors Fannie Mae and Freddie Mac) kept the "adjustment" process—that is, widespread asset devaluation—temporarily in check.

Apart from the U.S. financial crisis, there have been other "very long bouts of stagnant or even negative growth," according to the World Bank:

> The past 25 years have had numerous setbacks afflicting growth in the developing countries . . . Sub-Saharan Africa, the Middle East and North Africa, Latin America, and Europe and Central Asia . . . each had specific reasons for these periods of depressed growth ranging from Latin America's debt crisis in the 1980s, the Middle East and North Africa's (and, to a lesser extent, Africa's) energy decline, and Europe and Central Asia's emergence from its transition toward market-based economies. (2007, p. 56)

In each case, the Bank claims progress can be recorded in terms of improved macroeconomic conditions (such as less inflation and inflationary expectations), more sustainable debt levels (at least for developing countries on average), more diversified economies with less reliance on volatile commodities, a much greater role for services (which tend to be less volatile), much improved production management with lower inventories (which tended to be a major factor in past business cycles), and better macroeconomic management, particularly monetary policy (2007, p. 55). Nevertheless, as the Bank observes, "growing inequality, pressures in labor markets and threats to the global commons" are not only "evident in the current globalization" but "are likely to become more acute. If these forces are left unchecked, they could slow or even derail globalization" (2007, p. vii). The bank notes that threats from "environmental damage, social unrest, or new increases in protectionist sentiment are potentially serious," in part because "returns to skilled labor will continue to increase more quickly than those to unskilled labor, extending today's natural wage-widening tendencies evident in many, if not most, countries" (2007, p. vii, xxii).

Whether it is natural that the world is suffering the worst inequality in human history might be disputed. For example, one of the core arguments made by David Harvey is that neoliberalism is an explicit political project of "class war" (Harvey, 2003, 2007). That this war has generated vast inequalities between people in poor countries and people in rich countries is no longer in dispute (see Chapter 1, this volume), even if India and China complicate matters due to uneven development.

If the orthodox explanation for these durable economic problems is unsatisfactory, what do political economists have to offer instead?

STAGNATION, VOLATILITY, AND UNEVEN DEVELOPMENT

Contemporary political economy requires us to address not only volatility but also the long slowdown in economic growth. Global annual growth in GDP per capita fell from 3.6 per cent during the 1960s, to 2.1 per cent during the 1970s, to 1.3 per cent during the 1980s, to 1.1 per cent during the 1990s followed by a rise to 2.5 per cent for the first half of the 2000s (World Bank, 2005, p. 297). To be sure, the bundle of goods and services produced over time has changed. High technology products enjoyed today were not available in the last century, sometimes not in the last decade. Conversely, GDP fails to take into account natural resource depletion and many forms of environmental degradation (with the associated loss or endangerment of ecosystem services). We must also acknowledge the extremely uneven character of accumulation across the world, with some regions—especially Eastern Europe—having suffered substantial reductions in output during 1980s–90s downturns.

As for the poorest continent, outgoing chair of the IMF and World Bank Development Committee Trevor Manuel bragged, "Right now, the macroeconomic conditions in Africa have never been better. You have growth across the continent at 4.7%. You have inflation in single digits. The bulk of countries have very strong fiscal balances as well" (International Monetary Fund, 2005). Extractions of nonrenewable resources, however, were not included in Manuel's calculations; if they had been, Africa would have shown net *negative* savings (World Bank, 2005; Bond, 2006).

Even before the 2007–08 economic turbulence, several powerful analyses addressed the crisis faced by global, and especially US, businesses in their restructuring of production systems, social relations, and geopolitics (Brenner, 2002; Harvey, 2003; Pollin, 2003; Wood, 2005). From the standpoint of political economy, concerns have long been expressed about not only distorted US financial and trade accounts, but also underlying features of production, ecological destruction, and social degradation. The core ingredients in any explanation include worker-employer-employee class conflict (especially emanating from late 1960s Europe, but waning since the mid-1970s and at very low levels during the 1980s when nominal profits increased); international political conflict; energy and other resource constraints (especially looming oil shortages); and the tendency to overaccumulation (production of excess goods, beyond the capacity of the market to absorb).

For David Harvey, "Global capitalism has experienced a chronic and enduring problem of over-accumulation since the 1970s"(Harvey, 2003, p. 63). Robert Brenner finds evidence of this problem insofar as:

> costs grow as fast or faster in non-manufacturing than in manufacturing, but the rate of profit falls in the latter rather than the former, because the price increase is much slower in manufacturing than non-manufacturing. In other words, due to international overcapacity, manufacturers cannot raise prices sufficiently to cover costs. (personal communication, November 9, 2004)

That overcapacity has continued, and even at the height of the West's devalorization stage of overaccumulation during the 1980s, other political economists (Clarke, 1988, pp. 279–360; Harvey, 1989, pp. 180–97; Mandel, 1989, pp. 30–58) showed how deindustrialization and intensified uneven development were correlated to overaccumulation. Subsequently, evidence of the ongoing displacement of economic crisis to the low-to-middle-income countries and via other sectors was documented by Harry Shutt (1999, pp. 34–45) and Robert Biel (2000, pp. 131–89).

The intensification of uneven development between and within advanced and low-to-middle-income countries is a feature of this overaccumulation crisis. Amplification of uneven development has been obvious insofar as some poles of the world economy grew far faster than others, and the Gini coefficient measure between countries rose dramatically from the early 1980s. Within countries, as well, inequality rose, due particularly to rapid trade-related integration. As the World Bank's main econometrician of inequality, Branco Milanovic, noted, "at very low average income levels, it is the rich who benefit from openness . . . It seems that openness makes income distribution worse before making it better" (2005). China and India are often cited as examples of globalization's ability to spread wealth, but in reality their extreme rise in internal income inequality has generated mass protests (85,000 in 2005, the last time police released data) and tens of thousands of rural suicides, respectively. This is classic uneven development.

The "combined" feature of uneven and combined development (Bond & Desai, 2006) occurred especially in specific peripheral or semiperipheral settings where the market mode of production depends upon earlier modes of production for an additional superexploitative subsidy—extraeconomic coercion—in part by virtue of reducing the costs of labor power reproduction (Wolpe, 1980). Women, particularly, are compelled to take on additional burdens through not only patriarchy but a neoliberal policy shift, as Isabella Bakker and Stephen Gill have shown:

> Reprivatization of social reproduction involves at least four shifts that relate to the household, the state and social institutions, and finally the basic mechanisms of livelihood, particularly in poorer countries:
>
> 1) Household and caring activities are increasingly provided through the market and are thus exposed to the movement of money.
> 2) Societies seem to become redefined as collections of individuals (or at best collections of families), particularly when the state retreats from universal social protection.
> 3) Accumulation patterns premised on connected control over wider areas of social life and thus the provisions for social reproduction.
> 4) Survival and livelihood. For example, a large proportion of the world's population has no effective health insurance or even basic care. (2003, p. 36)

Environmentally, too, the penetration of the market into every sphere of life—even the privatization of air, via carbon trading (that alleged solution to the climate crisis)—was theorized at the peak of proglobalization hubris: "I've always thought that under-populated countries in Africa are vastly UNDER-polluted, their air quality is probably vastly inefficiently low" (Summers, 1991). Also according to Larry Summers, then the World Bank's chief economist, later the Clinton administration's treasury secretary and president of Harvard, "I think the economic logic behind dumping a load of toxic waste in the lowest-wage country is impeccable and we should face up to that" (1991). Despoliation of the environment has worsened via the combination of market and nonmarket processes, as increasingly desperate productive capital seeks to compete with hyperprofitable financial capital through appropriation of ecological resources at little or no cost.

The overall logic of uneven and combined development also entails differential (or "disarticulated") production and consumption along class lines (de Janvry, 1981), so that internal balance within economies degrades. Likewise, national economies have suffered worsening discrepancies between capital goods and consumer goods, and between different circuits and fractions of capital. For example, the rise of financial markets during periods of over-production crisis means that, as Michel Aglietta showed, "Uneven development creates artificial differences in the apparent financial results of firms, which are realized only on credit. These differences favor speculative gains on the financial market" (1979, p. 359). And yet the rise of financial bubbles far beyond the underlying values in the real economy must come to an end at some point, as witnessed so vividly in the 2007–2008 devalorization of speculative real estate markets. Unlike economists who argue the merits of markets as *equilibrating* forces (i.e., always self-correcting the over- or underpricing of assets), the recent turmoil caused by uneven development and witnessed in financial market expansion could better be described as systematic *dis*equilibration.

Hence, tendencies towards sectoral and spatial unevenness are also manifest periodically in the sort of financial crises that have characterized the world economy in recent years, and that worsen relative power of asset creation especially in an era in which exchange controls were lifted and vast flows of portfolio capital cross the world in search of momentary gains through currency speculation. Although unevenness has been associated with theories of unequal exchange and forms of core dominance and peripheral dependency for many years, these analyses have had the effect of overemphasizing interstate relations and underemphasizing the flows of capital and social struggles that have more decisively shaped local "underdevelopment." It is here that the articulation of the market and premarket modes of production generate a combined development between wealthy and poor countries, which feeds into the overall unevenness of the world economy, appropriately named by the South African president Thabo Mbeki "global apartheid" (see Bond, 2003).

David Harvey has argued that the process of generating unevenness should be understood in more general ways, as "different places compet[ing] endlessly with one another to attract investment. In the process they tend to amplifying unevenness, allowing capital to play one local or regional or national class configuration off against others" (1996, p. 295). While comprehending the uneven development of sector, space, and scale is ambitious enough, there must be, as well, future opportunities to explore systematic unevenness in spheres as diverse as the production and destruction of the environment, social reproduction, and human domination along lines of class, gender, and race/ethnicity. Such an exercise would bring to the fore the many ways that health has both reflected and contributed to inequality—and ways to reverse unevenness in access to healthcare across the world and within countries.

CONCLUSION: IMPLICATIONS FOR PUBLIC HEALTH AND PUBLIC POLICY

What, finally, are the strategic lessons of the foregoing discussion, for contemporary politics and public policy, and for public health? While the latter point is largely beyond the scope of a short chapter, we can posit trends that have some important lessons for future strategies to promote health care and mitigate disease burdens.

The problems of health care associated with and largely caused *by* globalization follow from the volatile political economic processes (including South-North resource drain) and hostile geopolitical environments discussed previously. To be sure, however, there are defenders of globalization, such as the World Bank's David Dollar (2001, p. 827), whose arguments concerning globalization's positive effects on developing country growth, poverty reduction, and health (via liberalization) were discussed, and rebutted, in Chapter 1. Dollar, however, did recognize that global economic integration also carried with it adverse health effects: the transmission of AIDS through migration and travel is a dramatic recent example. However, both relatively closed and relatively open developing countries have severe AIDS problems. The practical solution lies in health policies as well as strong commitments by states to provide compulsory licenses to manufacture medicines, as permitted by exemptions to the Agreement on Trade Related Intellectual Property Rights agreed in Doha at a 2001 WTO ministerial summit, not in policies that force faster economic integration. Likewise, free trade in tobacco will lead to increased smoking unless health-motivated disincentives are put in place, one of the reasons behind the creation of the Framework Convention on Tobacco Control (see Chapter 12, this volume).

Dollar's argument, furthermore, is that the international architecture can be improved so that it is more beneficial to poor countries. For example, with regard to intellectual property rights, it may be practical for pharmaceutical innovators to choose to have intellectual property rights in either rich country markets or poor country ones, but not both. In this way, incentives could be strong for research on diseases in both rich and poor countries. Yet not only is there little evidence of this (aside from the exemption noted previously) given the adverse balance of forces at the global scale, his prescriptions for both of these health issues are problematic. Effecting adequate access to AIDS medicines, for example, relied upon active civil society resistance to commodification and corporate power, as illustrated in the ferocious battle that South Africa's Treatment Action Campaign was compelled to join against Big Pharma, the US government, and especially the South African government from 1998 to 2003.

In sum, the neoliberal policy ascendancy seemed to have occurred through important power shifts reflected in roughly a dozen major moments of crisis, as noted earlier. But these crises, in turn, reflected underlying structural dynamics that emerged during the 1970s: stagnation, financial volatility, and uneven development. The public health sector is adversely affected by each of these. Directly, there have been cuts in state resources for health care (or imposition of cost recovery which lowered low-income people's utilization rates) and structural adjustment's early and indeed ongoing orientation to privatization of state services (see Chapter 8, this volume). Indirectly there are worsening health conditions associated with unevenly experienced unemployment, income inequality, and workplace conditions which are the result of global capital's mobility and the limited scope for state employment-generation policies. Although this chapter does not have scope to draw these links explicitly, one of the key insights from the literature on political economy and geopolitics is the problem of coercive "extraeconomic" extraction of surpluses beyond the purview of the market, in part through gendered and environmental power relations. This problem follows from market interrelationships with nonmarket social and ecological systems, and has implications for resources that might otherwise have been channeled into building strong public services.

Politically, the stress caused by stagnation and volatility has been exacerbated by the conjoining of neoliberal and neoconservative forces. In Table 3.1, the five major ideological orientations of contending forces are considered. Although these ideologies seemed to have firmed over the past decade, none of the five orientations has overcome internal contradictions sufficiently so as to represent an unproblematic approach to public policy. To illustrate, the US neoconservatives are, in 2008, on the defensive not only because of military defeats, political unpopularity, and economic stress, but also because of sociocultural features such as divergent religious influences and disputes over how to best protect culture, patriarchy, and state sovereignty. The neoliberal bloc, stretching from Washington through most of Europe's major capitals to Japan, has also suffered from an inability to overcome the durable economic crisis on its own terms. There have, as well, been differing reactions to the US imperial agenda, due to divergent national-capitalist interests and domestic political dynamics. And yet the neoconservatives and neoliberals have generated a working partnership on most multilateral matters that, in turn, has foiled global-scale reforms necessary for human health and welfare, not to mention the environment.

The reform-oriented post-Washington Consensus agents and key personalities (Joseph Stiglitz, Jeffrey Sachs, George Soros, etc.) have, indeed, failed to achieve meaningful gains in global governance venues, since the last moment of success, the 1996 chlorofluorocarbon ban in Montreal. Largely because of the adverse power relations that follow from the economic and geopolitical processes discussed earlier, the world's reformers face several daunting problems:

1. In relation to geopolitical tension, the lack of peace settlements (or indeed prospects) in the Middle East, Gulf, central Asia, central Africa, and the Horn of Africa, with a looming war involving the United States, Iran, and probably Israel, and oft-predicted long-term interimperial conflicts between the United States and China.

2. On United Nations democratization, the inability to expand the Security Council in recent heads-of-state summits, notwithstanding pressure from aspirant members Japan, Germany, India, Brazil, Nigeria, and South Africa.
3. On trade, repeated delays in concluding the Doha Round of WTO negotiations.
4. In international finance, ongoing contagion of turbulence (including bursting market bubbles, bankruptcies and volatile currencies), extremely high—and growing—current account deficits in the United States and other countries, World Bank legitimacy crisis, worsening IMF financial deficits, and US/European Union (EU) resistance to Bretton Woods reform as witnessed by the leadership appointments in 2007 of two men from the neoconservative/neoliberal power structure, Robert Zoellick (World Bank) and Dominique Strauss-Kahn (IMF).
5. Environmentally, the failure of the EU and supportive low/middle-income states to defend, much less decisively expand, the Kyoto Protocol, as the 2007 Bali and 2008 G8 meetings failed to make sufficient breakthroughs to halt and reverse potentially catastrophic climate change (and with respect to other global ecological management problems arising in freshwater, maritime resources, trade in toxics, species extinction, and the like, there has been very little or no progress.)
6. An overall "global apartheid" structure in terms of economics, political power, culture, public health, and social services, through which most measures of inequality and genuine progress continue worsening, making mockery of the (already relatively unambitious) Millennium Development Goals.

The more radical forces in world politics are the Third World nationalists and the global-justice movements. Emanating, respectively, from national sites like Cuba, Venezuela, Bolivia, Ecuador, and Paraguay, and from civil society settings such as the Zapatistas' Chiapas province of Mexico, or occupied factories of Buenos Aires, or health clinics with AIDS medicines catalyzed by the South African Treatment Action Campaign, or the anti-dam encampments in India's Narmada Valley, to give a few prominent examples, these progressive nationalists and global-justice advocates may have the will and vision to advance the required far-reaching reforms. Whether they have the capacity and support depends upon politics, but the past three and a half decades of elite mismanagement described earlier should alert us to the dire consequences of top-down strategies for improved health and social determinants of health. The future will be forged where neoconservative/neoliberal globalization-from-above is countered by globalization-from-below.

Table 3.1 Five Geopolitical Currents

Political current:	Global Justice	Third World Nationalism	Post-Wash. Consensus	Washington Consensus	Resurgent Right Wing
Tradition	*socialism, anarchism*	*national capitalism*	*(lite) social democracy*	*Neoliberalism*	*Neoconservatism*
Main agenda	"deglobalization" of *capital* (not *people*); "globalization-from-below," international solidarity; antiwar; antiracism; indigenous rights; women's liberation; ecology; "decom-modified" state services; participatory democracy	increased (but fairer) global integration via reform of interstate system, based on debt relief and expanded market access; reformed global governance; regionalism; rhetorical anti-imperialism; and Third World unity	fix "imperfect markets"; add "sustainable development" to existing capitalist framework via UN and similar global state-building; promote a degree of global Keynesianism; oppose US unilateralism and militarism	reform neoliberalism with provisions for "transparency"; self-regulation and bailout mechanisms; co-opt potential emerging-market resistance; offer financial support for US-led empire	unilateral petro-military imperialism; crony deals, corporate subsidies, protectionism and tariffs; reverse globalization of people via racism and xenophobia; religious extremism; patriarchy and biosocial power
Leading institutions	social movements; environmental justice activists; indigenous people; autonomists; radical activist networks; leftist labor movements; liberation theology; radical think tanks (e.g., Focus on the Global South, Global Exchange, IBASE, IFG, IPS, Nader centers, TNI)[c]; radical media (*GreenLeft Weekly*, Indymedia Pacifica, Pambazuka, zmag.org); semiliberated zones (Bolivaran projects, Kerala); sector-based or local coalitions in the WSF (World Social Forum)	Non-Aligned Movement, G77 and South Center; self-selecting regimes (often authoritarian): Argentina, Brazil, China, Egypt, India, Indonesia, Kenya, Libya, Malaysia, Nigeria, Pakistan, Palestine, Russia, South Africa, Turkey, Uganda, Zimbabwe with a few—Bolivia, Cuba, Ecuador and Venezuela—that lean left; *Aljazeera*, supportive NGOs (e.g., Seatini, Third World Network)	some UN agencies (e.g., UNICEF, WIDER);[b] some INGOs (e.g, CARE, CIVICUS, IUCN, Oxfam, TI);[c] large enviro. groups (e.g., Sierra Club and World Wildlife Federation); big labor (e.g., ICFTU and AFL-CIO;[c] liberal foundations (Carnegie, Ford, MacArthur, Mott, Open Society, Rockefeller); Columbia U. economics department; the Socialist International; Norway	US State (Fed, Treasury, USAID); corporate media, IT (information technology)and financiers; World Bank, IMF, WTO; elite clubs (Bilder-bergers, Trilateral Commission, World Economic Forum); some UN agencies (UNDP, UNCTAD, United Nations Global Compact); universities and think tanks (U. of Chicago economics, Cato Institute, Council on Foreign Relations, Adam Smith Inst., Inst. of International Economics, Brookings); BBC, CNN,[d] and Sky; most G8 states	Republican Party populist and libertarian wings; Project for a New American Century; right-wing think tanks (AEI, CSIS, Heritage Foundation, Manhat-tan Institute)[e]; Christian right institutions and media; petro-military complex and industrial firms; the Pentagon; right-wing media (Fox, *National Interest, Weekly Standard, Washington Times*); *proto-fascist European parties—but also Zionism and Islamic extremism*

Notes: [a]Instituto Brasileiro de Analises Sociais e Economicas, International Forum on Globalization, Institute for Policy Studies, Transnational Institute; [b]UN Research Institute for Social Development, World Institute for Development Economics Research, International Union for the Conservation of Nature, Transparency International; c International Confederation of Free Trade Unions, American Federation of Labor and Congress of Industrial Organizations; [d]British Broadcasting Corporation, Cable News Network; [e]American Enterprise Institute.

NOTES

1. As the Jubilee South movement described the problem (Focus on the Global South, 1999).
2. A "run" refers to the sudden and rapid withdrawal of investment in a country's financial markets, generally by foreign speculative investors. This causes the traded value of the country's currency to decline. In an attempt to stabilize its currency, the country uses its foreign currency reserves to purchase back its own currency to "signal" its value to other currency traders.

REFERENCES

Aglietta, M. (1979). *A theory of capitalist regulation*. London: New Left Books.
Bakker, I., & Gill, S. (2003). Ontology, method and hypotheses. In I. Bakker & S. Gill (eds.), *Power, production and social reproduction*. Basingstoke, UK: Palgrave Macmillan.
Bank for International Settlements. (2005). *75th annual report: 1 April 2004–31 March 2005*. Basel: Bank for International Settlements. Retrieved from: http://www.bis.org/publ/arpdf/ar2005e.pdf?noframes=1.
Biel, R. (2000). *The new imperialism*. London: Zed Books.
Bond, P. (2003). *Against global apartheid: South Africa meets the World Bank, IMF and international finance* (2nd ed.). London: Zed Books.
———. (2006). *Looting Africa: The economics of exploitation*. London and Pietermaritzburg: Zed Books/University of KwaZulu Natal Press.
Bond, P., & Desai, A. (2006). Explaining uneven and combined development in South Africa. In B. Dunn & H. Radice (eds.), *100 years of permanent revolution*. .London: Pluto Press.
Brenner, R. (2002). *The boom and the bubble: The US in the world economy*. London: Verso Press.
Clarke, S. (1988). *Keynesianism, monetarism and the crisis of the state*. Aldershot, UK: Edward Elgar.
de Janvry, A. (1981). *The agrarian question and reformism in Latin America*. Baltimore: Johns Hopkins University Press.
Dollar, D. (2001). Is globalization good for your health? *Bulletin of the World Health Organization, 79*, 827–33.
Eichengreen, B. (2006). The blind men and the elephant. *Issues in Economic Policy.*
Gérard, D., & Lévy, D. (2004). *Capital resurgent: Roots of the neoliberal revolution*. Cambridge, MA: Harvard University Press.
Greenhill, R., & Watt, P. (2005). *Real aid: An agenda for making aid work*. Johannesburg: Action Aid International. Retrieved from: http://www.actionaid.org.uk/wps/content/documents/real_aid.pdf.
Harvey, D. (1989). *The condition of postmodernity*. Oxford: Basil Blackwell.
———. (1996). *Justice, nature and the geography of difference*. Oxford: Basil Blackwell.
———. (2003). The "new" imperialism: Accumulation by dispossession. In L. Panitch & C. Leys (eds.), *Socialist register 2004: The new imperial challenge* (pp. 63–87). London: Merlin Press. Retrieved from: http://socialistregister.com/recent/2004.
———. (2007). Neoliberalism as creative destruction. *The Annals of the American Academy of Political and Social Science, 610*, 21–44.

International Monetary Fund. (2005). Transcript of a Joint IMF/World Bank Town Hall with civil society organizations: Washington, DC, September 22, 2005. Retrieved from: http://www.imf.org/external/np/tr/2005/tr050922a.htm.

Mandel, E. (1989). Theories of crisis: An explanation of the 1974–82 cycle. In M. Gottdiener & N. Komninos (eds.), *Capitalist development and crisis theory: Accumulation, regulation and spatial restructuring.* London: Macmillan.

Milanovic, B. (2005). Can we discern the effect of globalization on income distribution? Evidence from household surveys. *The World Bank Economic Review,* 19, 21–44.

Pollin, R. (2003). *Contours of descent: U.S. economic fractures and the landscape of global austerity.* London: Verso.

Shutt, H. (1999). *The trouble with capitalism.* London: Zed Books.

Summers, L. H. (1991). Memo. The Whirled Bank Group [online]. Retrieved from: http://www.whirledbank.org/ourwords/summers.html.

Wolpe, H., ed. (1980). *The articulations of modes of production.* London: Routledge & Kegan Paul.

Wood, E. M. (2005). *Empire of capital.* London: Verso.

World Bank. (2005). *World Bank World Development Report 2006: Equity and development.* New York: World Bank and Oxford University Press.

———. (2007). *Global economic prospects 2007: Managing the next wave of globalization.* Washington, DC: World Bank.

4 Labor Markets, Equity, and Social Determinants of Health

Ted Schrecker[1]

[T]he usual argument in favour of globalisation—that it will make most workers better off, with only a few low-skilled ones losing out—has not so far been borne out by the facts. Most workers are being squeezed. (Woodall, 2006, p. 6)

INTRODUCTION

As the World Bank notes in its 2006 *World Development Report*, on the theme of equity and development: "For most of the world's people, economic opportunities are primarily determined, or at least mediated, by the labor market—in formal and informal work. . . . The functioning of the labor market has a profound effect on equity—across workers, in patterns of access to work, and between workers and employers" (World Bank, 2005, pp. 185–86). The relation between labor-market outcomes and poverty is especially dramatic. The World Bank's "$1/day" and "$2/day" poverty lines have been widely criticized as underestimating the true extent of poverty,[2] yet even using these measures the working poor are numerous: "There are still 486.7 million workers in the world," including those in both formal and informal sectors, "who do not earn enough to lift themselves and their families above the US$1 a day poverty line and 1.3 billion workers do not earn enough to lift themselves and their family above the US$2 a day line" (International Labour Organization, 2008, p. 10), in part because of the pernicious effects of underemployment (Felipe & Hasan, 2005, p. 11). An additional 190 million are classified by the International Labour Organization (ILO) as unemployed. The work that may be available is often hazardous to health and safety; workers in the developing world are routinely exposed to hazards similar to those eliminated from most workplaces in high-income countries generations ago.[3] A further influence involves the connection between labor markets and the consequences of illness. This connection is evident in countries as diverse as the United States, where insurance coverage for much of the privately insured population is provided by employers and more than 40 million people lack any insurance coverage, and Viet Nam, where limited compulsory insurance coverage for a minority of workers employed in the formal economy coexists with a high proportion of private, out-of-pocket health expenditure that pushes large numbers of people into poverty every year (Sepehri, Chernomas, & Akram-Lodhi, 2003; United Nations Country Team Viet Nam, 2003; van Doorslaer et al., 2006; Huong et al., 2007; Ekman, Liem, Duc, & Axelson, 2008)

What happens in labor markets thus influences material deprivation, access to medical progress, acute psychosocial stress, income inequality, and social disintegration: four of the five pathways identified by Cornia et al. (this volume) linking social conditions with mortality. Stated in terms of a different but compatible conceptual framework, labor markets have powerful effects on social stratification, differential exposure (to hazards or risk factors), differential vulnerability, and differential consequences (e.g., of illness): the four generic mechanisms identified by Diderichsen, Evans, & Whitehead (2001) as contributing to social disparities in health. A sanguine view is that labor-market opportunities presented by globalization offer the potential for improving social determinants of health (SDH) by reducing poverty and inequality and improving living standards in a way that is possible only through higher incomes. There are reasons to accept this proposition in some country contexts, but for many of the employed (and of course for the unemployed) it is only part of the story and largely irrelevant to their short-term situations. Notably, worldwide progress in poverty reduction as measured using the World Bank thresholds has been modest: although some countries (such as China and Viet Nam) have made impressive strides (Chen & Ravallion, 2007) poverty has (for instance) increased substantially in sub-Saharan Africa (Chen & Ravallion, 2007) and remained stubbornly high in south Asia (Felipe & Hasan, 2005).

With respect to labor markets as in other areas, generalizations about globalization's impacts are precarious and the relevant research literature is huge. This chapter identifies a number of broad trends, and then describes some generic policy implications for advocates for health equity regardless of their institutional location, national and subnational governments, and multilateral institutions for global governance (on these last see Chapter 12, this volume). The analysis presented here does not and cannot substitute for historically informed study of specific countries, specific sectors of national economies, and the production networks that are characteristic of specific industries.

NEW INTERNATIONAL DIVISION(S) OF LABOR

A detailed study published in 1977 described a "new international division of labor" exemplified by the relocation of labor-intensive production in the textile and garment industries to sites in the developing world selected on the basis of low wages and minimal protections for workers. These sites were usually in export processing zones (EPZs) established by national governments, offering relaxed or nonexistent regulation of wages and working conditions as well as other incentives to investors in production for export (Fröbel, Heinrichs, & Kreye, 1980). According to the ILO, as of 2007 more than 66 million workers were employed in 3,500 EPZs worldwide, as compared with 845 EPZs and 22.5 million workers a decade earlier. Of these, approximately 40 million workers are in China, more than five million in Central America and Mexico, and 3.2 million in bonded factories in Bangladesh (Boyenge, 2007).

The international division of labor has both deepened and become more complicated in the course of a global reorganization of production across multiple national borders (Dicken, 2007). Many industries are now characterized by global commodity or value chains (the terms are used here interchangeably), in which multiple discrete elements of the production process are located where returns can be maximized and risks minimized (Gereffi & Korzeniewicz, 1994; Kaplinsky, 2004; Schrank, 2004; Bair, 2005). In the words of two leading researchers on commodity chains: "Globalization entails uneven development for firms and workers both within and across regions and nations, and viewing the process through the lens of the commodity chains framework contributes to our understanding of who wins and who loses, and why" (Bair & Gereffi, 2003, p. 165). In many instances, production networks and intrafirm trade that involve multiple subsidiaries of a transnational corporation (TNC) are being supplemented or replaced by contractual relationships with external suppliers and service providers ("outsourcing"), with the latter expanding rapidly in importance (Milberg, 2004; Edwards, 2004). These suppliers are often in direct competition with one another. It may be useful to think of this as the Nike model, after the athletic shoe firm (which actually owns almost no factories) that pioneered it (Donaghu & Barff, 1990; Rothenberg-Aalami, 2004). The case of Nike is an early example of a "buyer-driven" commodity chain: one in which the control exercised by brand-name manufacturers or retail chains (such as the supermarkets that dominate many segments of the global agri-food system; see Chapter 10, this volume) enables them to capture much of the value added in the production process, while exercising relentless pressure on producers farther down the chain to cut costs and shifting production among contractors and jurisdictions where profitable. The ability of Wal-Mart to do this in the retail sector is particularly noteworthy because of its sheer size (*Economist*, 2004; Appelbaum & Lichtenstein, 2006).

The distribution of globalization's gains and losses often depends on the niches that individual workers and firms are able to carve out in global value chains. Recent case studies applying commodity chain analysis to industries such as horticulture, textile manufacturing, and garment production in Kenya, South Africa, Bangladesh, and Vietnam (Nadvi, 2004; Jenkins, 2005) found that substantial opportunities for employment and income gains for some workers, although not all, were associated with integration into global value chains and the resulting access to export markets. Conversely: "Global value chain pressures are . . . associated with increasing casualization of labor and excessive hours of work" (Nadvi, 2004, p. 25). These pressures are familiar from studies of the footwear and clothing industries in many jurisdictions (e.g., Ross, 1997; Gereffi, Spener, & Bair, 2002). A case study of grape production in Brazil for northern supermarkets found that workers were able to achieve substantial gains in wages and working conditions because of their potential ability to disrupt the commodity chain, but the author admits that this finding is exceptional (Selwyn, 2007). Over the longer term, ability to capture gains from globalization is critically dependent on the ability of firms to move up the global value chain from component supply or assembly to become original equipment manufacturers or full-package producers and, ultimately, to develop their own brands (Arrunada & Vazquez, 2006; Tokatli, 2007): a process exemplified by some sectors of Asian manufacturing but also evident in other industries.

Gereffi and colleagues (Bair & Gereffi, 2002; Gereffi & Memedovic, 2003) are cautiously optimistic about the ability of manufacturers in textile and garment value chains to accomplish this, but they and others (e.g., Kaplinsky, 2004) emphasize that this is by no means certain and much depends on the structure of the particular value chain—a variable that may be outside the control of developing country firms or governments. A more pessimistic view is exemplified by a study of the Caribbean basin's emergence as a rival to Mexico for garment production: "While the manufacturers in my sample [from the Dominican Republic] hoped that full-package production would constitute an upgrading strategy, they increasingly view it as a survival strategy" (Schrank, 2004, p. 138); even full-package producers are facing intensive labor-cost competition (Schrank, 2004, p. 140). In the case of Mexico's *maquiladora* sector, which originated with the establishment of EPZs, cost containment by way of falling wages and deteriorating working conditions for many manufacturing workers (Alarcón-González & McKinley, 1999; Fussell, 2000; Cypher, 2001, 2004; Frey, 2003; Martínez, 2004) has failed to avoid the recent loss of an estimated 200,000 export production jobs to China. Weight is lent to the pessimistic view by such factors as the impact on employment of financial crises resulting from rapid disinvestment (see Chapter 5, this volume): such crises have resulted in the loss of millions of jobs in the formal sector, and employment tends to recover more slowly than gross domestic product (GDP) in the aftermath (van der Hoeven & Lübker, 2005). Writing mainly about sub-Saharan Africa, Collier makes a further point about the constraints on strategies of export-led development through integration into global value chains, even at the bottom. Asia, he points out, began industrializing without competition from other low-wage manufacturers, and with "a wage advantage over the existing competition (in Organization for Economic Cooperation and Development [OECD] countries) of around forty-to-one." However, because of the global reorganization of production, countries seeking to pursue a similar strategy today have no wage advantage over Asian manufacturers, which still rely in part on low labor costs as a source of comparative advantage (Collier, 2006, p. 1437).

GLOBAL LABOR MARKETS, "FLEXIBILIZATION," AND THE CHINA SYNDROME

The increasing importance of global commodity chains instantiates the gradual emergence of a genuinely global labor market (World Bank, 1995). Other things being equal, globalization tends to increase inequalities between "skilled" and "unskilled" workers, both within national economies and across national borders (see, e.g., Rama, 2003, pp. 169–71; Somavia, 2006). In industrialized countries, perhaps the most conspicuous manifestation of this phenomenon has been a precipitous drop in the demand for, and the labor incomes of, "unskilled" workers (Nickell & Bell, 1995; Wood, 1998).[4] Much debate among economists has surrounded the relative contributions of globalization (sometimes, although not always, equated with openness to trade) and technological change (for a review, see Chusseau, Dumont, & Hellier, 2008). The emerging consensus is that the answer is "both," with the specific contributions depending on the country or regional context (International Monetary Fund, 2007, p. 179). Indeed, it would seem analytically difficult to distinguish these relative contributions, as noted in a *Business Week* feature on the job losses associated with corporate downsizing in the 1990s: "A global economy, rousting American employers from business-as-usual management, demands such change; rapidly evolving technology allows it" (Hammonds, Kelly, & Thurston, 1994, p. 77). Recognizing this point, the World Bank now identifies technological diffusion as one of the four channels of globalization (World Bank, 2007).

Meanwhile, inflation-adjusted manufacturing wages adjusted for differences in purchasing power in some Asian economies (most notably South Korea, Singapore, and Thailand), but *not* in Latin America, have risen toward US levels between 1970 and 2000 (International Monetary Fund, 2007, p. 172). Manufacturing employment is only a small proportion (and especially in the high-income countries a declining proportion) of total employment, so almost nothing can be inferred about overall labor income patterns from this figure. Meanwhile, in some, although not all, high-income countries, rising inequality in market incomes is being driven by increases at the very top of the income scale, among those described as the working rich by Duménil & Lévy (2004).[5] A similar pattern is now emerging in India (Felipe & Hasan, 2005, p. 24). In Canada and the United States, even when one descends from the commanding heights of the income pyramid, a strong tendency exists for disparities in labor income to widen because of growth near the top of the distribution, and stagnation or decline elsewhere (Mishel, Bernstein, & Allegretto, 2007; Yalnizyan, 2007). This divergence is at least partly explained by the fact that in rich and poor countries alike, the working poor are normally price-takers in labor markets (Cormier & Craypo, 2000); what they have to offer is in abundant supply relative to the demand. During certain historical periods, this disadvantage has been off-set by the ability to organize and bargain collectively. As shown later in the chapter, many aspects of globalization neutralize or undermine this abil-ity. Meanwhile, globalization provides new opportunities for those labor-market participants with highly marketable skills ("human capital"), often acquired through advanced education, the financial cost of which creates a formidable barrier to entry. This segment of the labor market is character-ized not by competition among workers for jobs but rather by competition among employers for talent that can move with relative ease across national borders, at least within multinational organizations.

Global economic integration and the expansion of the global labor force are almost certainly combining to generate increased pressures for labor-market "flexibility," with negative effects on economic security for many workers. International relations scholar Robert Cox (1999) argues that glo-balization leads to a division among integrated, precarious, and excluded forms of employment—a typology that is valuable because it focuses on the character of the employment relationship, rather than its geographical situ-ation within production networks that are often in continuous flux. Within the industrialized world, Cox's typology is validated by research on US cor-porate downsizing in the 1990s, and the associated rise in temporary or contractual employment relationships (Hammonds et al., 1994; Uchitelle et al., 1996; DiTomaso, 2001). For example, General Motors replaced fac-tory workers in Detroit with home-based workers in two towns in the US Midwest, who earned far lower wages and minimal benefits doing piece-work (Gringeri, 1994). More recently, firms in the southern United States are finding a source of competitive advantage in the low-wage and almost infinitely flexible labor of Latino immigrants (Smith & Winders, 2008). In Latin America the typology is validated by 1997 survey data from Brazil, Chile, Colombia, Costa Rica, El Salvador, Mexico, Panama, and Venezu-ela showing that "the occupational structure has become the foundation for an unyielding and stable polarization of income," with lower-income per-sonal service, agricultural, commercial, and industrial workers making up 74 percent of the working population; an intermediate stratum of technicians and administrative employees 14 per cent; and higher-income professionals, employers, and managers just 9 per cent (United Nations Economic Com-mission for Latin America and the Caribbean, 2000, pp. 61–91; for a similar analysis of South Africa, see Webster, 2005). Although the connections with globalization will vary among countries and regions, interpretation of these data by the United Nations Economic Commission on Latin America and the Caribbean (ECLAC) links "the need to participate competitively in the world economy" to labor-market deregulation, increased flexibility, and the growth of economic insecurity (United Nations Economic Commission for Latin America and the Caribbean, 2000, pp. 93–102). Labor markets are clearly contributing to levels of income inequality that, in many Asian economies, are rising toward Latin America's, despite what appears to be widespread underreporting of labor incomes by higher-income households in Asian surveys (Development Indicators and Policy Research Division, 2007).

Globalization's impact on labor-market incomes will almost certainly be increased as integration of India, China, and the transition economies into the global economy roughly doubles the global labor force relative to its size before 1990 (Freeman, 2007). The research literature offers conflicting interpretations of the effects. Some commentators argue that it will exert long-term worldwide downward pressure on wages, indeed is already doing so (Woodall, 2006; Freeman, 2007). An alternative perspective is that wage inflation in economies like China's, which is already being observed among certain categories of workers, "will create space for low-income countries to move into the lowest-skill activities vacated by producers in the large emerging countries" (World Bank, 2007, p. 102). Arguably, this is already happening, as evidenced by the shift of manufacturing employment from Mexico to China and the emergence of Viet Nam as a lower-cost alternative to China for the location of manufacturing operations (York, 2005; Bradsher, 2008). However, in the former case at least, it is far from clear that Mexican producers have actually "vacated" the field of so-called low-skill activities by moving up the value chain; many Mexican workers may simply be priced out of the relevant global labor markets (Parrado, 2005).

The World Bank's 2007 *Global Economic Prospects* report predicted that labor-market trends will fuel the expansion of a global middle class, yet at the same time anticipated that labor market effects of globalization will increase economic inequality in countries accounting for 86 per cent of the developing world's population over the period until 2030, with the "unskilled poor" being left farther behind (World Bank, 2007, pp. 67–100). This is almost certainly an understatement of the true increase in economic inequality that can be anticipated over the period in question, since the World Bank does not consider the potential impact of shifts in the distribution of income from labor to capital, within and across national borders. The International Monetary Fund (IMF) has described a clear decline in labor's share of national income in the high-income countries since the early 1980s as a consequence of globalization (International Monetary Fund, 2007, pp. 166–69). Between the early 1980s and 2006, corporate profits in the G7 countries rose from just over 11 per cent of national income to 15.5 percent (Woodall, 2006, pp. 6–7) while real labor incomes for most workers have flatlined or declined. Outside the industrialized world in Mexico, the proportion of GDP going to wages fell from 40 per cent in 1976 to 18.9 per cent in 2000, during a period of rapid integration into the global economy and two major economic crises (Palma, 2006, pp. 15–16). The Mexican case is perhaps extreme, but it is what one might expect given the increasing mobility, and therefore bargaining power, of capital relative to most forms of labor.

GENDER AND INFORMALIZATION

As with other aspects of macroeconomic policy (Elson & Cagatay, 2000), men and women experience globalization's effects on labor markets differently. In general, globalization has been accompanied by the reproduction of gender hierarchies (Mills, 2003) in which women tend to occupy lower paid, less desirable, and less secure jobs. In some cases globalization has led to economic gains and social empowerment for women, for instance, by creating new employment opportunities in export-oriented industries. "The reality is that, for many women, working in exports is better than the alternatives of working (or being unemployed) in the domestic economy" (Barrientos, Kabeer, & Hossain, 2004, p. 2; see also Kabeer, 2004a, 2004b; Chen, Vanek, Lund, & Heintz, 2005). A comparative study of export-oriented employment and social policy in South Korea, China, Mexico, Mauritius, South Africa, and India, where economic policies have supported expansion of export employment (often in EPZs), identified economic gains for women in terms both of labor incomes and of work-related entitlement to benefits (Razavi, Pearson, & Danloy, 2004). However, these gains are disproportionately vulnerable both to economic crises and to systemic, globalization-related pressures for "labor market 'flexibility' and fiscal restraint" (Razavi & Pearson, 2004, p. 25). It is important, as well, to consider the difference between situations in which the emergence of new forms of employment creates opportunities for women, and situations in which women have no alternative but to take jobs in export production because of declining real wages, rising economic insecurity, and new financial demands on the household in the form, for instance, of user fees for health care and children's education (Shaw, 2007; Razavi, 2007). The health effects of the work itself are another issue: women in Bangladesh, for instance, "do not necessarily expect to work in garment factories for a prolonged period. Indeed, given the toll taken on their health by long working hours, it would not be possible to undertake such work for an extended period of time" (Kabeer & Mahmud, 2004, p. 151).

A further manifestation of gender hierarchy is the emergence of "global care chains" that are analogous to commodity chains in terms of their fragmentation of tasks as highly unequal distribution of benefits. The indispensable work in such global care chains is overwhelmingly done by women (Yeates, 2004, 2005). "The same processes that increase cross-border supply through the disembodied export of labor in EPZs or outsourcing of information technology service work also promote the embodied supply of care work through transnational migration" (Summerfield, Pyle, & Desai, 2006, p. 281; see also Ehrenreich & Hochschild, 2002; Misra, Woodring, & Merz, 2006; Pyle, 2006b), often with highly destructive effects on the health of female migrants and their own families (Pyle, 2006a). The extreme example is what appears to be an expanding, and increasingly lucrative, trade in trafficked sex workers (Hughes, 2000; Drevland, 2004).

Sassen makes a strong case that, whether or not it is coerced in a sense recognizable to television viewers, such migration instantiates a "survival circuit" driven not only by "the deepening misery of the global south" but also by the pull factor of an expanding demand for low-wage work in the "global cities" that are the command centers of the world economy (Sassen, 2002; for background see Sassen, 2006). The jobs in question involve not only care work, but also such activities as changing hotel linens, preparing and serving restaurant meals, and cleaning office buildings and airports for globalization's winners (Winerip, 1998; Herod & Aguilar, 2006; McDowell, Batnitzky, & Dyer, 2008).

Discussion of globalization and labor markets often concentrates on employment in the formal, waged economy. However, in many low- and middle-income labor markets the majority of the working population derives its livelihood in other ways (Garcia, 2004; Chen, Vanek, & Heintz, 2006). In India, for example, 92 per cent of workers are engaged in informal employment, either self-employed or in waged employment but without contracts or social protection (Chen et al., 2006; see also Unni & Rani, 2003; Lerche, 2007). In the developing world as a whole, "fully 50 to 80 per cent of non-agricultural employment is informal" (Chen et al., 2005, p. 8). "Growing labor market informalization amounts to a regressive process of redistribution" (Benería & Floro, 2005, p. 12) driven by competition to lower production costs through labor-market flexibility, by financial crises (as noted earlier), and by import liberalization that wipes out livelihoods in formerly protected sectors. Far from disappearing as part of the process of modernization, informal work is increasing in importance; the boundaries between formal and informal sectors are blurring, especially at the "bottom end" of global commodity chains; and policies adopted by national governments in order to accelerate integration into the global economy often actively encourage informalization (Lund & Nicholson, 2003; Kudva & Beneria, 2005; Benería & Floro, 2005). In most regions of the world, gender hierarchies in labor markets extend to the informal sector: women are disproportionately likely to engage in informal employment, disproportionately vulnerable to the effects of structural economic changes such as financial crises that drive people into the informal economy, and, within the informal sector, likely to have lower wages and less legal and social protection.

Meanwhile, and crucially, women in countries rich and poor alike continue to bear most of the burden of unpaid care work in the household. A review of gender dimensions of the globalization of production carried out for the ILO concluded: "The single most important factor which acts as a barrier to women's ability to participate as full economic actors in the global economy is their domestic responsibilities, and for a large subgroup, their childcare responsibilities. The childcare constraint appears to operate across contexts which are otherwise very different" (Barrientos et al., 2004, p. 13). This conclusion is supported by other research, notably Heymann's findings from surveys of 55,000 households and more that 1,000 in-depth interviews in eight countries (Heymann, 2006). Admittedly, improving women's ability to participate in the labor market will not eliminate gender hierarchies, and the issue may not be one of "participation" in the global economy but rather one of how gender hierarchies structure the terms of that participation (see, e.g., Buechler, 2002; Sassen, 2002). It is therefore best to view policies that address the domestic labor/childcare constraint as necessary but by no means sufficient conditions for reducing gender inequities in access to work in the formal economy and the associated benefits.

GLOBALIZATION AND LABOR STANDARDS

Findings that seemingly contradict the analysis so far presented emerge from a series of cross-national comparative studies by Neumayer and De Soysa, who considered the relation between globalization and compliance with the core labor standards set out in the ILO's 1998 Declaration on Fundamental Principles and Rights at Work: freedom of association and collective bargaining, abolition of child labor, elimination of forced or compulsory labor, and elimination of discrimination in employment and occupation.[6] These studies generally failed to find negative effects of global economic integration, as measured by openness to trade and foreign direct investment (FDI) (Neumayer & De Soysa, 2005, 2006, 2007). Openness to trade was in fact associated with higher respect for women's economic rights, a lower prevalence of forced labor (Neumayer & De Soysa, 2007), and higher respect for free association and collective bargaining (Neumayer & De Soysa, 2006); higher levels of FDI were associated with lower prevalence of child labor (Neumayer & De Soysa, 2005); and no statistical support was found for the "race to the bottom" hypothesis that globalization leads to a lowering of labor standards. At the same time, the authors are emphatic about the limited inferences with respect to causation that can be drawn from their findings, *and* that the findings cannot be used to infer that globalization is beneficial in terms of labor outcomes as distinct from process-related variables such as free association and collective bargaining. According to Neumayer and De Soysa: "It is entirely possible, of course, perhaps even likely, that globalization boosts the bargaining power of capital at the expense of labor, which would put downward pressure on outcome-related labor standards such as wages, working times and other employment conditions. . . ." (2007, p. 1532).

A similar caveat applies to another cross-national study of the relation between FDI and respect for collective labor rights in ninety developing countries between 1986 and 2002. The study found a positive correlation between FDI inflows and respect for labor rights, but (unlike the Neumayer and De Soysa study) partial support for the race-to-the-bottom hypothesis with respect to trade liberalization. It also found a positive regional effect stronger than the effects of either FDI or trade: in other words, the level of respect for labor rights tends to be similar among developing countries in the same region (Mosley & Uno, 2007). This is what one might expect given the regional rather than truly global character of competition for investment and production in many commodity chains. The study's value is limited inter alia by a scoring system in which multiple violations of labor standards of any given type count as a single violation. The authors themselves note multiple data limitations and the need for more specific descriptions of how individual nations are integrated into the world economy. Finally, none of the studies addresses the possibility that neither the ILO's core labor standards nor other labor-market policy initiatives will be sufficient in many contexts to counter the "disequalizing" (Birdsall, 2006, p. 8) dynamic of the global labor market.

Cross-national studies of labor-market outcomes, notably Rudra's (2005) study of manufacturing in 59 developing countries between 1972 and 1997, and a number of country- and region-specific studies lend support to this last hypothesis (see also Rama, 2003, pp. 169–71). Globalization in South Korea, and in particular the effects of the 1997–98 financial crisis, led to intensification of union activity and an eventual increase in labor's bargaining power and associated rapid expansion of labor rights and social-protection programs (Kim & Kim, 2003; Lee, 2004). Another observer (Kong, 2005) notes a similar pattern of labor-market reform in Taiwan, but emphasizes that Taiwan and Korea have accommodated neoliberalism rather than challenging it,[7] and wonders whether the experience of either country is widely generalizable.[8] As noted earlier, whatever policy shifts have taken place have not halted the rise of economic inequality in many Asian economies. It has been observed that prolabor changes to labor law in Latin America, even when they were belatedly accompanied by an increase in resources directed to enforcement, failed to offset the difficulties for labor mobilization created by globalization—notably the outsourcing, pressures for flexibility and fragmentation of production characteristic of global commodity chains (Anner, 2007, 2008; Hershberg, 2007). As a result, the percentage of workers represented by a union has been falling sharply even in manufacturing—as in the high-income countries, at least according to Lee (2005), as a consequence of the reorganization of industrial production. Furthermore, the "regime of flexible labor . . . operates in stark tension with the traditional model of labor as a solidaristic collective actor" (Hershberg, 2007, p. 170).[9] Similarly, union effectiveness and formal employment have declined, and privatization has proceeded apace, even in African countries like Mozambique, Zambia, and South Africa with historical legacies of trade union action (Pitcher, 2007). This is far from an exhaustive review, but it does suggest the extent to which labor-market outcomes that undermine social determinants of health originate with basic "asymmetries" in the global economic system, as outlined in the introductory chapter to this volume, and will be highly resistant to policy intervention.

IMPLICATIONS FOR PUBLIC POLICY AND ADVOCACY

If it is assumed that poverty, however measured, must be reduced as part of the process of reducing health inequities, then labor-market issues must be central to any analysis of globalization's effects on the social determinants of health, and must be explicitly addressed in development and health policy alike. Yet employment is not high on the international agenda for poverty reduction. Notably, employment is neither a target nor an indicator under the first Millennium Development Goal of eradicating extreme poverty and hunger. It is necessary to "bring employment back in" as a central concern of economic and development policy. In many cases, this will require challenging elements of the international economic policy environment that lead even governments that are rhetorically concerned with equity and poverty reduction to pursue policies that lead to "dismal development and excellent macroeconomic outcomes," in the words of one observer of South Africa (Streak, 2004). These pressures include not only lender conditionalities, such as the IMF's insistence on primary budget surpluses and very low inflation rates even at the cost of growth, but also threats of disinvestment and capital flight (see Chapter 5, this volume). The former constraint is more readily amenable to policy intervention than the latter. "[T]he case for locking capital down" (Bond, 2001, ch.12) is intuitively compelling, but a country adopting this approach risks the destructive consequences of isolating itself in a world of global production networks and competition for FDI.[10]

There are, however, policy instruments that can be used to shift the balance in favor of labor market outcomes that are more favorable from an equity perspective. One of these is the Poverty Reduction Strategy Papers (PRSP) process that national governments must undertake as a precondition for debt relief under the Multilateral Debt Relief Initiative (see Chapter 7, this volume) and for other forms of development assistance. The United Nations Development Fund for Women reported in 2005 that it had reviewed forty-one PRSPs (most of the ones that had then been prepared) and found that while 23 incorporated some form of employment indicator, the indicators might not be the most appropriate ones for the majority of nonagricultural workers in the informal economy and "only five . . . set any kind of explicit target for employment" (Chen et al., 2005, p. 20). Above and beyond employment targets, it is important explicitly to incorporate the interests and situations of the working poor in PRSPs. A related policy focus involves childcare. Crucially, in view of all that is known about how (lack of) access to childcare affects women's abilities to take advantage of labor-market opportunities, priority must be given to providing all women with access to childcare, free or at minimal cost. Depending on the country context, this can be achieved through an appropriate combination of labor standards (where applicable) and direct expenditure by national governments and development assistance providers. Childcare must, in turn, be just one element of a complex of interventions aimed at improving women's access to employment in global production, as well as the *terms* of that access (Barrientos & Kabeer, 2004).

Another set of policy instruments derives from the ILO's set of core labor standards, referenced earlier. The fact that these standards, at least according to Alston (2004), represent a retreat from the more explicit focus on labor *rights* in the conventions from which the standards are drawn is probably less important than the fact that disregard for the standards remains widespread. Many countries have only a limited incentive to ensure compliance—and indeed, a strong incentive not to do so in cases where their competitors for markets and investment cannot be relied upon to comply. At the same time, proposals to internationalize the implementation of labor standards are contentious: Basu (2005), for instance, warns darkly against "wanton interventionism." Based partly on her field research in Bangladesh's export-oriented garment industry, Kabeer (2004b, p. 12) argues eloquently that linking labor standards to market access by way of "social clauses" in trade agreements may in fact hurt precisely those workers they are purportedly designed to help, penalizing poor workers "for their poverty or for the poverty of their country." Broadly similar claims about the adverse consequences of linking market access to labor standards have been made with respect to child labor (Cigno, Rosati, & Guarcello, 2006).

A separate claim has to do with the purported ineffectiveness of labor standards, for instance in reducing inequality (Rama, 2003). However, the data set used by Rama in the cited study makes no distinction between ratification of ILO conventions and their effective implementation. His conclusion that the standards embodied in such conventions do little or nothing to reduce inequality, while the "traditional instruments of social protection" do, must be treated with caution, although it certainly supports the more extensive and equity-focused use of those instruments (see Chapter 6, this volume). Similarly, Kabeer (2004b, p. 5) argues that "the spirit of global solidarity," which she acknowledges as a motivation for proposing such clauses, "would be better served if the international labor movement were to campaign for a universal social floor that would protect the basic needs of all citizens, regardless of their labor market status."

Social floors and labor standards are not mutually exclusive, and it is likely that "[t]he debate on linkage [of trade policy with labor standards] has been overly narrow due to a lack of institutional imagination" (Barry & Reddy, 2006, p. 627). In a detailed reply to the objections just cited and others, Barry and Reddy concede that the unilateral imposition of labor standards (through, e.g., trade sanctions) is illegitimate, but argue (a) that linkage of market access with labor standards following a system of fair negotiation among countries is legitimate, and (b) that it is administratively feasible to design an institutional framework involving the World Trade Organization (WTO)[11] that would overcome objections having to do with feasibility and effectiveness. To be both legitimate and feasible, such a framework would inter alia guard against opportunistic use of labor standards as a protectionist strategy by high-income countries, and incorporate mechanisms whereby the rich countries would share the burdens imposed on poor ones by compliance with core labor standards. Space does not permit adequate treatment either of the richness of their argument or of objections rooted in political economy, specifically the likelihood that elites in developing countries would have a great deal to lose from such a mechanism and would resist efforts to build political support domestically (see, for example, Wise & Cypher, 2007). It suffices to say that their argument is strong enough to support renewed attention to such linkages based on their potential contribution to reducing health inequity through labor markets.

Debates about these and other policy directions are usefully understood with reference to the values underpinning two distinct, although not mutually exclusive, approaches to labor markets and their effects. One approach treats the primary objective of intervening in labor markets, directly or indirectly (e.g., in the form of public spending on education), as correcting for market failures. This approach is exemplified by recent World Bank inventories (World Bank, 2005, pp. 186–93; World Bank, 2007, pp. 125–33) of measures that national and subnational governments can take to make labor markets function more equitably. Although these inventories represent a useful starting point, they often state objectives too narrowly and neglect the potential importance of equity objectives apart from considerations of market failure. In other words, the objectives might be important and demand policy attention even if markets were functioning perfectly.

A second approach explicitly incorporates equity objectives and views labor-market policies as part of a much larger set of interventions directed at reducing inequalities in access to social determinants of health. This is, in fact, the approach implicitly adopted by the World Bank in its 2006 *World Development Report*, where (for instance) early childhood development programs, public expenditure on health care to improve equity in access to treatment, and public works programs to provide employment incomes are viewed in terms of their ability to improve human capacities (World Bank, 2005, pp. 132–55). Viewing labor-market and social-protection policies as complementary parts of a whole is especially important, for instance, with respect to the large numbers of workers in the informal sector. Providing effective social protection for such workers—who, as noted earlier, comprise a majority of the working population in some developing countries and tend to be disproportionately female—represents a formidable challenge even for well-intentioned governments, and also for organized labor (Gallin, 2001).

CODA: WHAT ROLE FOR THE HEALTH POLICY COMMUNITY?

The influence of labor markets on SDH is typical of a class of policy challenges that are big, untidy, complicated, largely outside the remit (and often beyond the professional competence) of heath ministries, yet must be addressed in order to achieve widely shared and equitable improvements in population health. Health ministries, health professionals, and agencies with a health mandate must become engaged in the relevant policy debates. This is a challenge in itself, and at the national level requires confronting the "unequal structure of representation" (Mahon, 1977) within state institutions, where health is often marginalized relative to concerns like providing a favorable investment climate. Globalization generates a variety of pressures to make those concerns even more central to policy and the intrastate distribution of power and resources (Cerny, 2000). A further obstacle is presented by domestic elites that may have an interest in resisting the directly or indirectly redistributive effects of policies that improve SDH, and may be able either to block the emergence of decisive pluralities in support of those policies (in formally democratic jurisdictions) or exercise a veto in other ways, for example, by way of actual or anticipated capital flight. Although a satisfactory comparative exploration of the domestic politics of labor-market policy requires its own discussion, it should be noted that conflicts between labor and capital over economic distribution in today's high-income countries, and in some others, were historically resolved by various forms of "social contracts" or class compromises delimited by national boundaries. The effect of globalization has been decisively to increase the ease with which capital (but not most workers) can take advantage of the "exit" option (see, e.g., Bronfenbrenner, 2000).

Even before these challenges are confronted, the health policy community must clearly understand how policies related (for instance) to labor markets influence health outcomes. Based on the amount of time I have spent, during thirty months' involvement in the work of the World Health Organization Commission on Social Determinants of Health, slowly and carefully explaining to various audiences how and why poverty is hazardous to health, this must be counted as a formidable task. It is formidable despite the strength of the evidence that poverty, and in particular the relation between poverty and other forms of social marginalization, wears people out in biologically measurable ways even in the richest societies in the world (Geronimus, Hicken, Keene, & Bound, 2006). Achieving a thorough understanding—preferably, visceral as well as intellectual—of these relations on the part of the health policy community is not a sufficient condition for the relevant policy changes, but it is most certainly a necessary one, and must be ranked as a top priority for all those concerned with such matters, critically including the World Health Organization itself.

NOTES

1. I am grateful for the research assistance of Daniel Poon.
2. For a detailed critique and a proposal for a (higher) poverty threshold more closely related to the cost of basic needs, see Woodward & Abdallah, 2008.

3. For example, the Triangle Shirtwaist Factory fire in the United States in 1911, in which 148 workers died, led to a public outcry and eventually to improved safety standards; similar fires occur with some frequency today in Bangladeshi garment factories (Brooks, 2007, p. 85). For additional examples and a detailed discussion of the relation between working conditions and health, see Employment Conditions Knowledge Network, 2007.

4. Although it is widely used in the literature, the distinction between skilled and unskilled workers is problematic for at least two reasons: (a) in conventional usage it does not appear to have any clear relation to the complexity of the tasks involved (an exception is Grossman & Rossi-Hansberg, 2006), and (b) it implicitly situates the locus of responsibility for declining wages and employability at the level of the individual, rather than directing attention to characteristics of the production system and the influences on those characteristics.

5. For discussions of labor income trends that reach similar conclusions, see also Kerstetter, 2002; Saez & Veall, 2005; Saez, 2005.

6. A useful introduction to these standards is provided by Asian Development Bank, 2006, and a critical review of their historical background by Alston, 2004.

7. Indeed, much Korean economic policy immediately post-1997 was driven by the requirements of IMF conditionalities (Crotty & Lee, 2005; Hundt, 2005; Moore, 2007, ch. 4).

8. It is also worthwhile to note that postdemocratization increases in labor activism in these two countries were preceded by a long period of authoritarian government during which capital accumulation was facilitated, in part, by ruthlessly repressive policies toward labor (see, e.g., Deyo, 1989; Amsden, 1990; Minns, 2006; Moore, 2007, ch. 3).

9. Veteran Belgian politician Frank Vandenbroucke suggests that a similar dynamic may be under way in high-income countries: "To the extent that skill has become more important as an explanatory factor of quite visible wage inequalities, such inequalities come to have a more 'biographical' character: they seem to be more related to personal history and qualifications than to class as traditionally understood" (Vandenbroucke, 1998, p. 47).

10. Cf. on this point the economic policy dilemma identified by Crotty, Epstein, & Kelly (1998, p. 121): "[P]rogressives often criticize FDI as a destructive force while at the same time decrying the fact that many poor countries can't seem to attract any. It may be that the only thing worse than engaging in this bidding war and getting FDI is engaging in it and not getting any."

11. And thereby reducing the potential for destructive free riding, since most of the world's economies are now WTO members.

REFERENCES

Alarcón-González, D., & McKinley, T. (1999). The adverse effects of structural adjustment on working women in Mexico. *Latin American Perspectives, 26,* 103–17.

Alston, P. (2004). "Core labour standards" and the transformation of the international labour rights regime. *European Journal of International Law, 15,* 457–521.

Amsden, A. (1990). Third World industrialization: "Global Fordism" or a new model. *New Left Review, 182,* 5–31.

Anner, M. (2008). Meeting the challenges of industrial restructuring: Labor reform and enforcement in Latin America. *Latin American Politics and Society, 50,* 33–65.

———. (2007). Forging new labor activism in global commodity chains in Latin America. *International Labor and Working-Class History, 72,* 18–41.

Appelbaum, R., & Lichtenstein, N. (2006). A new world of retail supremacy: Supply chains and workers' chains in the age of Wal-Mart. *International Labor and Working-Class History, 70,* 106–25.

Arrunada, B., & Vazquez, X. H. (2006). When your contract manufacturer becomes your competitor. *Harvard Business Review, 84,* 135.

Asian Development Bank (2006). *Core labor standards handbook.* Manila: Asian Development Bank. Retrieved from: http://www.adb.org/Documents/Handbooks/Core-Labor-Standards/default.asp.

Bair, J. (2005). Global capitalism and commodity chains: Looking back, going forward. *Competition and Change, 9,* 153–80.

Bair, J., & Gereffi, G. (2002). NAFTA and the apparel commodity chain: Corporate strategies, interfirm networks, and industrial upgrading. In G. Gereffi, D. Spener, & J. Bair (eds.), *Free trade and uneven development: The North American apparel industry after NAFTA* (pp. 23–50). Philadelphia: Temple University Press.

———. (2003). Upgrading, uneven development, and jobs in the North American apparel industry. *Global Networks, 3,* 143–69.

Barrientos, S., & Kabeer, N. (2004). Enhancing female employment in global production. *Global Social Policy, 4,* 153–69.

Barrientos, S., Kabeer, N., & Hossain, N. (2004). *The gender dimensions of the globalization of production,* Working Papers No. 17. Geneva: Policy Integration Department, World Commission on the Social Dimensions of Globalization, International Labour Office.

Barry, C., & Reddy, S. G. (2006). International trade and labor standards: A Proposal for linkage. *Cornell International Law Journal, 39,* 545–640.

Basu, K. (2005). Global labour standards and local freedoms. In UNU-WIDER (ed.), *WIDER perspectives on global development* (pp. 175–200). London: Palgrave Macmillan.

Benería, L., & Floro, M. (2005). Distribution, gender, and labor market informalization: A conceptual framework with a focus on homeworkers . In N. Kudva & L. Beneria (eds.), *Rethinking informalization: Poverty, precarious jobs and social protection* (pp. 9–27). Ithaca, NY: Cornell University Open Access Repository. Retrieved from: http://hdl.handle.net/1813/3716 .

Birdsall, N. (2006). *The world is not flat: Inequality and injustice in our global economy,* WIDER Annual Lectures. Helsinki: World Institute for Development Economics Research. Retrieved from: http://www.wider.unu.edu/publications/annual-lectures/annual-lecture-2005.pdf.

Bond, P. (2001). *Against global apartheid: South Africa meets the World Bank, IMF and international finance.* Cape Town: University of Cape Town Press.

Boyenge, J. P. S. (2007). *ILO database on export processing zones* (revised), Working Papers No. WP 251. Geneva: International Labour Office. Retrieved from: http://www.ilo.org/public/english/dialogue/sector/themes/epz/epz-db.pdf.

Bradsher, K. (2008, June 18). Labor costs rise, and manufacturers look beyond China. *New York Times.*

Bronfenbrenner, K. (2000). *Uneasy terrain: The impact of capital mobility on workers, wages, and union organizing.* Ithaca, NY: New York State School of Industrial and Labor Relations, Cornell University.

Brooks, E. (2007). *Unraveling the garment industry: Transnational organizing and women's work.* Minneapolis: University of Minnesota Press.

Buechler, S. J. (2002). *Enacting the global economy in São Paulo, Brazil: The impact of labor market restructuring on low-income women.* PhD Graduate School of Arts and Sciences, Columbia University.

Cerny, P. G. (2000). Restructuring the political arena: Globalization and the paradoxes of the competition state. In R. D. Germain (ed.), *Globalization and its critics: Perspectives from political economy* (pp. 117–38). Houndmills, UK: Macmillan.

Chen, M., Vanek, J., & Heintz, J. (2006). Informality, gender and poverty: A global picture. *Economic and Political Weekly*, 41, 2131–39.

Chen, M., Vanek, J., Lund, F., & Heintz, J. (2005). *Progress of the world's women 2005: Women, work and poverty.* New York: United Nations Development Fund for Women (UNIFEM). Retrieved from: http://www.unifem.org/attachments/products/PoWW2005_eng.pdf .

Chen, S., & Ravallion, M. (2007). *Absolute poverty measures for the developing world, 1981–2004,* World Bank Policy Research Working Papers No. WPS4211. Washington, DC: World Bank. Retrieved from: http://d.repec.org/n?u=RePEc:wbk:wbrwps:4211&r=ltv.

Chusseau, N., Dumont, M., & Hellier, J. (2008). Explaining rising inequality: Skill-biased technical change and North-South trade. *Journal of Economic Surveys*, 22, 409–57.

Cigno, A., Rosati, F. C., & Guarcello, L. (2006). Globalisation and child labour. In G. A. Cornia (ed.), *Harnessing globalisation for children: A report to UNICEF.* Florence: UNICEF Innocenti Research Centre. Retrieved from: http://www.unicef-irc.org/research/ESP/globalization/.

Collier, P. (2006). Why the WTO is deadlocked: And what can be done about it. *The World Economy*, 29, 1423–49.

Cormier, D., & Craypo, C. (2000). The working poor and the working of American labour markets. *Cambridge Journal of Economics*, 24, 691–708.

Cox, R. W. (1999). Civil society at the turn of the millennium: Prospects for an alternative world order. *Review of International Studies*, 25, 3–28.

Crotty, J., Epstein, G., & Kelly, P. (1998). Multinational corporations in the neoliberal regime. In D. Baker, G. Epstein, & R. Pollin (eds.), *Globalization and progressive economic policy* (pp. 117–43). Cambridge: Cambridge University Press.

Crotty, J., & Lee, K. (2005). From East Asian "miracle" to neo-liberal "mediocrity": The effects of liberalization and financial opening on the post-crisis Korean economy. *Global Economic Review*, 34, 415–34.

Cypher, J. M. (2001). Developing disarticulation within the Mexican economy. *Latin American Perspectives*, 28, 11–37.

———. (2004). Development diverted: Socioeconomic characteristics and impacts of mature maquilization. In K. Kopinak (ed.), *The social costs of industrial growth in Northern Mexico* (pp. 343–82). La Jolla, CA: Centre for US-Mexican Studies, University of California–San Diego.

Development Indicators and Policy Research Division, E. a. R. D. A. D. B. (2007). *Key indicators 2007: Inequality in Asia.* (vol. 38). Manila: Asian Development Bank. Retrieved from: http://www.adb.org/Documents/Books/Key_Indicators/2007/default.asp.

Deyo, F. C. (1989). *Beneath the miracle: Labor subordination in the new Asian industrialism.* Berkeley: University of California Press.

Dicken, P. (2007). *Global shift: Reshaping the global economic map in the 21st century* (5th ed.). New York: Guilford Press.

Diderichsen, F., Evans, T., & Whitehead, M. (2001). The social basis of disparities in health. In M. Whitehead, T. Evans, F. Diderichsen, A. Bhuiya, & M. Wirth (eds.), *Challenging inequities in health: From ethics to action* (pp. 13–23). New York: Oxford University Press.

DiTomaso, N. (2001). The loose coupling of jobs: The subcontracting of everyone? In I. Berg & A. L. Kalleberg (eds.), *Sourcebook on labor markets: Evolving structures and processes* (pp. 247–70). New York: Plenum.

Donaghu, M., & Barff, R. (1990). Nike just did it: International subcontracting and flexibility in athletic footwear production. *Regional Studies, 24,* 537–52.

Drevland, R. A. J. (2004). *Trafficked women/fractured women: Russian women surviving in the "new global order."* M.A. thesis, University of Northern British Columbia, Canada.

Duménil, G., & Lévy, D. (2004). Neoliberal income trends: Wealth, class and ownership in the USA. *New Left Review,* new series, 105–33.

Economist. (2004, April 17). How big can it grow?, pp. 67–69.

Edwards, B. (2004, November 13). A world of work: A survey of outsourcing. *The Economist.*

Ehrenreich, B., & Hochschild, A., eds. (2002). *Global woman: Nannies, maids, and sex workers in the new economy.* New York: Metropolitan Books.

Ekman, B., Liem, N. T., Duc, H. A., & Axelson, H. (2008). Health insurance reform in Vietnam: A review of recent developments and future challenges. *Health Policy and Planning, 23,* 252–63.

Elson, D., & Cagatay, N. (2000). The social content of macroeconomic policies. *World Development, 28,* 1347–64.

Employment Conditions Knowledge Network. (2007). *Employment conditions and health inequalities: Final report to the WHO Commission on Social Determinants of Health (CSDH).* Barcelona: Health Inequalities Research Group, Occupational Health Research Unit, Department of Experimental Sciences and Health, Universitat Pompeu Fabra. Retrieved from: http://www.who.int/social_determinants/resources/articles/emconet_who_report.pdf .

Felipe, J., & Hasan, R. (2005). Special chapter—labor markets in Asia: Promoting full, productive, and decent employment. In *Key indicators 2005: Labor markets in Asia: Promoting full, productive, and decent employment* (pp. 1–108). Manila: Asian Development Bank. Retrieved from: http://www.adb.org/documents/books/key_indicators/2005/default.asp.

Freeman, R. B. (2007). The challenge of the growing globalization of labor markets to economic and social policy. In E. Paus (ed.), *Global capitalism unbound: Winners and losers from offshore outsourcing* (pp. 23–40). Houndmills, UK: Palgrave Macmillan.

Frey, R. S. (2003). The transfer of core-based hazardous production processes to the export processing zones of the periphery: The maquiladora centers of northern Mexico. *Journal of World-Systems Research, 9,* 317–54.

Fröbel, F., Heinrichs, J., & Kreye, O. (1980). *The new international division of labour.* Cambridge: Cambridge University Press. (Original German publication 1977)

Fussell, E. (2000). Making labor flexible: The recomposition of Tijuana's maquiladora female labor force. *Feminist Economics, 6,* 59–79.

Gallin, D. (2001). Propositions on trade unions and informal employment in times of globalisation. *Antipode, 33,* 531–49.

Garcia, N. E. (2004). Growth, competitiveness and employment in Peru, 1990–2003. *CEPAL Review, 83,* 81–100.

Gereffi, G., & Korzeniewicz, M., eds. (1994). *Commodity chains and global capitalism.* New York: Praeger.

Gereffi, G., & Memedovic, O. (2003). *The global apparel value chain: What prospects for upgrading by developing countries?* Vienna: United Nations Industrial Development Organization.

Gereffi, G., Spener, D., & Bair, J., eds. (2002). *Free trade and uneven development: The North American apparel industry after NAFTA.* Philadelphia: Temple University Press.

Geronimus, A. T., Hicken, M., Keene, D., & Bound, J. (2006). "Weathering" and age patterns of allostatic load scores among blacks and whites in the United States. *American Journal of Public Health, 96,* 826–33.

Gringeri, C. E. (1994). Assembling "genuine GM parts": Rural homeworkers and economic development. *Economic Development Quarterly,* 8, 147–57.

Grossman, G., & Rossi-Hansberg, E. (2006). *Trading tasks: A simple theory of off-shoring.* Retrieved from: http://www.princeton.edu/~grossman/offshoring.pdf.

Hammonds, K., Kelly, K., and Thurston, K. (1994, October 17). The new world of work. *Business Week,* pp. 76–86.

Herod, A., & Aguilar, L., eds. (2006). The dirty work of neoliberalism: Cleaners in the global economy. *Antipode,* 38, 3.

Hershberg, E. (2007). Globalization and labor: Reflections on contemporary Latin America. *International Labor and Working-Class History,* 72, 164–72.

Heymann, J. (2006). *Forgotten families: Ending the growing crisis confronting children and working parents in the global economy.* New York: Oxford University Press. Retrieved from: http://www.oup.com/us/catalog/general/subject/Sociology/OrganizationsOccupationsWork/~~/cHI9MTAmcGY9MCZzcz1-wdWJkYXRlLmFzYyZzZj1jb21pbmdzb29uJnNkPWFzYyZaWV3PXVzYZ-jaT0wMTk1MTU2NTk1Tk1.

Hughes, D. M. (2000). The "Natasha" trade: The transnational shadow market of trafficking in women. *Journal of International Affairs,* 53, 625–51.

Hundt, D. (2005). A legitimate paradox: Neo-liberal reform and the return of the state in Korea. *The Journal of Development Studies,* 41, 242–60.

Huong, D. B., Phuong, N. K., Bales, S., Jiaying, C., Lucas, H., & Segall, M. (2007). Rural health care in Vietnam and China: Conflict between market reforms and social need. *International Journal of Health Services,* 37, 555–72.

International Labour Organization. (2008). *Global employment trends—January 2008.* Geneva: ILO. Retrieved from: http://www.ilo.org/public/english/employ-ment/strat/download/get08.pdf.

International Monetary Fund. (2007). *Spillovers and cycles in the global economy: World economic outlook April 07.* Washington, DC: IMF. Retrieved from: http://www.imf.org/external/pubs/ft/weo/2007/01/index.htm.

Jenkins, R. (2005). *Globalization, production and poverty,* Research Paper No. 2005/40. Helsinki, Finland: The World Institute for Development Economics Research.

Kabeer, N. (2004a). Labor standards, women's rights, basic needs. In L. Beneria & S. Bisnath (eds.), *Global tensions: Challenges and opportunities in the world economy* (pp. 173–92). New York and London: Routledge.

———. (2004b). Globalisation, labour standards and women's rights: Dilemmas of collective (in)action in an interdependent world. *Feminist Economics,* 10, 3–35.

Kabeer, N., & Mahmud, S. (2004). Rags, riches and women workers: Export-oriented garment manufacturing in Bangladesh. In M. Carr (ed.), *Chains of fortune: Linking women producers and workers with global markets* (pp. 133–64). London: Commonwealth Secretariat. Retrieved from: http://www.divinechocolate.com/shared_asp_files/uploadedfiles/F7284775-DFCD-447D-B79F-0CCE784FD654_ChainsofFortune.pdf.

Kaplinsky, R. (2004). Spreading the gains from globalization: What can be learned from value-chain analysis? *Problems of Economic Transition,* 47, 74–115.

Kerstetter, S. (2002). *Rags and riches: Wealth inequality in Canada.* Vancouver: Canadian Centre for Policy Alternatives. Retrieved from: http://www.policy-alternatives.ca/documents/National_Office_Pubs/rags_riches.pdf.

Kim, D. O., & Kim, S. (2003). Globalization, financial crisis, and industrial relations: The case of South Korea. *Industrial Relations,* 42, 341–67.

Kong, T. Y. (2005). Labour and neo-liberal globalization in South Korea and Taiwan. *Modern Asian Studies,* 39, 155–88.

Kudva, N., & Beneria, L., eds. (2005). *Rethinking informalization: Poverty, precarious jobs and social protection.* Ithaca, NY: Cornell University Open Access Repository. Retrieved from: http://hdl.handle.net/1813/3716.

Lee, C. S. (2005). International migration, deindustrialization and union decline in 16 affluent OECD countries, 1962–1997. *Social Forces, 84*, 71–88.

Lee, H. K. (2004). Welfare reforms in post-crisis Korea: Dilemmas and choices. *Social Policy and Society, 3*, 291–99.

Lerche, J. (2007). A global alliance against forced labour? Unfree labour, neo-liberal globalization and the International Labour Organization. *Journal of Agrarian Change, 7*, 425–52.

Lund, F., & Nicholson, J., eds. (2003). *Chains of production, ladders of protection: Social protection for workers in the informal economy*. Durban, South Africa: School of Development Studies, University of Natal. Retrieved from: http://www-wds.worldbank.org/servlet/WDSContentServer/WDSP/IB/2004/0 6/23/000160016_20040623105223/Rendered/PDF/28116.pdf.

Mahon, R. (1977). Canadian public policy: The unequal structure of representation. In L. Panitch (ed.), *The Canadian state: Political economy and political power* (pp. 165–98). Toronto: University of Toronto Press.

Martínez, M. (2004). Women in the maquiladora industry: Toward understanding gender and regional dynamics in Mexico. In K. Kopinak (ed.), *The social costs of industrial growth in Northern Mexico* (pp. 65–95). La Jolla, CA: Centre for US-Mexican Studies, University of California–San Diego.

McDowell, L., Batnitzky, A., & Dyer, S. (2008). Internationalization and the spaces of temporary labour: The global assembly of a local workforce. *British Journal of Industrial Relations, 46*, 750–770.

Milberg, W. (2004). The changing structure of trade linked to global production systems: What are the policy implications? *International Labour Review, 143*, 45–90.

Mills, M. B. (2003). Gender and inequality in the global labour force. *Annual Review of Anthropology, 32*, 41–62.

Minns, J. (2006). *The politics of developmentalism: The Midas states of Mexico, South Korea and Taiwan*. Houndmills, UK: Palgrave Macmillan.

Mishel, L., Bernstein, J., & Allegretto, S. (2007[prepublication version]). *The state of working America 2006/07*. Ithaca, NY: Cornell University Press. Retrieved from: http://www.stateofworkingamerica.org/.

Misra, J., Woodring, J., & Merz, S. N. (2006). The globalization of care work: Neo-liberal economic restructuring and migration policy. *Globalizations, 3*, 317–32.

Moore, P. (2007). *Globalisation and labour struggle in Asia: A neo-Gramscian critique of South Korea's political economy*. London: Tauris Academic Studies.

Mosley, L., & Uno, S. (2007). Racing to the bottom or climbing to the top? Economic globalization and collective labor rights. *Comparative Political Studies, 40*, 923–48.

Nadvi, K. (2004). Globalization and poverty: How can global value chain research inform the policy debate? *IDS Bulletin, 35*(1), 20–30.

Neumayer, E., & De Soysa, I. (2005b). Trade openness, foreign direct investment and child labor. *World Development, 33*, 43–63.

———. (2006). Globalization and the right to free association and collective bargaining: An empirical analysis. *World Development, 34*, 31–49.

———. (2007). Globalisation, women's economic rights and forced labour. *The World Economy, 30*, 1510–35.

Nickell, S., & Bell, B. (1995). The collapse in demand for the unskilled and unemployment across the OECD. *Oxford Review of Economic Policy, 11*, 40–62.

Palma, J. G. (2006). *Globalizing inequality: "Centrifugal" and "centripetal" forces at work, ST/ESA/2006/DWP/35*, DESA Working Papers No. 35. New York: United Nations Department of Economic and Social Affairs. Retrieved from: http://www.un.org/esa/desa/papers/2006/wp35_2006.pdf.

Parrado, E. A. (2005). Economic restructuring and intra-generational class mobility in Mexico. *Social Forces, 84*, 733–57.

Pitcher, M. A. (2007). What has happened to organized labor in southern Africa? *International Labor and Working-Class History, 72,* 134–60.

Pyle, J. L. (2006a). Globalization and the increase in transnational care work: The flip side. *Globalizations, 3,* 297–315.

———. (2006b). Globalization, transnational migration, and gendered care work: Introduction. *Globalizations, 3,* 283–95.

Rama, M. (2003). Globalization and the labor market. *The World Bank Research Observer, 18,* 159–86.

Razavi, S. (2007). Does paid work enhance women's access to welfare? Evidence from selected industrializing countries. *Social Politics: International Studies in Gender, State Society, 14,* 58–92.

Razavi, S. & Pearson, R. (2004). Globalization, export-oriented employment and social policy: Gendered connections. In S. Razavi, R. Pearson, & C. Danloy (eds.), *Globalization, export-oriented employment and social policy: Gendered connections* (pp. 1–29). Houndmills, UK: Palgrave Macmillan.

Razavi, S., Pearson, R., & Danloy, C., eds. (2004). *Globalization, export-oriented employment and social policy: Gendered connections.* Houndmills, UK: Palgrave Macmillan.

Ross, A., ed. (1997). *No sweat: Fashion, free trade, and the rights of garment workers.* London: Verso.

Rothenberg-Aalami, J. (2004). Coming full circle? Forging missing links along Nike's integrated production networks. *Global Networks—A Journal of Transnational Affairs, 4,* 335–54.

Rudra, N. (2005). Are workers in the developing world winners or losers in the current era of globalization? *Studies in Comparative International Development, 40,* 29–64.

Saez, E. (2005). Top incomes in the United States and Canada over the twentieth century. *Journal of the European Economic Association, 3,* 402–11.

Saez, E., & Veall, M. R. (2005). The evolution of high incomes in northern America: Lessons from Canadian evidence . *American Economic Review, 95,* 831–49.

Sassen, S. (2002). Global cities and survival circuits. In B. Ehrenreich & A. Hochschild (eds.), *Global woman: Nannies, maids, and sex workers in the economy* (pp. 254–74). New York: Metropolitan Books.

Sassen, S. (2006). *Cities in a world economy* (3 ed.). Thousand Oaks, CA: Pine Forge Press.

Schrank, A. (2004). Ready-to-wear development? Foreign investment, technology transfer, and learning by watching in the apparel trade. *Social Forces, 83,* 123–56.

Selwyn, B. (2007). Labour process and workers' bargaining power in export grape production, North East Brazil. *Journal of Agrarian Change, 7,* 526–53.

Sepehri, A., Chernomas, R., & Akram-Lodhi, A. (2003). If they get sick, they are in trouble: Health care restructuring, user charges, and equity in Vietnam. *International Journal of Health Services, 33,* 137–61.

Shaw, J. (2007). "There is no work in my village": The employment decisions of female garment workers in Sri Lanka's export processing zones. *Journal of Developing Societies, 23,* 37–58.

Smith, B. E., & Winders, J. (2008). "We're here to stay": Economic restructuring, Latino migration and place-making in the US South. *Transactions of the Institute of British Geographers, 33,* 60–72.

Somavia, J. (2006). *Decent work in the Americas: An agenda for the hemisphere, 2006–2015 (Report of the Director-General).* Geneva: International Labour Office. Retrieved from: http://www.summit-americas.org/IV%20Summit/Publicaciones/Eng/dwork.pdf.

Streak, J. C. (2004). The GEAR legacy: Did gear fail or move South Africa forward in development? *Development Southern Africa, 21,* 271–88.

Summerfield, G., Pyle, J. L., & Desai, M. (2006). Preface to the symposium: Globalizations, transnational migration, and gendered care work. *Globalizations, 3,* 281–82.

Tokatli, N. (2007). Asymmetrical power relations and upgrading among suppliers of global clothing brands: Hugo Boss in Turkey. *Journal of Economic Geography, 7,* 67–92.

Uchitelle, L., Kleinfield, N. R., Bragg, R., Rimer, S., Johnson, K., Kolbert, E., et al. (1996). *The downsizing of America.* New York: Times Books.

United Nations Country Team Viet Nam. (2003). *Health care financing for Viet Nam,* Discussion Paper No. 2. Hanoi: United Nations Viet Nam. Retrieved from: http://www.un.org.vn/undocs/healthcare/HealthcareFinancing.pdf.

United Nations Economic Commission for Latin America and the Caribbean. (2000). *Social panorama of Latin America 1999–2000.* Santiago: ECLAC. Retrieved from: http://www.cepal.cl/cgi-bin/getProd.asp?xml=/publicaciones/xml/2/6002/P6002.xml&xsl=/dds/tpl-i/p9f.xsl&base=/tpl-i/top-bottom.xsl.

Unni, J., & Rani, U. (2003). Social protection for informal workers in India: Insecurities, Instruments and institutional mechanisms. *Development and Change, 34,* 127–61.

van der Hoeven, R., & Lübker, M. (2005). Financial openness and employment: A challenge for international and national institutions. In *2006 Meeting, Global Development Network,* St. Petersburg. Geneva: International Policy Group, International Labour Office. Retrieved from: http://ctool.gdnet.org/conf_docs/Hoeven_Paper_Lunch%20Time%20Session_ILO.pdf

van Doorslaer, E., O'Donnell, O., Rannan-Eliya, R. P., Somanathan, A., Adhikari, S. R., Garg, C., et al. (2006). Effect of payments for health care on poverty estimates in 11 countries in Asia: An analysis of household survey data. *The Lancet, 368,* 1357–64.

Vandenbroucke, F. (1998). *Globalisation, inequality and social democracy.* London: Institute for Public Policy Research.

Webster, E. (2005). Making a living, earning a living: Work and employment in southern Africa. *International Political Science Review, 26,* 55–71.

Winerip, M. (1998, June 7). The blue-collar millionaire. *New York Times Magazine,* pp. 72–76.

Wise, R. D., & Cypher, J. M. (2007). The strategic role of Mexican Labor under NAFTA: Critical perspectives on current economic integration. *The ANNALS of the American Academy of Political and Social Science, 610,* 119–42.

Wood, A. (1998). Globalisation and the rise in labour market inequalities. *The Economic Journal, 108,* 1463–82.

Woodall, P. (2006, September 16). The new titans: A survey of the world economy. *Economist, 380.*

Woodward, D., & Abdallah, S. (2008). *How poor is "poor"? Towards a rights-based poverty line (technical version).* London: New Economics Foundation.

World Bank. (1995). *World Development Report 1995: Workers in an integrating world.* New York: Oxford University Press.

World Bank. (2005). *World Bank World Development Report 2006: Equity and development.* New York: World Bank and Oxford University Press.

World Bank. (2007). *Global economic prospects 2007: Managing the next wave of globalization.* Washington, DC: World Bank.

Yalnizyan, A. (2007). *The rich and the rest of us: The changing face of Canada's growing gap.* Ottawa: Canadian Centre for Policy Alternatives. Retrieved from: www.growinggap.ca.

Yeates, N. (2004). Global care chains. Critical reflections and lines of enquiry. *International Feminist Journal of Politics, 6,* 369–91.

———. (2005). A global political economy of care. *Social Policy and Society, 4,* 227–34.

York, Geoffrey. (2005, April 29). Is Vietnam destined to become the next China? *The [Toronto] Globe and Mail.*

5 Globalization and Policy Space for Health and Social Determinants of Health

Meri Koivusalo, Ted Schrecker, and Ronald Labonté

INTRODUCTION

Policy space can be defined in different ways depending on context. In this chapter we focus on policy space defined as the freedom, scope, and mechanisms that governments have to choose, design, and implement public policies to fulfill their aims. Our concern is with how globalization and the processes that comprise it are influencing the availability of such space.

Globalization-related restrictions on policy space are not necessarily inimical to improvements in health equity. Agreements entered into by governments, such as human rights treaties, core standards in labor conventions, and environmental protocols can all contribute to improvements in social determinants of health (SDH). Prevention of conflicts and maintenance of peace can have a profound influence on health and SDH and, again, may require restricting a nation's ability to act unilaterally (e.g., in the case of United Nations [UN]-sanctioned peace-keeping efforts). At the same time, the policy space that is available for protecting or improving health and SDH may not be used by governments for a variety of reasons that may be unrelated to globalization per se. For example, even without external pressure governments may make choices in macroeconomic policy, trade, agriculture, or other sectors that restrict policy space for protecting and enhancing health and SDH. Policy space for health thus differs from national policy space as governments may choose, for example, to favor their industrial or agricultural priorities in trade negotiations rather than health and SDH. While the preceding points are important in understanding policy space more generally, the particular focus of this chapter is on the constraining effects of globalization on policy space for health and its social determinants.

The structure of the chapter is as follows. We first elaborate on the importance of the concept of policy space for discussions of SDH. We then identify several respects in which the current structure of international trade policy and law generates constraints on the policy space that is available for protecting health and maintaining or enhancing equity in access to SDH.

Similar constraints arising from the operation of financial markets are next identified, followed by a discussion of a further dimension of the problem: the globalization of ideas about what is feasible or desirable in the realm of national or subnational social and macroeconomic policy. We conclude with a few necessarily generic recommendations for policy directions.

POLICY SPACE IN THE GLOBAL ENVIRONMENT: TERMINOLOGY AND CONTEXT

The concept of national policy space was used, although not precisely defined, in the São Paulo Consensus document that emerged from the 2004 United Nations Conference on Trade and Development (UNCTAD), which recognized that:

> The increasing interdependence of national economies in a globalizing world and the emergence of rule-based regimes for international economic relations have meant that the space for national economic policy, i.e. the scope for domestic policies, especially in the areas of trade, investment and industrial development, is now often framed by international disciplines, commitments and global market considerations (2004, p. 8).

A subsequent UNCTAD report emphasized the contraction of national policy space related for development as a consequence of the growing number of trade treaties, noting that such agreements "could rule out the very policy measures that were instrumental in the development of today's mature economies and late industrializers" (United Nations Conference on Trade and Development, 2006, p. xii).

A frequently stated concern is that World Trade Organization (WTO) disciplines either already in place or under negotiation will restrict the ability of developing country governments to utilize a range of policies that favor domestic producers and industries with the potential for rapid growth. This point is relevant to SDH because of the possibilities that rapid growth creates for poverty reduction and social provision in low-income countries, and because historical evidence shows that such policies, including (but not limited to) highly flexible intellectual property protection regimes, were routinely used by today's high-income countries during their process of industrializing. For this reason, Chang describes the foreclosing of such options by today's trade policy disciplines as "kicking away the ladder" and warns of the impact of ongoing WTO negotiations that could further limit developing countries' remaining flexibilities (Chang, 2005).

In parallel with these developments, the term *fiscal policy space* has emerged in the first instance in the context of sound macroeconomic policies as defined by the International Monetary Fund (IMF). Heller describes fiscal space in its broadest sense as "the availability of budgetary room that allows a government to provide resources for a desired purpose without any prejudice to the sustainability of government's financial position" (2005, p. 3). When dramatic increases occurred in HIV/AIDS financing in the early 2000s, a briefing paper for the Overseas Development Institute warned about the potential conflict between the ability to receive such funds, given fiscal spending constraints imposed by the IMF (deRenzio, 2005). This issue has since been raised by a variety of other actors who argue that IMF public expenditures ceilings have reduced public spending on health and social sectors in several countries (e.g., Ooms & Schrecker, 2005; Wood, 2006). Although these criticisms were disputed by the World Bank and IMF (Sarbib & Heller, 2005), a March 2007 report by the IMF's Independent Evaluation Office on IMF programs in 29 countries in sub-Saharan Africa found that evaluation of "aid absorptive capacity" focused on macroeconomic variables with "almost no attention to sectors such as education, health and infrastructure" (Independent Evaluation Office, 2007, p. 10)—in other words, confirming much of the external critiques.

GLOBALIZATION, POLICY SPACE, AND SOCIAL INEQUALITY

The debate on globalization and social inequalities is embedded within a longer and broader one concerning the impact of global economic and trade policies on poverty reduction (see, e.g., Birdsall, 2006a, 2006b). In the late 1990s, for example, it was claimed that trade liberalization is beneficial for poverty reduction based on the now well-known Dollar and Kraay studies (Dollar & Kraay, 2002). These studies, however, have been critiqued in terms of methods, data, choice of countries, and timeframe (Lubker, Smith, & Weeks, 2002; Nye, Reddy, & Watkins, 2002; Milanovic, 2003); some of these critiques were touched on in this book's introductory chapter. More generally, even the proponents of trade liberalization, who argued that poverty would be reduced, conceded that economic inequality would increase.

Birdsall (2006b, p. 18) makes the point even more emphatically, stating that "A fundamental challenge posed by the increasing reach of global markets (globalization) is that global markets are inherently disequalizing, making rising inequality within developing countries more rather than less likely." This disequalizing effect, according to Birdsall (2006b, p. 22), exists because:

1. Global markets reward more fully those countries and individuals with more of the most productive assets (call this, for simplicity, the market works).

2. In the global economy, negative externalities raise new costs for the vulnerable and compound the risks faced by the already weak and disadvantaged (call this, for simplicity, the market fails).
3. In the global economy, existing rules tend to benefit most those countries and individuals who already have economic power. It is natural that the richer and more powerful manage to influence the design and implementation of global rules—even those rules meant to constrain them—to their own advantage.

This advantage extends beyond "hard" legal and economic influences, such as trade treaties or conditionalities associated with loans or aid, to "softer" influences: what is assumed as possible in the context of globalization and the imperative of maintaining national competitiveness. Thus, as the 2005 report of the United Nations Department of Economic and Social Affairs concluded, the current international trade and financial system is exerting at least some constriction on policy space, in part because "decisions or actions required to advance social policies and social equality are usually perceived as unnecessary costs . . . in conflict with the preservation of a country's international competitiveness," a perception the report further noted as "mistaken" (p. 105).

THE ROLE OF TRADE POLICIES, TRADE AGREEMENTS, AND TRADE NEGOTIATIONS

National governments' trade policies define the context in which trade negotiations take place and what rules different governments may seek to establish in trade agreements. Trade agreements, in turn, form a part of what has been called the "legalization" or "constitutionalization" of global governance in the economic sphere (Goldstein, Kahler, Keohane, & Slaughter, 2001; Coicaud & Heiskanen, 2001; Gill & Bakker, 2006, p. 36) and describe the trade, investment and intellectual property rights agreements that set these rules as institutional elements of a "new constitutionalism" that "seeks," in the terminology used by the World Bank, to "lock in" the rights and freedoms of capital (or large property owners), and to extend and to secure those rights from political threats, such as nationalization of efforts to socialize control over property. They further point out that this new constitutionalism involves interrelated legal and political measures to minimize investor uncertainty across different jurisdictions and, more fundamentally, to expand the scope of operation of corporations and investors to new markets. The reference to trade agreements as part of the global governance's new "constitutionalization" gains further support from the existence of the dispute-settlement process used to enforce trade rules under the WTO.[1]

Although the only truly global trade treaty body, the WTO is only one part of a larger international trade regime. Bilateral and regional agreements, often between industrialized and developing countries, are increasing in number and importance, particularly as they generally go beyond requirements within WTO agreements. This is notably the case with respect to intellectual property rights (Fink & Reichenmiller, 2005; Roffe & Spennermann, 2006; Krikorian & Szymkowiak, 2007; and see Chapter 11, this volume). By late 2004, approximately 230 regional trade agreements (RTAs) were in place, with trade between RTA partners making up nearly 40 per cent of total global trade in 2004 (World Bank, 2004, p. 27; see generally pp. 27–56). By the end of 2002 more than 2,200 bilateral investment agreements were also in place (Choudry, 2005). In a study of agreements between the United States and developing countries, Shadlen (2005b) contrasts the industrial policy flexibility that developing countries still retain as members of the WTO with much more restrictive provisions in such areas as investment and intellectual property found in such bilateral and regional agreements.

Several trade agreements contain text affirming a government's right to regulate for the purpose of achieving set aims. Such assurances, however, need to be set in the context of other WTO requirements that such regulations be otherwise consistent with the agreements, which limits the ways in which these aims can be met. Some agreements, such as the General Agreement on Trade in Services (GATS), give substantial initial leeway in how far and which sectors governments might to wish cover. Others, such as the Agreement on Trade-Related Aspects of Intellectual Property Rights (TRIPS), provide some latitude for exceptions and flexibilities through mechanisms such as compulsory licensing. But in contrast to lowering tariffs, enhancing services trade and protecting intellectual property rights do extend much further into national policy space. The very purpose of trade agreements is to regulate government actions so as to liberalize trade and ensure protection of intellectual property rights. Thus, by necessity, government commitments made within the scope of trade agreements do restrict how they can regulate and subsidize markets, or limit market access of foreign goods or service providers.

Tariff reductions, a basic requirement of trade liberalization, can also have implications for national policy space (or more accurately, the capacity to use policy space). Tariffs remain an important source of public revenue for many low- and middle-income countries, as they once were for high-income countries in the early stages of their industrialization. Alternative revenue streams (e.g., via income or consumption taxes) have proved difficult to create and administer, with best available research finding that many middle-income countries, and especially low-income countries, have been unable to replace most or even all of the tariffs revenues lost from trade liberalization (Baunsgaard & Keen, 2005; see also Aizenman & Jinjarak, 2006). This revenue loss reduces the potential resources available for public spending on health, education, other forms of social protection, and SDH more generally.

Trade negotiations processes themselves can be important in maintaining or reducing national policy space, in three main aspects. First, when negotiations take place as "single undertakings,"[2] health or social services that are not economically important enough to attract the attention of negotiators may become scheduled more extensively for liberalization than would have otherwise been intended. Second, negotiation practices involving so-called mini-Ministerials or other negotiating sessions restricted to participation by more powerful WTO member nations can affect trade treaty outcomes with negative health or development prospects for poorer countries (see, e.g., Jawara & Kwa, 2003).

Third, the use of specific negotiation mechanisms may lead countries to include sectors inadvertently or to make more and deeper commitments than had been anticipated or than they might otherwise have made based on a fuller understanding of the regulatory implications. Such mechanisms include negotiations carried out on the basis of existing legislation, and commitments that are horizontal (applying to all sectors) or made in blocks covering more than one sector. One example is the European Union (EU)-Mexico Free Trade Agreement, which covers government procurement (contracting and purchasing) and investment, neither of which are presently covered by WTO agreements. This agreement also commits the EU and Mexico to not enact legislation that would be more trade restrictive than what is presently in force in their services sectors, referred to as a "standstill" horizontal commitment (European Union–Mexico Free Trade Agreement, 2001). Yet a country's existing services legislation may be more open to foreign providers than what governments might want to bind within a trade agreement, which restrains their future ability to reinstate public provision or expand regulation should such actions harm the commercial interests of foreign providers.

Trade negotiations that simultaneously cover several sectors can lead easily to more extensive commitments than were intended. This contributes to what one of us (M.K.) has termed "outside own priority setting" (OOPS) commitments, where the scope and extent of commitments are not realized by those to whom they will at the time when they are made. Strong and explicit trade policy guidance on health and social development could reduce future OOPS commitments that arise from insufficient prioritization of health issues in trade negotiations. While particular attention needs to be drawn to the negotiation capacities of smaller and poorer countries (South Centre, 2004), the OOPS mistakes take place across countries (see later in this chapter).

TRADE TREATY CONSTRAINTS ON HEALTH-RELATED REGULATION AND STANDARD-SETTING

The impact of trade agreements on national and global health-and-safety-standard-setting mechanisms remains contested. Standards purportedly set in order to protect health and safety are sometimes viewed as disguised protectionist measures against imports from low-income countries; they may involve not only intranational conflicts between industrial or commercial and public health interests but also commercial tensions between high-income countries. Such was the case against legislation banning products containing asbestos brought by Canada against the EU (World Trade Organization, 2000, 2001). Canada claimed that the EU Member states' asbestos ban was against trade rules, since these countries permitted the use of glass fiber insulation, which is a "like" product to asbestos and so covered by the nondiscrimination principle of all WTO agreements. The EU lost the initial case in the dispute settlement, but the WTO's Appellate Body (which must authorize dispute panel decisions), after receiving many complaints about the dispute panel's decision, allowed the EU to maintain its asbestos ban (World Trade Organization, 2001).

GATS Article XX does allow measures to protect public health (and was invoked by the EU in the asbestos case), but is limited by a "chapeau": a leading sentence or preambular text that sets the context and basis for interpreting and using a particular stipulation. The use of this chapeau was further elaborated in Article XX (b) in the Agreement on Sanitary and Phytosanitary Measures (SPS) in 1994, which sets the context in which measures to protect public health can take place. The SPS requires a country using this right to show that its regulations are based on a full scientific risk assessment and do not result in discrimination against members where identical or similar conditions prevail. These requirements formed the basis of the WTO dispute, persisting for over a decade, concerning hormone-treated meat products (World Trade Organization, 1998, 2008). The EU bans the use of certain hormones in cattle rearing within its borders and so in nondiscriminatory fashion, applied this ban to imported meat. The United States and other countries, however, argued successfully that the EU had not carried out sufficient risk assessment studies (as required by the SPS) to warrant their more stringent standards than those applying in the United States, considered a "like" country (World Trade Organization, 1998).

Governments can have clear aims to restrict and limit marketing and consumption of particular goods known to be harmful to health, such as tobacco and alcohol. Public policies in relation to alcohol and tobacco products have already been the subject of several trade disputes concerning national policies to tax or limit availability (World Trade Organization, 1999, 2005a, 2006) with direct constraints on national policy space. The Chilean case, for example, dealt with how taxation limits on the basis of alcohol content gave more beneficial tax treatment to the local product (Pisco) with lower alcohol content in comparison to imported alcohol products (World Trade Organization, 1999). While restriction of availability and taxation are known to be effective strategies to reduce consumption of health-damaging products, such policy measures are also more vulnerable to challenge in the context of trade policies in comparison to more individualized and less market restrictive forms of intervention (see, e.g., Yach & Bettcher, 2000; Babor et al., 2003; Shaffer, Brenner, & Houston, 2005).

WTO agreements are also shifting decision-making power on standards away from national governments. Particular attention has been drawn to the International Organization for Standardization (ISO), a nongovernmental body with strong industry involvement but weak government participation, especially by developing countries (see, e.g., Mattli & Buthe, 2003; Yeates & Murphy, 2007; Nadvi, 2008). The expanding role of ISO standards in the field of environment, services and occupational health and safety has implications for how standards are set (Braithwaite & Drahos, 1999; International Organization for Standardization, 2006). In health, particular attention has been drawn to tobacco and the role of the tobacco industry in determining the evidence and standard setting on their products in the ISO, including the measurement of cigarette tar and nicotine yield (Bialious & Yach, 2001).

Two WTO agreements, the SPS and the Agreement on Technical Barriers to Trade (TBT), defer to the Codex Alimentarius Commission, a joint Food and Agricultural Organization of the United Nations (FAO), and World Health Organization (WHO) food standard-setting organization and a reference body for international food standards. This deference by the WTO changed the global relevance of the Codex substantially as previously it had dealt only with voluntary standards. Veggeland and Borgen (2005) point out that, while national and economic interests have always been part of the Codex decision-making process, since the establishment of the WTO, countries have argued more strongly in favor of norms compatible with their national interests as expressed in WTO negotiations. They note further that this development may actually conflict with the mandate of Codex (Veggeland & Borgen, 2005). This raises two issues related to national policy space: the increasing relevance of standards set by Codex[3] and the ways in which the Codex process is itself becoming increasingly shaped by trade policy interests.

WTO agreements are concerned about the cross-border trade in goods and services and not with their production practices. This is a more widely recognized issue in global labor and occupational safety policies, but bears relevance also to health policies (for employment and labor issues, see Chapter 4, this volume). Global trade-related standard setting and regulatory work in other "nontrade" substantive areas have also surfaced in relation to multilateral environmental agreements (MEAs) and human rights treaties (Dommen, 2002; Cottier, Pauwelyn, & Burgi, 2005; World Trade Organization, 2007), concluding that, in the event of conflict involving WTO provisions, WTO provisions may not always prevail, including before a WTO panel. Being a framework agreement, the WTO and its provisions will often have to give way to, for example, MEAs or other conventions that impose obligations or grant explicit trade restriction rights applied to specific products or for particular reasons (Pauwelyn, 2003). The successful negotiation of the United Nations Educational, Scientific, and Cultural Organization (UNESCO) Convention on the Protection and Promotion of the Diversity of Cultural Expression is one example where governments have sought to retain policy space in light of obligations under trade agreements (UNESCO, 2005).

SCOPE OF PUBLIC POLICIES AND
REGULATION OF PUBLIC SERVICES

In the context of trade agreements and SDH, particular attention needs to be drawn to public services. The General Agreement on Trade in Services (GATS), for example, includes a commitment towards progressive liberalization of services. While GATS allows member countries to specify which service sectors and under what conditions they will open their borders for trade, the commitment towards progressive liberalization envisions a future in which *all* service sectors would eventually be open for global trade. There is an exclusion for public services in GATS, although it is expressed narrowly in the form of "a service supplied in the exercise of governmental authority," defined as applying only to services supplied neither on a commercial basis nor in competition with one or more service suppliers. Since publicly funded services in most countries usually include some contracted arrangements with the private sector (including here NGOs or not-for-profit organizations), these services cannot simply be assumed to be outside of the scope of GATS commitments (Krajewski, 2003; Luff, 2003; Fidler, Correa, & Aginam, 2005).

GATS Article VI on domestic regulation also has relevance to regulatory measures and, according to Delimatsis (2008), touches the interface of services trade liberalization and domestic autonomy. The legal mandate contained in this Article seeks to guarantee that licensing and qualification requirements or technical standards do not constitute unnecessary barriers to trade in services. According to Luff (Harvey, 2003), these are likely to cover all rules relating to the opportunities for doctors or hospitals to provide their services. In practice the supply of these services is subject to rather severe requirements and authorization procedures within countries, which generally create obstacles to trade by excluding or complicating entry of foreign services or services providers who do not comply with them. These stringent requirements could be constrained by the outcome of current negotiations to strengthen GATS disciplines for domestic regulations. Other GATS provisions with respect to monopolies and exclusive service suppliers (Luff, 2003; Fidler et al., 2005) and subsidies (Gauthier, O'Brien, & Spencer, 2000; Adlung, 2006) could also affect public financing and support to service provision in poorer areas.

Negotiations in services trade have proved to be particularly complex, making it difficult for governments to know exactly the scope and nature of commitments they are making, and what restrictions they might like to apply to these commitments. Although countries can stipulate restrictions in committed sectors, it is expected that such restrictions will not be permanent and will be removed during future GATS negotiating rounds. The recent WTO dispute settlement case on online gambling provides an example of an OOPS commitment discussed earlier (World Trade Organization, 2004, 2005b). While Antigua and Barbuda successfully claimed that the United States had scheduled online gambling services as part of market access commitments in "other recreational services (except sporting)," the United States considered that it had made no such commitments since it believed that gambling and betting services fell within sporting services, which it had excluded (World Trade Organization, 2004; Ortino, 2006). Similarly, in 1994 Canada unintentionally committed trade in private health insurance since this fell under the financial services sector (to which it did commit) and not under the health services sector (in which it made no commitments) (Campbell et al., 2003).

The Antigua and Barbuda case highlights another problematic issue for policy space. The dispute panel ruled that prohibiting all online gambling (that is, treating both foreign and local providers the same) would still violate United States GATS commitments, since it constituted a "zero quota" limitation on any potential foreign provider (Pauwelyn, 2005a; World Trade Organization, 2005b; Pauwelyn, 2005b). The appellate body did state that the United States could violate this rule as a measure "necessary to protect public morals or to maintain public order" (one of the exceptions allowed under GATS). But if this interpretation prevails within WTO, it means that when governments commit a service sector in GATS in which certain activities are prohibited for both domestic and foreign providers (that is, the prohibition is nondiscriminatory) they could still lose a trade dispute simply because the prohibition reduces market access for foreign providers.

The more commercialized and globalized service provision becomes, the more GATS and its disciplines will matter. Particular focus needs to be put on how policies intended to contain costs could become problematic under GATS. It is unlikely, for example, that denying patients the freedom to choose their doctors would be accepted under full GATS commitments to trade in health services (Luff, 2003), yet most health systems in practice limit this freedom for various sound policy reasons. The complexity of regulatory needs in the health sector, as well as the necessity of knowing everything before scheduling services, implies that the most secure regulatory option is not to make services commitments in the health sector. While this would address concerns within health systems, it would not, however, cover all those in relation to SDH.

Finally, while particular sectors at present can be kept outside GATS, this is affected by the practice of revisiting commitments under GATS with the aim of more and deeper commitments being made during each negotiation round. While commitments already made are not necessarily permanent or totally "locked in"—they can be altered or removed—this can become costly for countries since in exchange for limiting or removing commitments in one area they must expand commitments in another.

POLICY SPACE FOR HEALTH AND INTELLECTUAL PROPERTY RIGHTS

A broader literature describes the relationship between trade-related intellectual property rights (IPRs) and development via industrial policy strategies (see, e.g., Lall, 2003; Shadlen, 2005a; United Nations Conference on Trade and Development, 2007b), and in regards to patenting of genes, plants, life-forms, and regulation of bioprospecting (Shiva, 2001; Commission on Intellectual Property Rights, 2002; Jaffe & Lerner, 2004; Koo, Nottenburg, & Pardey, 2004; Jensen & Murray, 2005; Sampath, 2005; Correa, 2006; Howse, 2007). Because the TRIPS agreement is dealt with in another chapter in this volume (Chapter 11), we cover here only trade-related IPRs issues that pertain to national policy space for health, specifically those limiting the scope of options in pharmaceutical policies. A key issue in this regard is bilateral treaties that include restrictive measures going well beyond those contained in the TRIPS agreement, directly affecting national reimbursement and pricing policies in developed as well as developing countries (Drahos & Henry, 2004; Doran & Henry, 2008). One example of this expansion is reflected in the United States 301 trade-watch list of countries considered to threaten its IPR interests, which states explicitly that "even when a country's IPRs regime is adequate, price controls and regulatory and other market access barriers can serve to discourage the development of new drugs. These barriers can arise in a variety of contexts, including reference pricing, approval delays and procedural barriers to approvals, restrictions on dispensing and prescribing, and unfair reimbursement policies" (United States Trade Representative, 2006). Norway has been added to the U.S. watch-list due to its pharmaceutical pricing policies, and the pharmaceutical industry has threatened Finland with a similar fate should it implement TRIPS consistent reference pricing policies (United States Trade Representative, 2008; Anonymous, 2008).

The strong protection of IPRs as a core element of innovation strategies also has implications for national health-policy space both in pricing and rational use of pharmaceuticals and in access to knowledge and or development of research policies. IPRs, trade agreements, and industrial policy-related pressures are not only an issue of differing priorities between poor and rich countries, but of differing, if not conflicting, priorities between particular corporate sectors and health ministries. Common interests can be found across countries in drug-pricing policies and measures that ensure sufficient research and development in particular areas important for health but which lack sufficient commercial margins, such as research on new generations of antibiotics (Wenzel, 2004; Norrby, Nord, & Finch, 2005; see also Chapter 11, this volume).

LENDERS, INVESTORS, AND POLICY SPACE[4]

Trade treaties are not alone in imposong constraints on policy space; international lending and investing practices also exert a powerful influence. The role of the World Bank and the IMF has been a central feature of the social and economic policy context in many developing countries over the past twenty-five years. They are closely identified with structural adjustment, a term that entered the international development lexicon in 1980, when the World Bank and IMF began lending to countries needing to reorganize their economies in order to repay external creditors (Kahler, 1992). Background on this lending, and the structural adjustment conditionalities associated with it, was provided in the introductory chapter. Suffice it to say here that lender conditionalities create constraints on the policy space available to national governments; like trade agreements, that is their intent. However, several evidentiary problems complicate assessment of the severity and impact of those constraints. Conditionalities have often been implemented imperfectly, or resisted for substantial periods of time (Kahler, 1992; Killick, 2004). For analytical purposes, it is difficult to separate the effects of conditionalities from those of the economic crises that preceded structural adjustment. Any assessment of their effects presupposes one or more counterfactuals—assumptions about what would have been the case if no intervention by the World Bank and the IMF had been undertaken, or if some other set of interventions had been chosen (Huber & Solt, 2004). In many countries lender conditionalities have contributed to the reorganizing of national economies in ways that did not reflect popular or electoral priorities, and indeed provoked widespread popular resistance (Walton & Seddon, 1994). In at least a few cases, the constraints associated with lender conditionalities were also intended by national governments, which pursued agreements with the IMF so that they could create an aura of inevitability about policy changes that they might otherwise not have been able to implement (Vreeland, 2003).

The new Poverty Reduction Strategy Papers (PRSPs) have broadened participatory aspects, but still share many similarities with structural adjustment policies and conditionalities related to these. PRSPs must be approved by the World Bank and IMF as a condition for receiving debt relief under the Heavily Indebted Poor Countries Initiative (now the Multilateral Debt Relief Initiative), and increasingly determine eligibility for other forms of development assistance as well (see also Chapter 7, this volume). Griesgraber and Ugarteche (2006) point out that while many middle-income countries in

Asia and Latin America are now largely beyond the potential reach of IMF conditionality because of their large foreign exchange reserves[5] and early repayment of their debts to the fund, low-income countries "remain bound to the IMF" through the PRSP process and the new conditionalities associated with the Multilateral Debt Relief Initiative (MDRI) announced by the G8 in 2005. Further, the influence of the IMF in practice extends beyond formal conditionalities, because private investors view IMF approval of a country's macroeconomic policies as a seal of approval (Woods, 2006b, pp. 375–76) and, indeed, the resources at their disposal have been needed to complement those of the IMF (Gould, 2003).

"Financialization" has been among the dominant trends in the operation of many national economies, and especially the global economic system, over the past few decades (Epstein, 2005). While the total value of foreign direct investment (to build new production facilities or acquire existing assets) in 2006 was $1.2 trillion, the *daily* value of "traditional" foreign exchange transactions on the world's financial markets is now estimated at $3.2 trillion, not including a variety of financial derivatives, the market for which is growing even more rapidly (Bank for International Settlements, 2007; United Nations Conference on Trade and Development, 2007a).

Short-term flows of hypermobile investment can lead to financial crises that push millions into poverty and economic insecurity, with resulting negative health outcomes.[6] This happened, for instance, when disinvestment halved the value of the Mexican peso relative to the US dollar between December 1994 and March 1995 (US General Accounting Office, 1996). Immediate damage to Mexicans' purchasing power was compounded by the wage reductions, workforce cutbacks, and public-sector austerity measures needed to restore investor confidence (Grinspun & Cameron, 1993; Dussel Peters, 2000; Cypher, 2001). The Asian financial crisis of 1997–1998 involved comparable depreciation of the Thai and Korean currencies, and an even more drastic depreciation of Indonesia's (Martinez, 1998), again with effects on the economically vulnerable that were compounded by austerity measures needed to restore "investor confidence." The damage done by financial crises in terms of lost gross domestic product (GDP) (hence, government revenue) and employment can be substantial; Griffith-Jones and Gottschalk (2006) estimate the cost of the Asian financial crisis to the affected economies at US$917 billion over the period 1997–2002, and a comparison of financial crises in ten countries by van der Hoeven and Lübker (2005) showed that employment tends to recover much more slowly than GDP in the aftermath of financial crises. A further effect is that the value of external debt obligations denominated in dollars or other hard currency climbs with any devaluation, creating additional economic constraints on domestic public-sector budgets (Koelble & Lipuma, 2006).

The power dynamic underlying financial crises created by large flows of short-term capital was described by Michel Camdessus, then managing director of the International Monetary Fund, in the aftermath of the collapse of the Mexican peso in 1994–95:

> Countries that successfully attract large capital inflows must also bear in mind that their continued access to international capital is far from automatic, and the conditions attached to that access are not guaranteed. The decisive factor here is market perceptions: whether the country's policies are deemed basically sound and its economic future, promising. The corollary is that shifts in the market's perception of these underlying fundamentals can be quite swift, brutal, and destabilizing (Camdessus, 1995).

This blunt observation about the power of markets is notable for its author as much as for its content, which is now almost universally acknowledged.

Griffith-Jones and Stallings (1995) have described the constraint on policy space created by financial markets as "implicit conditionality," as contrasted with the explicit conditionality attached to lending from multilateral financial institutions. Like other constraints on policy space, implicit conditionality often operates by way of the mechanism of anticipated reaction: even governments committed to improving access to basic health-related needs are reluctant to risk the effects of displeasing the financial markets, just as they may be reluctant to implement policies that might be viewed negatively by sources of foreign direct investment. Investor concern about policies that might be adopted by the Workers' Party in Brazil (in advance of the 2002 elections) or the African National Congress in South Africa (after democratization) reduced the value of the country's currency by roughly 40 per cent in each case, arguably leading the governments in question at least temporarily to accept high unemployment and limited social expenditure rather than risk further depreciation of their currencies (Evans, 2005; Koelble & Lipuma, 2006). In South Africa, the result was "dismal development and excellent macroeconomic outcomes" (Streak, 2004) with the former including negative employment growth in every year between 1996 and 2000 and an official unemployment rate of over 30 percent; unofficial unemployment rates, using a broader measure, were and are considerably higher (Kingdon & Knight, 2005).

Writing about Latin America, economist John Williamson argues that "levying heavier taxes on the rich so as to increase social spending that benefits disproportionately the poor" is conceptually attractive, but "it would not be practical to push this very far, because too many of the Latin rich have the option of placing too many of their assets in Miami" (Williamson, 2004, p. 13). This is an illustration of the constraint created for public policy by capital flight: the process in which the wealthy shift their assets abroad in order to avoid "social control" (such as taxation) or risks of devaluation (Ndikumana & Boyce, 1998, p. 199; see also Beja, 2006, p. 265). The resource flows in question are substantial. Ndikumana and Boyce (2003) estimated the value of capital flight from sub-Saharan Africa—a region that includes many of the world's poorest countries—between 1970 and 1996 at $186.8 billion (in 1996 dollars), noting that during the period "roughly 80 cents on every dollar that flowed into the region from foreign loans flowed back out as capital flight *in the same year*" (Ndikumana & Boyce, 2003, p. 122; emphasis added). They have also concluded that the accumulated value of capital flight from 25 African countries between 1970 and 1996, plus imputed interest earnings, was considerably *higher* than the entire value of the combined external debt of those 25 countries in 1996 (Boyce & Ndikumana, 2001). Using a similar methodology, Beja (2006) estimates the accumulated value of capital flight from Indonesia, Malaysia, the Philippines, and Thailand over the period 1970–2000 at US $1 trillion. And at the end of 2001, while Argentina was undergoing an economic collapse that saw the value of the peso lose more than 60 per cent of its value against the U.S. dollar and GDP decline by 11 per cent in 2002, it was estimated that the value of assets held abroad by Argentine residents equaled the total value of the country's foreign debt (Centro de Estudios Legales y Sociales, 2003).

Understanding the constraints that contemporary financial markets create on national policy space requires recognition that those markets do not operate in isolation. Rather, they reinforce pressures to compete for FDI and outsourced production by way of policy convergence toward what Cerny has called a competition state: "The main focus of the competition state is the promotion of economic activities, whether at home or abroad, which will make firms and sectors located within the territory of the state competitive in international markets" (Cerny, 2000, p. 136). Often, as a consequence, the formal operations of democracy coexist with more or less severe limits on the content of public policy. Sassen describes the constraints in terms of "a sort of global, cross-border economic electorate," whose power over governments derives not from formal political participation but rather from the ownership of mobile assets (Sassen, 1996, p. 40). The extent to which this constraint operates will vary depending on a country's or a region's position in the world economic system, and it is by no means absolute—as suggested, for instance, by the Malaysian government's successful resistance to IMF prescriptions in the immediate aftermath of the Asian financial crisis. Its decision instead to impose capital controls is credited by many observers with both reducing the impacts of the crisis and speeding up the Malaysian economy's subsequent recovery. However, the constraint should not be underestimated. One of the most accomplished investigators of how global financial markets actually work (Mosley, 2003) has warned, for instance, that "those societies most in need of egalitarian redistribution may have, in terms of external financial market pressures, the most difficulty achieving it" (Mosley, 2006, p. 90).

GLOBALIZATION OF IDEAS

Ideas matter in public policy and globalization is also about the worldwide diffusion of assumptions about what is feasible and possible in economic policy—in particular, neoliberal or market-oriented policy perspectives (Deacon, Stubbs, & Hulse, 1997; Scholte, 2000; Gill & Bakker, 2006). Przeworski et al. noted in the foreword to their report on the sustainability of democracy that the embrace of rapid economic liberalization, "particularly but not only in Eastern Europe," represents the implementation of a neoliberal ideology "developed within the walls of the North American academia and shaped by international financial institutions. . . . For the first time in history capitalism is being adopted as an application of a doctrine, rather than evolving as a historical process of trial and error" (1995, p. viii).

The World Bank and the IMF have played important roles in this process; they exercise influence not only in their role as lenders, but also in the realm of ideas as well-funded definers of conventional wisdom, knowledge producers (Mehta, 2001; Wade, 2002; Broad, 2006), and nodes in transnational networks of professionals who share assumptions (mostly those of neoclassical economics), training experiences (notably in the economics departments of US and British universities), and career paths (Lee & Goodman, 2002; Woods, 2006a, pp. 53–56). The Organization for Economic Cooperation and Development (OECD) has also been identified as a key actor in globalization of health system reforms (Moran & Wood, 1996). Outside the health sector, the World Bank's influence was evident for instance in advocacy of pension privatization in Latin America, following the lead of Chile under Pinochet. Although the Bank sometimes made loans contingent on pension "reform," its major effect was rather as a "teacher of norms" and as a promoter of economic liberalization more generally (Mesa-Lago & Müller, 2002, pp. 709–12; Brooks, 2004, pp. 54–65). World Bank documents tend to become important sources amongst policy actors and consultancy companies in aid policies, and hence highly influential in the policy choices made by many aid-dependent countries, even decades after these documents and their basic assumptions first appear. Many of these assumptions also find renewed voice; thus, the emphasis on priority of market-based mechanisms remained prominent in the World Bank 2000 *Social Protection Sector Strategy*. This document invoked the need for "[a] new conceptualization of social protection that is better aligned with current worldwide realities" in support of the position that, "[i]n an ideal world with perfectly symmetrical information and complete, well-functioning markets, all risk management arrangements can and should be market-based (except for the incapacitated)" (Holzmann & Jörgensen, 2001, p. 16). The Social Protection Sector Strategy, in particular, is also an example of how globalization-driven distributions of economic power and property rights also *create* the "worldwide realities" that globalization is claimed to invoke.

CONCLUSION: CREATING AND PROTECTING POLICY SPACE

At the national and subnational level, substantial space exists for policies that support health and SDH, despite the context created by globalization. The extent of that policy space depends on a country's position in the world economy, as reflected (for instance) in its bargaining power in trade negotiations and in its relation to the global financial marketplace. Policy choices are framed by assumptions about what is economically sound, effective, feasible or possible. Whether this space is used for health is further dependent on national policy, choices, and politics in relation to health and other priorities. However, both formal and informal constraints associated with globalization are limiting the range of policy measures governments can use to reduce social inequalities, many of which themselves arise from globalization (see also Chapter 2, this volume).

Governments need to understand better the potential health-policy implications of commitments that increase the mobility of capital or limit the ability of governments to exert "social control" over investors. Required, as well, are global level actions that focus on international financial institutions and multilateral, regional, and bilateral trade negotiations, specifically drawing attention to the importance of the decisions made in these fora on the capacities of countries to address distributional issues within their borders important for social cohesion.

International trade agreements are designed to limit national policy space. Health-policy makers need to understand what implications—in particular regulatory and cost implications—trade agreements have for national policy space for health. They will also need to be able to articulate their own priorities in relation to trade and economic policy negotiations at the national level to ensure either that their priorities are not compromised by trade agreements or, where compromises are made, that these are accompanied by sufficient compensatory mechanisms.

Because trade negotiation practices may lead to inadvertent OOPS commitments, explicit and clear guidance on national trade policy priorities could help to maintain policy space for health during negotiations. There is also a case to be made for removing all policies affecting health systems from the scope of commercial multilateral, regional, and bilateral trade agreements. Other options could include specific regional or global cooperation arrangements or agreements based upon health, rather than trade, policy priorities and needs, and under WHO or, where appropriate, other competent agencies' aegis. However, while such measures could address some concerns with health systems, they would not address issues of relevance to SDH.

Addressing the ways in which financial markets limit the ability of national governments to pursue equity-oriented health and social policies presents formidable challenges, yet is likely to be essential as a counterforce to the interests of the "cross-border economic electorate" described by Sassen (1996). Broad policy directions that would carry forward this ambitious project by way of "redistribution, regulation and rights" are outlined in Chapter 13.

Finally, there is a need to confront the globalization of ideas, notably those concerning what is feasible, desirable, and possible in the context of pressures for policy convergence created by the imperative of maintaining national economic competitiveness. It is thus important to draw attention not only to the implications of globalization for development and the limits to the range of economic and industrial policies at governments' disposals; but also the ways in which globalization is changing the scope and capacities of governments to undertake regulatory and redistributive policies, notably those concerning health, health systems, and social security.

NOTES

1. Not all that is traded is affected by multilateral agreements under WTO, or even regional or bilateral agreements. The migration of health professionals from low- to high-income countries, a health equity issue of increasing global importance, for example, has so far had little to do with trade agreements (see Chapter 9, this volume).
2. This describes the "all-or-nothing process" used in WTO negotiations, where consensus must be reached in all agreements under negotiation to complete one round of trade talks, and before commencing a new round. This process presumably allows countries to trade off losses in one area of trade with the prospect of gains in another.
3. The fact that Codex had set acceptable levels for five of the six hormones in the WTO beef-hormone case played a role in the dispute ruling against the EU. Determination of safety, while informed by scientific evidence, is ultimately made through voting by individual nations. The five hormones in question were voted safe by a margin of 33-39, with seven abstentions (Labonté & Sanger, 2006).
4. A more extensive discussion of the issues raised in this section is provided by Schrecker (forthcoming).
5. The accumulation of foreign exchange reserves that has reduced the vulnerability of some economies to the threat of financial crisis has not come without costs. Accumulation of foreign exchange reserves has contributed to net financial outflows from the developing world, primarily from Asian countries, of more than US$480 billion in 2005 (United Nations Department of Economic and Social Affairs, 2006, pp. 65–88). This loss is partly explained by

the fact that governments receive very low interest rates on these reserves (e.g., when held in U.S. treasury bills) while having to borrow domestically at higher rates—thus, in effect, poor countries are lending to rich ones at a net loss, losing opportunities for domestic investment and growth in the process.

6. For a description of the relevant pathways, see Hopkins (2006).

REFERENCES

Adlung, R. (2006). Public Services and the GATS. *Journal of International Economic Law, 9*, 455–85.

Aizenman, J., & Jinjarak, Y. (2006). *Globalization and developing countries—a shrinking tax base?* No. 11933. Cambridge, MA: UCSC and the National Bureau of Economic Research BER NTU Economics Department, E2 Division of Economics. Retrieved from: http://www.nber.org/papers/w11933.

Anonymous (2008). Mitä Norja edellä sitä Suomi perässä. Tiedote. Press Release [*What Norway does first, Finland will follow*]. Lääketeollisuus [online]. Retrieved from: http://www.laaketeollisuus.fi/page.php?page_id=99&offset=0&news_id=28.

Babb, S. (2005). The social consequences of structural adjustment: Recent evidence and current debates. *Annual Review of Sociology, 31*, 199–222.

Babor, T. F., Caetano, R., Casswell, S., Edwards, G., Giesbrecht, N., Graham, K., et al. (2003). *Alcohol: No ordinary commodity. Research and public policy.* Oxford: Oxford University Press.

Bank for International Settlements. (2007). *Triennial central bank survey: Foreign exchange and derivatives market activity in 2007.* Basel: BIS. Retrieved from: http://www.bis.org/publ/rpfxf07t.htm.

Baunsgaard, T., & Keen, M. (2005). *Tax Revenue and (or?) trade liberalization,* IMF Working Papers No. WP/05/112. Washington, DC: International Monetary Fund. Retrieved from: http://www.imf.org/external/pubs/ft/wp/2005/wp05112.pdf.

Beja, E. L. (2006). Was capital fleeing Southeast Asia? Estimates from Indonesia, Malaysia, the Philippines, and Thailand. *Asia Pacific Business Review, 12*, 261–83.

Bialious, S. A., & Yach, D. (2001). Whose standard is it anyway? How the tobacco industry determines the International Organisation for Standardisation (ISO) standards for tobacco and tobacco products. *Tobacco Control, 10*, 96–104.

Birdsall, N. (2006a). *Stormy days on an open field: Asymmetries in the global economy,* Research Papers No. 2006/31. Helsinki: World Institute for Development Economics Research. Retrieved from: http://www.wider.unu.edu/publications/rps/rps2006/rp2006–31.pdf.

———. (2006b). *The world is not flat: Inequality and injustice in our global economy,* WIDER Annual Lectures. Helsinki: World Institute for Development Economics Research. Retrieved from: http://www.wider.unu.edu/publications/annual-lectures/annual-lecture-2005.pdf.

Boyce, J. K., & Ndikumana, L. (2001). Is Africa a net creditor? New estimates of capital flight from severely indebted sub-Saharan African countries, 1970–96. *Journal of Development Studies, 38*, 27–56.

Braithwaite, J., & Drahos, P. (1999). Ratcheting up and driving down global regulatory standards. *Development, 42*, 109–14.

Broad, R. (2006). Research, knowledge, and the art of' "paradigm maintenance": The World Bank's development economics vice-presidency (DEC). *Review of International Political Economy, 13*, 387–419.

Brooks, S. M. (2004). International financial institutions and the diffusion of foreign models for social security reform in Latin America. In K. Weyland (ed.), *Learning from foreign models in Latin American policy reform* (pp. 53–80). Washington, DC: Woodrow Wilson Center Press.

Camdessus, M. (1995). *The IMF and the challenges of globalization—the fund's evolving approach to its constant mission: The case of Mexico.* Address at Zurich Economics Society No. 95/17. Washington, DC: International Monetary Fund. Retrieved from: http://www.imf.org/external/np/sec/mds/1995/mds9517.htm.

Campbell, B., Blouin, C., Foster, J., Labonté, R., Lexchin, J., Sanger, M., et al. (2003). *Putting health first: Canadian health care, trade treaties and foreign policy.* Ottawa: Canadian Centre for Policy Alternatives. Retrieved from: www.policyalternatives.ca.

Centro de Estudios Legales y Sociales. (2003). Argentina: In the hands of the oligopoly of foreign capital. In Social Watch (ed.), *The poor and the market: Social watch report 2003* (pp. 82–83). Montevideo, Uruguay: Instituto del Tercer Mundo.

Cerny, P. G. (2000). Restructuring the political arena: Globalization and the paradoxes of the competition state. In R. D. Germain (ed.), *Globalization and its critics: Perspectives from political economy* (pp. 117–38). Houndmills, UK: Macmillan.

Chang, H. J. (2005). *Why developing countries need tariffs: How WTO NAMA negotiations could deny developing countries' right to a future.* Geneva: South Centre. Retrieved from: http://www.southcentre.org/publications/SouthPerspectiveSeries/WhyDevCountriesNeedTariffsNew.pdf.

Choudry, A. (2005). Corporate conquest, global geopolitics: Intellectual property rights and bilateral investment agreements. Asia-Pacific Research Network [online]. Retrieved from: http://www.aprnet.org/index.php?a=show&t=issues&i=53.

Coicaud, J. M. & Heiskanen, V., eds. (2001). *Legitimacy of international organisations.* Tokyo: United Nations University Press.

Commission on Intellectual Property Rights (CIPR). (2002). *Integrating intellectual property and development policy—report of the Commission on Intellectual Property Rights.* London: Commission on Intellectual Property Rights. Retrieved from: http://www.iprcommission.org/papers/pdfs/final_report/CIPRfullfinal.pdf.

Correa, C. (2006). *Guidelines for the examination of pharmaceutical patents: Developing a public health perspective—a working paper.* Geneva: ICTSD/UNCTAD/WHO. Retrieved from: http://www.iprsonline.org/unctadictsd/docs/Correa_Pharmaceutical-Patents-Guidelines.pdf.

Cottier, T., Pauwelyn, J., & Burgi, E. (2005). *Human rights and international trade.* Oxford: Oxford University Press.

Cypher, J. M. (2001). Developing disarticulation within the Mexican economy. *Latin American Perspectives, 28,* 11–37.

Deacon, B., Stubbs, P., & Hulse, M. (1997). *Global social policy.* London: Sage.

Delimatsis, P. (2008). Determining the necessity of domestic regulations in services. The best is yet to come. *European Journal of International Law, 19,* 365–408.

deRenzio, P. (2005). *Scaling up versus absorptive capacity: Challenges and opportunities in reaching the MDGs in Africa.* ODI briefing paper. London: Overseas Development Institute. Retrieved from: http://www.odi.org.uk/publications/briefing/bp_may05_absorptive_capacity.pdf .

Dollar, D., & Kraay, A. (2002). *Growth is good for the poor.* Washington, DC: World Bank. Retrieved from: www.worldbank.org/research.

Dommen, C. (2002). Raising human rights concerns in the World Trade Organisation: Actors, processes and possible strategies. *Human Rights Quarterly, 24,* 1–50.

Doran, E., & Henry, D. A. (2008). Australian pharmaceutical policy: Price control, equity, and drug innovation in Australia. *Journal of Public Health Policy, 29,* 106–20.

Drahos, P., & Henry, D. (2004). The free trade agreement between Australia and US undermines Australian public health and protects US interests in pharmaceuticals. *British Medical Journal, 328,* 1271–72.

Dussel Peters, E. (2000). *Polarizing Mexico: The impact of liberalization strategy.* Boulder, CO: Lynne Rienner.

Epstein, G. A. (2005). Introduction: Financialization and the world economy. In G. A. Epstein (ed.), *Financialization and the world economy* (pp. 3–16). Cheltenham, UK: Edward Elgar.

European Union–Mexico Free Trade Agreement. (2001). *Free trade agreement between the EFTA states and Mexico.* Retrieved from: http://www.worldtradelaw.net/fta/agreements/eftamexfta.pdf.

Evans, P. (2005). Neoliberalism as a political opportunity: Constraint and innovation in contemporary development strategy. In K. Gallagher (ed.), *Putting development first: The importance of policy space in the WTO and IFIs* (pp. 195–215). London: Zed Books.

Fidler, D. P., Correa, C., & Aginam, O. (2005). *Legal review of the General Agreement on Trade in Services (GATS) from a health policy perspective.* Geneva: World Health Organization. Retrieved from: http://www.who.int/trade/resource/GATS_Legal_Review_15_12_05.pdf.

Fink, C., & Reichenmiller, P. (2005). *Tightening TRIPS: The intellectual property provisions of recent US free trade agreements,* No. 20. Washington, DC: World Bank.

Gauthier, G., O'Brien, E., & Spencer, S. (2000). Déjà vu or new beginning for safeguards and subsidies rules in services trade. In P. Sauve & R. Stern (eds.), *GATS 2000: New directions in services trade liberalisation.* Washington, DC: Brookings Institution.

Gill, S., & Bakker, I. (2006). New constitutionalism and the social reproduction of caring institutions. *Theoretical Medicine and Bioethics, 27,* 35–57.

Goldstein, J., Kahler, M., Keohane, R., & Slaughter, A.-M., eds. (2001). *Legalisation and world politics.* Cambridge: MIT Press.

Gould, E. R. (2003). Money talks: Supplementary financiers and International Monetary Fund conditionality. *International Organization, 57,* 551–86.

Griesgraber, J. M., & Ugarteche, O. (2006). The IMF today and tomorrow: Some civil society perspectives. *Global Governance: A Review of Multilateralism and International Organizations, 12,* 351–60.

Griffith-Jones, S., & Gottschalk, R. (2006). Financial vulnerability in Asia: Paper for Session 2: Challenges and risks to development in Asia. In *Asia 2015: Promoting growth, ending poverty.* London. London and Sussex: Institute of Development Studies and Overseas Development Institute. Retrieved from: http://www.asia2015conference.org/pdfs/Griffith-Jones&Gottschalk.pdf.

Griffith-Jones, S. & Stallings, B. (1995). New global financial trends: Implications for development. In B. Stallings (ed.), *Global change, regional response: The new international context of development* (pp. 143–73). Cambridge: Cambridge University Press.

Grinspun, R., & Cameron, M. A. (1993). Mexico: The wages of trade. *NACLA Report on the Americas, 26,* 32–37.

Harvey, D. (2003). The "new" imperialism: Accumulation by dispossession. In L. Panitch & C. Leys (eds.), *Socialist register 2004: The new imperial challenge* (pp. 63–87). London: Merlin Press. Retrieved from: http://socialistregister.com/recent/2004.

Heller, P. S. (2005). *Understanding fiscal space.* IMF Policy Discussion Papers No. 05/4. Washington, DC: International Monetary Fund. Retrieved from: http://www.imf.org/external/pubs/ft/pdp/2005/pdp04.pdf.

Holzmann, R., & Jörgensen, S. (2001). *Social protection sector strategy: From safety net to springboard.* Washington, DC: World Bank. Retrieved from:

http://wbln0018.worldbank.org/HDNet/hddocs.nsf/2d5135ecbf351de6852566 a90069b8b6/1628e080eb4593a78525681c0070a518/$FILE/complete.pdf.

Hopkins, S. (2006). Economic stability and health status: Evidence from East Asia before and after the 1990s economic crisis. *Health Policy, 75,* 347–57.

Howse, R., ed. (2007). *Trade related aspects of intellectual property rights: A commentary on the TRIPS agreement.* Oxford: Oxford University Press.

Huber, E., & Solt, F. (2004). Successes and failures of neoliberalism. *Latin American Research Review, 39,* 150–64.

Independent Evaluation Office, I. M. F. (2007). *An evaluation of The IMF and aid to sub-Saharan Africa.* Washington, DC: IEO Publications. Retrieved from: http://www.imf.org/External/NP/ieo/2007/ssa/eng/index.htm.

International Organization for Standardization. (2006). *ISO in brief: International standards for a sustainable world.* Geneva: ISO.

Jaffe, A. B.. & Lerner, J. (2004). *Innovation and its discontents: How our broken patent system is endangering innovation and progress, and what to do about it.* Princeton, NJ: Princeton University Press.

Jawara, F., & Kwa, E. (2003). *Behind the scenes at the WTO: The real world of international trade negotiations.* London: Zed Books.

Jensen, K., & Murray, F. (2005). Intellectual property landscape of the human genome. *Science, 310,* 239–40.

Kahler, M. (1992). External influence, conditionality, and the politics of adjustment. In S. Haggard & R. B. Kaufman (eds.), *The politics of economic adjustment* (pp. 89–136). Princeton, NJ: Princeton University Press.

Killick, T. (2004). Politics, evidence and the new aid agenda. *Development Policy Review, 22,* 5–29.

Kingdon, G., & Knight, J. (2005). *Unemployment in South Africa, 1995–2003: Causes, problems and policies.* Oxford: Centre for the Study of African Economies, University of Oxford. Retrieved from: http://www.csae.ox.ac.uk/conferences/2006-EOI-RPI/papers/csae/Kingdon.pdf.

Koelble, T., & Lipuma, E. (2006). The effects of circulatory capitalism on democratization: Observations from South Africa and Brazil. *Democratization, 13,* 605–31.

Koo, B., Nottenburg, C., & Pardey, P. (2004). Plants and intellectual property: An international approach. *Science, 306,* 1295–97.

Krajewski, M. (2003). Public services and trade liberalisation: Mapping the legal framework. *Journal of International Economic Law, 6,* 341–67.

Krikorian, G. P., & Szymkowiak, D. M. (2007). Intellectual property rights in the making: The evolution of intellectual property provisions in US free trade agreements and access to medicines. *The Journal of World Intellectual Property, 10,* 388 Krajewski 418.

Labonté, R., & Sanger, M. (2006). Glossary of the World Trade Organisation and public health: Part 1. *Journal of Epidemiology and Community Health, 60,* 655–61.

Lall, S. (2003). *Reinventing industrial strategy: The role of government policy in building industrial competitiveness.* Prepared for the Intergovernmental Group on Monetary Affairs and Development (G-24). Oxford: International Development Centre, University of Oxford. Retrieved from: http://www.g24.org/slall-gva.pdf.

Lee, K., & Goodman, H. (2002). Global policy networks: The propagation of health care financing reform since the 1980's. In K. Lee, K. Buse, & S. Fustukian (eds.), *Health policy in a globalising world* (pp. 97–119). Cambridge: Cambridge University Press.

Lubker, M., Smith, G., & Weeks, J. (2002). Growth and the poor: A comment on Dollar and Kraay. *Journal of International Development, 14,* 555–71.

Luff, D. (2003). Regulation of health services and international trade law. In A. Mattoo & P. Sauve (eds.), *Domestic regulation and service trade liberalisation* (pp. 191–220). Washington, DC: World Bank and Oxford University Press.

Martinez, G. O. (1998). What lessons does the Mexican crisis hold for recovery in Asia? *Finance and Development, 35,* 6.

Mattli, W., & Buthe, T. (2003). Setting international standards: Technological rationality or primacy of power. *World Politics, 56,* 1–42.

Mehta, L. (2001). Commentary: The World Bank and its emerging knowledge empire. *Human Organization, 60,* 189–96.

Mesa-Lago, C., & Müller, K. (2002). The politics of pension reform in Latin America. *Journal of Latin American Studies, 34,* 687–715.

Milanovic, B. (2003). The two faces of globalization: Against globalization as we know it. *World Development, 31,* 667–83.

Milward, B. (2000). What is structural adjustment? In G. Mohan, E. Brown, B. Milward, & A. B. Zack-Williams (eds.), *Structural adjustment: Theory, practice and impacts* (pp. 24–38). London: Routledge.

Moran, M., & Wood, B. (1996). The globalisation of health care policy. In P. Gummett (ed.), *Globalisation and public policy.* Cheltenham, UK: Edward Elgar.

Mosley, L. (2003). *Global capital and national governments.* Cambridge: Cambridge University Press.

———. (2006). Constraints, opportunities, and information: Financial market-government relations around the world. In P. Bardhan, S. Bowles, & M. Wallerstein (eds.), *Globalization and egalitarian redistribution* (pp. 87–119). New York and Princeton, NJ: Russell Sage Foundation and Princeton University Press.

Nadvi, K. (2008). Global standards, global governance and the organization of global value chains. *Journal of Economic Geography, 8,* 1–21.

Ndikumana, L., & Boyce, J. K. (1998). Congo's odious debt: External borrowing and capital flight in Zaire. *Development and Change, 29,* 195–217.

———. (2003). Public debts and private assets: Explaining capital flight from sub-Saharan African countries. *World Development, 31,* 107–30.

Norrby, S., Nord, C., & Finch, R. (2005). Lack of development of new antimicrobial drugs: A potential serious threat to public health. *Lancet Infectious Diseases, 5,* 115–19.

Nye, H. L. M., Reddy, S. G., & Watkins, K. (2002). Dollar and Kraay on "trade, growth, and poverty": A critique. Retrieved from: http://www.maketradefair.com/assets/english/finalDKcritique.pdf.

Ooms, G., & Schrecker, T. (2005). Viewpoint: Expenditure ceilings, multilateral financial institutions, and the health of poor populations. *Lancet, 365,* 1821–23.

Ortino, F. (2006). Treaty interpretation and the WTO appellate body report in the US-gambling: A critique. *Journal of International Economic Law, 9,* 117–46.

Pauwelyn, J. (2003). *Conflict of norms in public international law. How WTO law relates to other rules of international law.* Cambridge: Cambridge University Press.

———. (2005a). Rien ne va plus? Distinguishing domestic regulation from market access in GATT and GATS. *World Trade Review, 4,* 131–70.

———. (2005b). WTO softens earlier condemnation of US ban on Internet gambling, but confirms broad reach to sensitive domestic regulation. ASIL Insight [online]. Retrieved from: www.asil.org/insights/2005/04/insights050412.html.

Przeworski, A., Bardhan, P., Bresser Pereira, L. C., Bruszt, L., Choi, J. J., Comisso, E. T., et al. (1995). *Sustainable democracy.* Cambridge: Cambridge University Press.

Roffe, P., & Spennermann, C. (2006). The impact of FTAs on public health policies and TRIPs flexibilities. *Journal of Intellectual Property Management, 1,* 75–93.

Sampath, P. G. (2005). *Regulating bioprospecting. Institutions for drug research, access and benefit sharing.* Tokyo: United Nations University Press.

Sarbib, J. L., & Heller, P. S. (2005). Fiscal space: Response from World Bank and IMF. *Lancet, 365,* 2085.

Sassen, S. (1996). *Losing control? Sovereignty in an age of globalization.* New York: Columbia University Press.

Scholte, J. A. (2000). *Globalization: A critical introduction.* Houndmills, UK: Palgrave.

Schrecker, T. (forthcoming). The power of money: Global financial markets, national politics, and how they interact to affect social determinants of health. In O. D. Williams & A. Kay (eds.), *The crisis of global health governance: Political economy, ideas and institutions.* Houndmills, UK: Palgrave Macmillan.

Shadlen, K. C. (2005a). *Policy space for development in the WTO and beyond: The case of intellectual property rights,* GDEI Working Papers No. 05–06. Medford, MA: Global Development and Environment Institute, Tufts University.

———. (2005b). Exchanging development for market access? Deep integration and industrial policy under multilateral and regional-bilateral trade agreements. *Review of International Political Economy, 12,* 750–75.

Shaffer, E. R., Brenner, J. E., & Houston, T. P. (2005). International trade agreements: A threat to tobacco control policy. *Tobacco Control, 14,* ii19–ii25.

Shiva, V. (2001). *Protect or plunder.* London: Zed Books.

South Centre. (2004). *Strengthening developing countries' capacity for trade negotiations: Matching technical assistance to negotiating capacity constraints.* Special paper prepared for the G77. Geneva: South Centre. Retrieved from: http://www.southcentre.org/index.php?option=com_content&task=view&id=358&Itemid=67.

Streak, J. C. (2004). The GEAR legacy: Did GEAR fail or move South Africa forward in development? *Development Southern Africa, 21,* 271–88.

UNESCO. (2005). Convention on the protection and promotion of the diversity of cultural expressions. UNESCO [online]. Retrieved from: http://unesdoc.unesco.org/images/0014/001429/142919e.pdf.

United Nations Conference on Trade and Development (UNCTAD). (2004). *São Paulo Consensus,* No. TD/410. Geneva: UNCTAD. Retrieved from: http://www.unctad.org/en/docs/td410_en.pdf.

———. (2006). *Trade and development report 2006: Global partnership and national policies for development.* New York and Geneva: United Nations. Retrieved from: http://www.unctad.org/Templates/Download.asp?docid=7183&lang=1&intItemID=2068.

———. (2007a). *Foreign direct investment surged again in 2006.* New York: UNCTAD. Retrieved from: http://www.unctad.org/en/docs/iteiiamisc20072_en.pdf.

———. (2007b). *The least developed countries report 2007: Knowledge, technological learning and innovation for development.* New York and Geneva: United Nations. Retrieved from: http://www.unctad.org/Templates/webflyer.asp?docid=8674&intItemID=4314&lang=1&mode=downloads.

United Nations Department of Economic and Social Affairs. (2005). *Report on the world social situation: The inequity predicament.* New York: United Nations Department of Economic and Social Affairs.

———. (2006). *World economic situation and prospects 2006.* New York: United Nations. Retrieved from: http://www.un.org/esa/policy/wess/wesp2006files/wesp2006.pdf.

United States Trade Representative. (2006). *2006 special 301 report.* Washington, DC: Office of the USTR. Retrieved from: http://www.ustr.gov/assets/Document_Library/Reports_Publications/2006/2006_Special_301_Review/asset_upload_file473_9336.pdf.

————. (2008). *2008 special 301 report*. Washington, DC: Office of the USTR. Retrieved from: http://www.ustr.gov/assets/Document_Library/Reports_Publications/2008/2008_Special_301_Report/asset_upload_file553_14869.pdf.

U.S. General Accounting Office. (1996). *Mexico's financial crisis: Origins, awareness, assistance, and initial efforts to recover*, GAO/GGD-96-56. Washington, DC: U.S. General Accounting Office.

van der Hoeven, R., & Lübker, M. (2005). Financial openness and employment: A challenge for international and national institutions. In *2006 meeting, global development network*, St. Petersburg. Geneva: International Policy Group, International Labour Office. Retrieved from: http://ctool.gdnet.org/conf_docs/Hoeven_Paper_Lunch%20Time%20Session_ILO.pdf

Veggeland, F., & Borgen, S. O. (2005). Negotiating international food standards: The World Trade Organisation's impact on the Codex Alimentarius Commission. *Governance: An International Journal of Policy, Administration and Institutions, 18*, 675–708.

Vreeland, J. R. (2003). Why do governments and the IMF enter into agreements? Statistically selected cases. *International Political Science Review/Revue Internationale de Science Politique, 24*, 321–43.

Wade, R. H. (2002). US hegemony and the World Bank: The fight over people and ideas. *Review of International Political Economy, 9*, 201–29.

Walton, J., & Seddon, D. (1994). *Free markets & food riots: The politics of global adjustment*. Oxford: Blackwell.

Wenzel, R. (2004). The antibiotic pipeline—challenges, costs and values. *New England Journal of Medicine, 351*, 523–26.

Williamson, J. (2004). *The Washington consensus as policy prescription for development, World Bank practitioners for development lecture*. World Bank Practitioners for Development lecture series. Washington, DC: Institute for International Economics. Retrieved from: http://www.iie.com/publications/papers/williamson0204.pdf.

Wood, A. (2006). *IMF macroeconomic policies and health sector budgets*. Amsterdam: Wemos Foundation. Retrieved from: http://www.wemos.nl/Documents/wemos_synthesis_report.pdf.

Woods, N. (2006a). *The globalizers: The IMF, the World Bank, and their borrowers*. Ithaca, NY: Cornell University Press.

————. (2006b). Understanding pathways through financial crises and the impact of the IMF: An introduction. *Global Governance: A Review of Multilateralism and International Organizations, 12*, 373–94.

World Bank. (2004). *Global economic prospects 2005: Trade, regionalism, and development*. Washington, DC: World Bank.

World Trade Organization. (1998). *European communities: Measures concerning meat and meat products (hormones)*. No. WT/DS26AB/R. Geneva: World Trade Organization.

————. (1999). *Report of the panel: Chile—taxes on alcoholic beverages*. No. WT/DS87/R. Geneva: World Trade Organization.

————. (2000). *European communities: Measures affecting asbestos and asbestos containing products*. No. WT/DS135/R. Geveva: World Trade Organization.

————. (2001). *European communities: Measures affecting asbestos and asbestos-containing products—report of the appellate body*. No. WT/DS135/AB/R World Trade Organization.

————. (2004). *United States: Measures affecting the cross-border supply of gambling and betting services*. No. WT/DS285/R. Geneva: World Trade Organization.

————. (2005a). *Dominican Republic: Measures affecting the importation and internal sale of cigarettes*. No. WT/D/DS302/AB/R. Geneva: World Trade Organization.

————. (2005b). *United States: Measures affecting the cross-border supply of gambling and betting services.* No. WT/DS285/AB/R. Geneva: World Trade Organization.

————. (2006). *India: Measures affecting the importation and sale of wines and spirits from the European Communities.* Geneva: World Trade Organization.

————. (2007). *Matrix on trade measures pursuant to selected multilateral environmental agreements.* No. WT/CTE/W/160/Rev.4 TN/TE/S/5/Rev.2. Geneva: World Trade Organization.

————.(2008). *United States: Continued suspension of obligations in the EC-hormones dispute—report of the panel.* World Trade Organization No. WT/DS320/R. Geneva. Retrieved from: http://72.14.205.104/search?q=cache:ze7gl0zdRYYJ:www.internationaltraderelations.com/WTO.Case.EU%2520—%2520U.S.%2520Hormone%2520Sanctions%2520(March%252031,%25202008)..doc+World+Trade+Organisation+(2008)+United+States+-+Continued+suspension+of+obligations+in+the+EC-+hormones+dispute.+WT/DS320/R&hl=en&ct=clnk&cd=2&gl=ca&client=firefox-a.

Yach, D., & Bettcher, D. (2000). Globalisation of tobacco industry influence and new global responses. *Tobacco Control, 9,* 206–16.

Yeates, J., & Murphy, C. (2007). *Coordinating international standards: The formation of the ISO,* MIT-Sloan Working Papers No. 4638–07. Cambridge, MA: Massachusetts Institute of Technology.

6 Liberalization "Shocks" and Social Protection Policies
Lessons from the East Asian Financial Crisis

Aniket Bhushan and Chantal Blouin

INTRODUCTION

Globalization generally and trade liberalization specifically create winners and losers in domestic economies and among countries. Domestically, workers and producers in the sectors protected from foreign competition may see revenues decrease or employment disappear when tariffs or regulatory barriers are removed. The negative impacts of liberalization are not limited to one-time adjustments to trade reforms. The dynamics of an open economy differ greatly from an economy that is relatively insulated from foreign competition. By definition, the frequency and scope of economic restructuring in an open economy is higher. For example, an International Labour Organization (ILO) study of manufacturing employment in 77 countries found that a higher level of international trade in a national economy is associated with greater movement of workers between sectors (Torres, 2001). Such intersectoral movement is not without consequences. Low-skilled workers in particular find it difficult to find new employment, as moving into a different sector usually requires a different set of skills (Torres, 2001) which can bring with it costs associated with retraining and relocation. While the weight of existing evidence generally supports the view that trade liberalization and openness increase economic insecurity (Rodrik, 1997, 1998; Garrett, 1998; Burgoon, 2001; Boix, 2002; Hayes, Ehrlich, & Peinhardt, 2002; Gunter & van der Hoeven, 2004), there is little consensus on this point (see Bourguignon & Goh, 2003, for a review of studies challenging this linkage).[1]

There is greater consensus in the research literature that financial liberalization and the movement of capital are more important determinants of economic instability than trade openness per se (Cornia, 2001; Scheve & Slaughter, 2004; van der Hoeven & Lübker, 2005). Trade liberalization, however, is usually accompanied by increased openness to foreign capital and liberalization of financial markets and services. The combined effects of trade and financial liberalization have been greater financial market volatility, increased frequency of external shocks and transmission of vulnerability across borders, and rapid changes in labor markets and employment. These translate into increased economic inse-curity for individuals. Economic insecurity is closely linked to many chronic stress-related diseases such as cardiovascular problems, and its impact on health outcomes can be direct (Cornia, Rosignoli, & Tib-erti, 2008). Moreover, economic insecurity can also mean that non-poor households become poor, affecting material conditions, such as nutri-tion and housing, in addition to psychosocial factors affecting health.

Based on these findings, this chapter reviews national policies that have been effective in reducing economic vulnerability arising from trade and financial liberalization in a small subset of developing coun-tries in one region (see Chapter 5, this volume, for a discussion of the more generic effects of liberalization on policy space for both developed and developing countries). While the literature on social safety nets in developing countries is vast, in this chapter we focus on the experience of the 1997 East Asian economic crisis and the years following. The Asian economic crisis has often been described as a "financial sector" crisis (which led to a currency crisis) and not a crisis induced by trade liberalization per se. However, structural imbalances were present in many East Asian countries by the late 1990s; Malaysia, Thailand, and Indonesia, for example, were running large current account deficits in the range of 4 to 5 per cent of the gross domestic product (GDP). The additional fact that these imbalances were being financed by foreign investments primarily in speculative sectors (such as construction and real estate) led to a further blurring of differences between trade and financial liberalization.

The Asian crisis highlights the importance of social protection strate-gies in developing countries. It offers various examples of what works, what does not and why, on various levels. The affected countries—from Korea to the Philippines—present a range of cases and indicate a broad range of coping strategies and policy options. The Asian crisis is instruc-tive because East Asia stands out among developing economies as an example of successful poverty reduction (see Figure 6.1 and Tables 6.1 and 6.2) via greater integration with the global economy. Further, the East Asian crisis provides a good illustration of how a relatively short-lived (though large) macroeconomic shock which originated in the finan-cial sector can lead to significant long term health impacts, through a number of channels of influence.

The remainder of this chapter focuses on the following questions:

1. How does a financial crisis trigger a health crisis? What was the health impact of the Asian crisis?
2. What policies, already in place at the time of the crisis, helped cushion the impact on vulnerable groups?

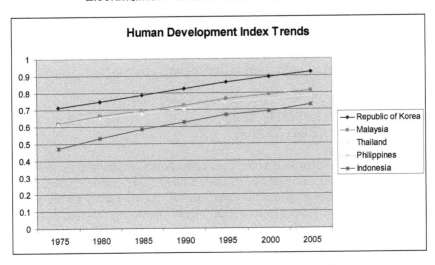

Figure 6.1   Poverty reduction in East Asian countries, 1975–2005.
Data source: UNDP, Human Development Report database (2007/08).

Table 6.1   Social Indicators for East Asian Countries

	Adult Illiteracy Rate (% Aged 15 and Older) (1995–2000)	Population Living Below $1 a Day (1995–2000)	Population Living Below $2 a Day (1995–2000)	Life Expectancy at Birth (years)		Infant Mortality Rate (per 1,000 live births)		Public Expenditure on Health (% GDP 2004)
				1970–1975	2000–2005	1970	2005	
Republic of Korea	1	< 2	< 2	62.6	77	43	5	2.9
Malaysia	11.3	< 2	9.3	63	73	46	10	2.2
Thailand	7.4	< 2	25.2	60.4	68.6	74	18	2.3
Philippines	7.4	14.8	43	58.1	70.3	56	25	1.4
Indonesia	9.6	7.5	52.4	49.2	68.6	104	28	1

Source: UNDP, Human Development Report, Statistical Database (2007/08).

Table 6.2   Growth Rates Across Developing Regions

	1960s	1970s	1980s	1990s–Present
East Asia & Pacific	3.77	7.21	7.72	8.03
Latin America & Caribbean	5.27	5.72	1.79	3.00
South Asia	4.22	2.98	5.55	6.25
Sub-Saharan Africa	4.63	4.07	2.18	3.93

Source: World Bank, World Development Indicators database.

3. What were some of the key emergency measures, new programs, and reforms to ongoing approaches, in response to the economic shock?
4. What are the main lessons to be drawn from the East Asian crisis regarding social protection in developing countries?

STATE OF SOCIAL PROTECTION: PRECRISIS AND CRISIS YEARS

In 1990, East Asia spent on average 1 per cent of total government expenditure on social protection and welfare, compared to 12.7 per cent in Organization for Economic Cooperation and Development (OECD) countries, 3.6 per cent in Latin America, and 2.2 per cent in South Asia (Armstrong, Viossat, & Flanagan, 1999, p. 7).[2] The openness of these economies is a further striking feature. In 1997, the value of trade as a percentage of GDP was 90 per cent in Malaysia, 45 per cent in Korea, and 30 per cent in the Philippines and Thailand.

The ratio of foreign direct investment (FDI) to GDP in the same year was 290 per cent in Malaysia, 117 per cent in Korea, 102 per cent in Thailand, 69 per cent in Indonesia, and 55 per cent in the Philippines (Armstrong et al., 1999, p. 12). The combined effect of low expenditures on social protection and high degrees of openness to foreign capital (especially in high employment-growth sectors like manufacturing and construction) by the mid-1990s had created in East Asia a situation particularly vulnerable to economic shocks.

Where wage flexibility was higher, for instance, in Indonesia, the rise in unemployment was less severe but the drop in real wages was high (34 per cent in Indonesia), coupled with a significant shift to underemployment and informal employment (Gough, 2001, p. 183). Thus, measures in place to respond to unemployment shocks, wage shocks, and the labor market in general have been a major source of debate in East Asia.

Table 6.3   Social Impact of East Asian Economic Crisis, 1998

Country	Real GDP Growth (%)	Poverty Incidence (Based on National Poverty Line, %)		Unemployment (%)		Real Wage (% Change)	CPI (% Change)
	1998	1997	1998	1997	1998	1998	1998
Korea	−5.8	9.0	19.0	2.1	8.7	−10.0	6.9
Thailand	−9.4	11.4	13.0	0.9	5.4	−6.0	7.0
Indonesia	−13.7	11.0	19.8	5.1	7.0	−35.0	82.4
Malaysia	−6.7	8.2	11.2	2.6	3.9	−10.0	5.5
Philippines	−0.5	38.0	...	7.7	11.8	−2.0	10.0

Source: Adapted from World Development Indicators and *Towards an East Asian Social Protection Strategy*, 1999.

The evolution of labor-market legislation, reforms, and new programs broadly parallels the levels of development of the various economies. At the top end we find Korea, Malaysia, and Thailand, with relatively developed employment protection and labor-market regulations. At the bottom are Indonesia and the Philippines, with little or no unemployment protection and weak labor laws in general.

HEALTH IMPACT OF THE EAST ASIAN ECONOMIC CRISIS

The financial crisis triggered a health crisis through a somewhat complex chain of influence. The initial impact involved a rapid shift to negative economic growth (economic contraction), increasing unemployment and inflation, and

Table 6.4 Impact of the Financial Crisis on Household Earnings, on Final Consumption Expenditure, on Health Care Provision, and on Health Outcomes

Country	Household Real Earnings (% Change), 1997–98	Household Final Consumption Expenditure (% Change), 1997–98	Key Country Specific Health Impacts
Indonesia	−27.0	−6.2	Increase in childhood anemia and maternal malnutrition; dramatic increase in price of prescription drugs; delays in seeking care, switching to cheaper forms of care, consumption of nutritionally inferior food, and declines in school retention rates
Malaysia	−1.0	−10.2	Reduction in diphtheria, polio, tetanus (DPT), and measles immunization rates; sharp increase in the proportion of people using public care facilities (substantial private-public switching due to financial impact of crisis on liberalized private sector); delays in seeking care, switching to cheaper forms of care, consumption of nutritionally inferior food, and declines in school retention rates
Thailand	−21.0	−11.5	Increase in underweight children; sharp increase in the proportion of people using public care facilities (substantial private-public switching due to financial impact of crisis on liberalized private sector); delays in seeking care, switching to cheaper forms of care, consumption of nutritionally inferior food, and declines in school retention rates

Source: Adapted from Hopkins, 2006.

a spate of public and private sector bankruptcies. These led to two further effects. First, reduced tax revenues led to short-term government scaling back of health and education expenditure. Simultaneously, a reduction in household real income due to contraction of real wages constrained household capacity to respond. Some of the key health impacts of this financial crisis are summarized in Table 6.4. The impacts that stand out are the following: delays in accessing health care; reduced food consumption and consumption of inferior food; switching to cheaper care; dramatic increases in the cost of prescription drugs; and large increases in the proportion of the population using public health care (due to the financial impact of the crisis on the liberalized private health care sector), thus overburdening inadequately funded public systems.

The preceding discussion is intended to demonstrate the ways in which increased openness can have important health impacts. However, this relationship is not a truism. The potential negative impacts of increased economic openness and volatility can be mitigated by coherent social protection strategies. East Asia's response to the crisis in the form of reforms and expansion of social protection strategies is one of the main lessons to be drawn from the crisis. The remainder of this chapter focuses on country-level responses.

THE REPUBLIC OF KOREA

Precrisis Republic of Korea (hereafter referred to as "Korea") had a relatively well-developed livelihood protection system as compared to the other East Asian newly industrialized countries (NICs). When the crisis hit, the Korean system was providing income support to 1.2 million persons.[3] Implementation of unemployment insurance and active labor-market policies was a recent development and coincided with Korea's entry into the OECD in 1996, which required a minimum level of social protection (Kapstein & Milanovic, 2003). In response to the insolvency of 3,323 small and medium enterprises in the first month of 1998 alone, the Tripartite Commission (business-labor-government) launched sweeping legislation extending unemployment insurance to all sections of the labor force. The Korean government developed the Temporary Livelihood Protection Program (TLPP) to absorb the newly unemployed, covering an additional 310,000 persons. TLPP eligibility provided four main benefits to the newly unemployed: direct cash transfer ($70/month), tuition fee waiver and lunch subsidies for school-aged children, and a 50 per cent reduction in medical insurance premiums for one year. The success of this program in cushioning the impact of the economic shock is evident in the Minimum Living Standards Security Act of 2000, which replaced and incorporated the TLPP into permanent legislation. The act provides for food, clothing, housing, education, and health care—subsidized through cash and in-kind transfers for households that otherwise would not meet the basic living standards guaranteed by the Korean government. Benefits are linked to participation in labor programs, such as public works and job training. The livelihood protection system and the minimum-living-standards legislation that followed stand out as effective strategies in response to the economic shock (Gough, 2001; United Nations Economic and Social Commission for Asia and the Pacific, 2001).

Korea's Employment Insurance System (EIS) and post-crisis reforms have been reviewed extensively. There are some criticisms of the employment insurance system, which include: the limited extent of overall coverage, highly selective eligibility criteria, low reemployment rates, and deadweight losses of "grants." The case has been made for more targeted measures. However, reviewers often view "aid for employment maintenance" and "employment facilitation assistance" more favorably. Korea epitomizes the "productivist" East Asian welfare regimes (Holliday, 2000) where investment in social protection, though limited as a percentage of the total official expenditure, is highly focused on education and health care (i.e., human capital development). Peng (2004) shows that "postindustrial" developments (such as the rise of the service sector and in particular the sharp increase in the participation of women in the workforce) have led to a coherent constituency that demands broader political reforms (such as reforms to divorce laws and increased childcare benefits). This has raised the important question of universality of coverage in Korea. A powerful argument can be made in favor of universality on the basis of the following facts:

1. Targeted coverage is exclusionary and reinforces existing social stratification and stigmatization.
2. Macroeconomic shocks are a reminder that in times of crisis there is little that separates middle from lower-middle income groups and those below the official income poverty line. This reinforces the claim that universality of coverage is inherently desirable, insofar as it forms the foundation of wider economic solidarity, indispensable in precarious times.
3. Targeted programs often involve greater administrative costs and are more likely to miss some eligible individuals ("leakage"), whereas universal coverage, such as unemployment insurance, is obliged to cover all equally.

In sum, post-crisis unemployment reforms in Korea followed a four-pillar approach: job security, job creation, training and placement, and livelihood care. While debate on Korea's social protection reforms continues, the measures described earlier played an important role in mitigating the negative health impact of the late 1990s crisis in Korea.

MALAYSIA

While not as advanced as Korea in terms of social protection preparedness, Malaysia had basic groundwork in place to meet the labor-market challenges of the economic shock. An important facet of Malaysian political history is the country's ethnic compromise between the various minorities. A long history of immigrant labor, mainly from India and China, has led to a tradition of well-organized labor and informal safety nets along ethnic lines to compensate for the low level of coverage of the formal safety nets. (Hashim & Shafruddin, 2002; Mansor & Awang, 2002). A strong trade union movement led to the setting up of Malaysia's Employee Provident Fund (EPF) in 1951, which forms the bulk of social protection in the country. The New Economic Policy of 1970 formally structured the ethnic compromise in Malaysia towards the goals of equality and poverty eradication. The EPF, the Employees Social Security Organization (SOCSO, 1971), and the Social Security Act (SSA, 1969) jointly laid the foundation for Malaysia's response to the economic shock. Along with the August 1998 amendment to the Employment Act (tougher legislation against unlawful dismissal) and the Employment Ordinance (1955), these policies resulted in coverage of two-thirds of Malaysian employees under one scheme or another at the time the crisis hit.[4] As a result, while unemployment increased threefold in Korea and Thailand in the crisis year, in Malaysia it was contained to between 2.7 and 3.2 per cent in the period 1997–1998.

The main response to the shock in Malaysia can be summarized as:

1. Reforms to existing provisions: In 1994 the EPF was made flexible by splitting each account into three, in which 60 per cent was held for retirement after age 55, (Account I), 30 percent for large one-time expenses such as housing (Account II), and 10 percent for medical emergencies (Account III). Account II was particularly important during the crisis year as housing interest rates rose rapidly, and flexibility in the EPF system made for better monitoring of withdrawals and expenditures.
2. Expansion of existing safety net provisions to cover retrenched workers entering the informal sector: Under the Amanah Ikhtiar Malaysia (AIM) revolving fund, RM300 million in interest-free loans were disbursed. The success of this strategy is evidenced by the 100 percent repayment of loan.[5]

Malaysian authorities used the crisis as an opportunity to strengthen entrepreneurial capacity in the informal sector by launching the Yayasan Tekun Nasional entrepreneurial loans scheme, the Graduate Entrepreneurs Scheme, and the Economic Business Group Fund, which provides assistance to women entrepreneurs. These initiatives are widely acknowledged as successful fiscal stimulation and crisis response measures (Whiteford, 2002).

THAILAND

With the exception of Malaysia, each of the East Asian crisis-hit countries (including Thailand) was forced to adopt a harsh set of International Monetary Fund (IMF) austerity measures. To simplify, the IMF recommended a highly deflationary approach in response to the crisis. This included raising interest rates, cutting public expenditure, closing down banks and investment houses, and letting asset markets (real estate, stocks, and currencies) find their own prices.[6] This strict austerity package further constrained policy space required to respond to the crisis effectively. Amid sharp civil society criticism of austerity policies recommended by the IMF, and as the full effects of the crisis unfolded, the Thai government introduced by 1999 four fiscal stimulation packages containing elements of social safety. These were an Unemployment Mitigation Plan, Social Investment programs (World Bank funded), a social sector program loan (Asian Development Bank funded), and loans under the Miyazawa Plan.[7]

In the 1990s, Thailand launched a concerted process of change with the 1997 People's Constitution and the Eighth National Economic and Social Development Plan. Together they signaled a shift from growth-centered to "a holistic people-centered developmental approach" (Pongsapich, 2001, p. 64). There was renewed emphasis on labor and social welfare, education, and health,[8] although Thailand still lacks universal unemployment insurance and health and education coverage. There are several social protection programs for government employees. The largest private sector program, as in Malaysia, is the provident fund system established by government decree. This fund includes the Civil Servants Pension Fund, Social Security Fund, and Provident Fund, which are the three largest formal social protection schemes in Thailand. Coverage of government employees is extensive and comprehensive. The Social Security Act (1990) and Labor Protection Act (1998—post-crisis) provide limited unemployment benefits for non-government employers and employees.[9]

The Unemployment Mitigation Program (1998) included several innovative measures such as the "Thai help Thai" social protection scheme, provisions for job creation, repatriation of workers, promotion of Thai workers working abroad, and employment of university graduates. The objectives of these programs were ambitious and reviews have been mixed. Common criticisms include: the need for better planning and coordination to avoid overlaps; targeting (especially wage setting for public works); and enforcement of laws (such as minimum-wage enforcement even when people are willing to work for much less).[10]

Early assessments of Thailand's post-crisis social protection emphasized two particular aspects, both of which were part of the Social Investment programs funded in large part by the World Bank. The two-channel strategy involved one channel which supported existing government programs and employment creation measures and another that focused on bottom-up local community building. This strategy has been widely lauded (Pongsapich, 2002) and points to the practical relevance of utilizing existing capabilities.

Historically, civil society organizations have played a crucial developmental role in Thailand.[11] In the early 1990s the Thai government set up the NGO Coordinating Committee on Development (NGO-COD). This community development department of the Ministry of Interior has supported community organizations, women's groups, and child development centers since the 1970s. The Social Investment Fund (SIF) and the Regional Urban Development Fund (RUDF) financed community-based, demand-driven projects that have attracted attention for their apparent success at various levels, including their support of community solidarity at the micro level. SIF and RUDF loans, for example, were administered at market rates directly to civil society organizations. To secure grants and loans, communities went through the experience of drawing up proposals and learned the value of borrowings and community debt. At the macro level, projects undertaken resulted in small irrigation and other infrastructure repairs and tourist facility improvements. These programs provided employment to groups, such as women, that labor intensive workfare programs otherwise neglect. The funds had a clear exit strategy (known to participants) and were terminated at the end of 1999. In this way, Thailand avoided the fiscal trap that often accompanies such programs.[12]

The experiences of the 1997 crisis spurred much talk of a "new social contract" across East Asia and Thailand in particular, where the Thai government was criticized for its uncritical acceptance of the IMF's emergency structural package. Various civil society groups, as well as the monarch of the country, came together to oppose the perceived loss of sovereignty evident in Thailand's forced adoption of harsh IMF austerity programs in the aftermath of the crisis (Hewison, 2006). This eventually brought Thaksin Shinawatra's TRT (or Thai Love Thai) party to power by 2001 in the first election under the new constitution. In principle, TRT stood for "social capitalism" or a renewed emphasis on the domestic capitalist class.

In the postcrisis years, Thailand has experimented with a number of universal schemes, the most prominent among them being the "30 baht scheme." Some of the universal programs have been criticized lately for being too expensive and unnecessary. These include the Universal Health Scheme (UHS), which provides universal health coverage at a set amount of 30 baht for all citizens, which has been relatively effective and has found international support, particularly from the WHO and the ILO (Hewison, 2006). Schemes such as the Village Community Fund, which provides low-interest loans of 20,000 baht to individuals in every village, have also received criticism (Whiteford, 2002).

As a number of studies have emphasized, the positive impact of UHS, particularly from the standpoint of health equity in a postcrisis situation, it is important to elaborate on the criticisms the scheme received, as these provide important lessons. At the time of inception, the political progress of UHS was controversial. While Thailand's health system had been considered successful in meeting the needs of the majority, health costs remained a significant expense for the poor. The crisis starkly brought out the divisions on access to health care. The UHS provided access to public hospital treatment for just "30 baht"; however, the government paid hospitals 1,252 baht per registered person in the scheme. The most obvious and immediate problem was that, while the scheme was expensive for the government, state hospitals complained that fixed government funding threatened their ability to provide adequate treatment. Media reports confirmed stories of patients being forced out of hospitals prior to the completion of their treatment. Health professionals argued that the scheme, with its emphasis on curative and institution-based health, was reversing gains that had been made in preventative healthcare, and was draining funds from health-promotion activities. The government tried to bolster funds available for UHS by merging it with existing programs like the Workers' Compensation and Social Security funds. This brought workers onto the streets in protest because they feared that their care would be downgraded once their funds were siphoned into the support of the scheme. Debate became increasingly polarized and much of the criticism came from medical professionals, including the Medical Council, the Thai Medical Association, and associations representing nurses, dentists, pharmacists, and private hospitals (Hewison, 2004, 2006).

It is important to point out that in recent years UHS has found broad political support and is presently an important element of Thailand's social protection framework. Similarly, another postcrisis scheme, the Voluntary and Low-Income Health Cards, though expensive, is believed to have genuinely facilitated the delivery of basic services in remote regions.

INDONESIA

In Indonesia, 1997 marked a sharp turnaround in economic performance, with GDP growth plummeting from 7 percent in 1997 to –13 percent in 1998. The main coping strategies employed by poor individuals and families were to reduce expenditures, to increase informal borrowing, and to raise their income through low-paying extra jobs. The government response included: securing affordable food supply, supplementing purchasing power, preserving access to health and education, and sustaining community activity through regional block grants and small-scale credit. Indonesia's experience in dealing with the crisis contrasts that of Thailand, where better-organized community involvement under the auspices of the NGO Coordinating Organization for Development (COD) played a more effective role in facilitating recovery.

Recovery in Indonesia was slow. The economic shock brought large numbers into what has been called "transient" poverty. The main reasons for the sharp spike in poverty numbers were skyrocketing prices of basic commodities, increased unemployment, and a decline in household incomes. The government's response was stymied by an inadequate bureaucracy, absence of early warning signals, and the lack of reliable and timely basic poverty data. Despite this, Indonesia has a long history of geographically and individually targeted poverty alleviation programs, such as the 1970s INPRES (Instruction of the President of the Republic of Indonesia) programs launched by a presidential decree and financed through windfall oil revenues. An important facet of the INPRES program was that it provided education for children who had never been to school through the building of some 60,000 schools in the mid-1970s alone (United Nations Economic and Social Commission for Asia and the Pacific, 2001, pp. 165–66; Puguh, 2001, p. 160). Common complaints in the health care initiatives, however, included poor targeting, lack of data, inconsistent data, and lack of administrative capacity.

The two most criticized programs were the public works program (Padat Karya) and the revolving-credit schemes (PDM-DKE). The main problem with the public works program was that wage rates were set above the minimum wage, creating distortions and diverting labor away from other sectors like harvesting food crops. PDM-DKE and other revolving-credit/cash-transfer schemes were criticized for being prone to corruption and cronyism (United Nations Economic and Social Commission for Asia and the Pacific, 2001).

THE PHILIPPINES

Of all the East Asian crisis-affected countries, the Philippines continues to be the least developed, both in general economic terms and in terms of social protection preparedness. Poverty is concentrated in rural areas. There was a downward trend in poverty figures until the crisis hit in 1997 (United Nations Economic and Social Commission for Asia and the Pacific, 2001, p. 3).[13] The impact was primarily the result of capital flight, a sharp decline in the exchange rate (peso to US$ dropping from 26.40 in 1997 to 42.70 in 1998), a considerable rise in interest rates, and significant negative impacts on dollar-dominated construction-sector firms, all combined with the El Niño drought. The response strategy can be summed up as a combination of food subsidies, public employment programs, and credit-based livelihood programs. However, by most accounts, the response to the social impact of the economic crisis has not been very effective (United Nations Economic and Social Commission for Asia and the Pacific, 2001, p. 4; Reyes & Manasan, 1999).[14]

In 1998, the main response was through the National Food Authority, which was mandated to set a floor price for rice to protect farmers and a ceiling price to ensure consumer welfare, and maintain a buffer stock. In 1998, the National Food Authority launched a two-pronged approach to food security. It imported rice and it set up Enhanced Retail Access for the Poor (ERAP), or *sari-sari,* stores intended to sell basic commodities (such as sugar, coffee, milk, cooking oil, sardines, and noodles) at below market prices. However, studies show it was overwhelmingly the nonpoor who benefited from these stores. As well, the National Food Authority was unable to prevent both high consumer and low producer prices (Bautista, Angeles, & Dionisio, 2000; Balisacan, Edillon, Brillantes, & Canlas, 2000).

In addition to direct subsidies, several microcredit programs and a comprehensive strategy formed the basis of the Philippines' response to the crisis. For instance, the Comprehensive and Integrated Delivery of Social Services (CIDSS), launched in 1994, has been praised as effective on several levels. The program facilitates consolidation and cooperation between government and civil society groups, delivering benefits using minimum basic needs indicators, community organizing, a total family approach, a community-based monitoring network, capability building, and resource mobilization. The focal programs of CIDSS include family and community welfare, women's welfare, child and youth welfare, emergency assistance, self-employment assistance (SEA-K), food and nutrition, health, water and sanitation, income security, basic education, and literacy. For instance, through the CIDSS self-employment programs, members were given small start-up capital with which they could set up ERAP stores. Nominal daily repayments were required, part of which was saved in bank accounts. These efforts are consistent with the long history of microcredit programs in the Philippines (84 were in operation when the crisis hit), which has the distinction of being the country that first pioneered the Grameen model outside Bangladesh. Collectively, the CIDSS and microcredit programs have had a significant (though incremental) positive effect on the poverty rate. During the crisis, participating families were better off than others because the culture of saving and community responsibility had already been well established. Some of the microcredit programs already in place but expanded when the crisis hit were:

1. Self-employment assistance through Kaunlaran People's Credit and Finance Corporation;
2. Production assistance guarantee funds of the Philippine Rural Reconstruction Movement (farmers' support in response to an El Niño–caused drought); and
3. The Grameen-based microcredit ASHI, the oldest one in place, expanded to include El Niño coverage.

Programs that received most criticism were the Food for Work initiatives and rural roads programs. Drawbacks of the former included the overlap of seasonal timing in agricultural harvesting, planting and cultivation, insufficient funds, and a bad law-and-order situation. The rural roads programs were found to be gender insensitive (United Nations Economic and Social Commission for Asia and the Pacific, 2001).

The Philippines' experience again points to the importance of community involvement. The main lesson is the importance of coordination when there are several programs in place across diverse regions. The CIDSS played this role in the Philippines. Moreover, this case shows that initiatives that require less outlay, are open to diverse funding sources, and are well coordinated can be far more beneficial than expensive public works programs. This is particularly the case in countries such as the Philippines, where labor is concentrated in the informal sector and poverty in rural areas. The long and successful history of microcredit initiatives and their role in responding to the crisis in the Philippines supports this perspective.

CONCLUSIONS: SOCIAL SAFETY NETS TO REDUCE ECONOMIC INSECURITY

This chapter has argued that trade and financial liberalization has increased economic insecurity and the vulnerability of households in developing countries, and therefore can pose a risk in terms of decline in health outcomes. In this context, we have examined how a number of middle-income countries have dealt with such economic insecurity by examining the policies in place and adopted during the Asia crisis of the late 1990s.

When thinking more generally about policy responses to economic insecurity in developing countries, it is important to distinguish recommendations for low- and middle-income countries. The former have limited financial resources to fund social protection and limited capacity to raise such funds because a large part of their economy is informal and/or based on subsistence agriculture. Given these limited resources, social protection should focus on interventions that contribute to long-term poverty reduction. They should also have multiplier effects (Smith & Subbarao, 2003), such as health insurance schemes that protect against unexpected medical expenses, which are major threats to household livelihood in low-income countries and a major source of impoverishment (so-called medical poverty) (Norton, Conway, & Foster, 2001; Wagstaff, Watanabe, & van Doorslaer, 2001). Protection against such insecurity is highly valued. However, social health insurance (i.e., insurance tied to employment) generally covers no more than 5 per cent of the workforce in low-income countries because of the low level of formal employment. In these conditions, the focus of the national government should be to enable an environment for the development of community-based health insurance schemes (Van Ginneken, 2003), or national health insurance schemes funded by progressive taxation. The latter is preferable because communities often lack sufficient savings for effective risk-pooling. Further, if there are large income inequalities between communities, community-based insurance may fail when measured against the WHO criteria for fairness in cross-subsidization, from rich to poor, and from healthy to sick (World Health Organization, 2000).

Middle-income countries have a wider range of instruments available to them than do low-income or least developed countries to reduce economic insecurity. A key policy issue becomes whether social protection should be targeted at particular groups or move towards universality of coverage. Targeted programs may be very attractive in terms of reducing the cost implications of social protection (Ravallion, 2003; Coady, Grosh, & Hoddinott, 2004; Prichett, 2005). Many middle-income countries, however, are now striving for universal coverage, realizing that there is a need "for broad-based social security systems that have the support of the majority of the population. Such schemes have a strong social insurance component, complemented by cost-effective tax-financed benefits" (Van Ginneken, 2003). Evaluative and policy studies offer powerful arguments in favor of universality. First, targeted coverage is exclusionary and reinforces existing social stratification and stigmatization. Second, macroeconomic shocks are a reminder that in times of systemic crisis there is little that separates middle from lower-middle classes, and even from those below the official poverty line. This reinforces the claim that universal coverage is inherently desirable insofar as it is the basis of a wider economic solidarity which is indispensable in precarious times. Third, targeted programs often involve greater administrative costs and are prone to leakage (errors in coverage) on many levels.

The financial and economic crisis that hit East Asia in 1997 generated responses in the form of social protection programs from which a number of lessons can be drawn. Even though the country experiences reviewed in this chapter vary in terms of the impact and the policies adopted, they are useful for thinking about the impact of liberalization on health in the context of other developing countries. A first lesson is that social protection programs should be designed in a flexible manner, allowing them to be easily scaled up in response to large economy-wide shocks. The cases of an employment guarantee scheme in India (see Box 6.1), or the scaling up of microcredit in the Philippines, provide examples of such flexibility. Even though it may be difficult to draw from this chapter broader generalizations and conclusions in terms of what specific types of social protection are the most effective to protect health in times of economic crisis, the findings strongly suggest the importance of having established social protection schemes before a crisis hits. The findings further emphasize the importance of having critical programs identified a priori with commitments for protection from budget cuts during a crisis. This forces recognition of policy/program priorities, institutionalizes the link between social and economic domains, and sends a clear message to donors when a crisis hits (Blomquist et al., 2002). The list of safeguarded programs should be guided by an overall strategy to prevent human development reversal, with a focus on preventing the long-term health impacts.

> *Box 6.1*   Alternative approaches to social protection through employment:
> Lessons from the Indian experience.
>
> Public works programs often serve as de facto social protection instruments in
> developing countries. Such programs are seen as dual purpose—on the one hand
> they help mitigate economic insecurity, while on the other hand they contribute to
> poverty alleviation through employment creation and development of community
> assets. India has a long history of such dual purpose public work programs; the one
> that stands out is the Maharashtra Employment Guarantee Scheme (M-EGS).
>   Certain areas of the Indian state of Maharashtra are particularly drought prone
> and arid. In response to a famine in 1972, the Maharashtra government launched
> a novel public works scheme in one such area, which has received much atten-
> tion on account of its use of the concept of guaranteed employment. Maharashtra
> became the first state in India to "guarantee" work to "every adult person (above
> 18 yrs), willing to do unskilled manual work on a piece-rate basis." M-EGS has
> attracted attention on account of its scale (approximately 200 million person-days
> of work are generated annually), longevity (33 years), and rights-based approach
> to social protection, which ensures "employment as an entitlement." Prospective
> workers are responsible for voluntarily registering in the scheme.

HOW AND WHY IT WORKS: "SOMETHING IN IT FOR EVERYBODY"

At the state level, an employment guarantee fund was established, which
receives proceeds primarily from urban taxes (professional-employment
tax, additional motor vehicle tax, sales tax, and a surcharge on land revenue), to which the state government contributes an equivalent amount.

It is widely believed that the reason behind M-EGS's endurance is that it
has "something in it for everybody"—urban middle-class and high-income
households pay for M-EGS (approximately 60 per cent of the funds come from
Mumbai urban taxes) because they want to reduce overcrowding and stem
rural-urban migration to Mumbai; high income groups in rural areas support the program because they benefit disproportionately from assets created.
Beyond physical assets like irrigation network repairs, the rural rich benefit
from not having to support off-season labor. Politicians support it because they
see it as a prestigious scheme and expect political mileage from it. Rural poor
benefit both directly (weekly wages) and indirectly (through public works such
as roads in remote areas). Women in particular have benefited from the scheme
because there is no gender-based wage differential, which is otherwise prevalent
in rural India (Herring & Edwards, 1983; Dev, 1995; Echeverri-Gent, 1998).

COUNTERCYCLICAL EFFECT AND NATIONAL COVERAGE

The real test of dual purpose public works schemes occurs in times of crisis.
The relevant question then becomes: how readily can such schemes be scaled
up in times of crisis? In this regard, M-EGS scores well in two respects. At one

time accounting for 12 per cent of state government expenditure, M-EGS was able to expand to 64 per cent in response to a drought in 1982 (Alderman & Haque, 2006), attesting to a favorable countercyclical role. While such expansion strains administration and dilutes quality, the general conclusions of several studies highlight the flexible management and targeting to low-income beneficiaries during the crisis. Moreover, a comparison of the 1974–75 famine in Bangladesh with the extended drought in Maharashtra (Cain & Lieberman, 1982) also underlines the importance of ex ante measures. Studies note that the frequency of land sales in Maharashtra remained low and relatively constant over the drought period, while it soared in Bangladesh, particularly in times of crisis. Ravallion, Datt, & Chaudhuri (1993, p. 166) further suggest that "from what we now know about the famine in Bangladesh during 1974, it is evident that if an effective rural public works scheme had existed, a great many people would have been saved from starvation and impoverishment."

The experience with the Maharashtra Employment Guarantee Scheme is widely seen as the impetus behind India's recent National Rural Employment Guarantee Act (2004), which aims to be a nationwide safety net for the country's rural poor, guaranteeing 100 days of work per year to one member of each poor family at a piece rate.

NOTES

1. Note that this literature does not simply apply to the East Asian region, but to all regions.
2. Social protection and welfare expenses do not include spending on education and health care services.
3. Concerted social policy reform had been ongoing in S. Korea, first and foremost under Park Chung-hee. One of the hallmarks of Park's regime was the 1977 Medical Insurance Law. As is well known, the Korean *chaebol* (business complex) best symbolizes Korea's phenomenal "state developmentalist" success. The big business-backed workers union Federation of Korean for years had opposed wage reforms and minimum wage legislation. Under Chun Doo-Hwan (1980–1988) in 1986, the landmark Minimum Wage Law was implemented (the first such legislation among the NICs, with the exception of Taiwan). For a review, see Joo, 1999, and for a review of program coverage, see World Bank, International Monetary Fund, Asian Development Bank, and Inter-American Development Bank, 2001.
4. The rest of the employed population is still not covered by any retirement scheme. These include the self-employed and informal sector dwellers. In fact, all the aforementioned schemes are applicable only to urban and industrial workers. Agricultural workers, who form 16 per cent of the workforce, are not included in the scheme. This suggests that while there is a huge amount of resources available that could be tapped, there is still a large number of employed persons who have to depend on their own savings for their old age. Not all workers retrenched during the economic crisis received termination benefits or benefited from the Voluntary Separation Scheme. There is no unemployment insurance or benefit in Malaysia that provides a cushion during the transition period (one criticism of Malaysia's response has been its programmatic ad hoc nature). With the resources at hand, a persuasive case

has been made for a state administered "Social Aid Fund" for employment; for a greater exposition of this and related recommendations, see Mansor & Awang (2002), p. 211–14.

5. For a discussion of Amanah Ikhtiar Malaysia in comparative review, see Mansor & Awang (2002), p. 199.

6. It is indeed remarkable that as we commit these words to paper, the global economy is again hit by a large-scale financial crisis; however, this time emerging from excesses in the developed world financial systems (primarily U.S. and Europe mortgage, restructured debt, and derivatives markets). It is interesting to note that so far the IMF has been all praises for the way developed-country central bankers and financial policymakers have handled this present crisis. In many ways, the policy tools used by the United States (for example, fiscal expansion through tax rebates, monetary laxity via large interest rate cuts, and large bailouts of Wall Street investment banks) follow the exact opposite approach to that of the IMF advice to East Asia about a decade ago. The irony is hardly lost among watchful observers.

7. The Miyazawa Plan is named for the Japanese finance minister at the time of the financial crisis who committed over US$30 billion in loans to the most affected countries in order to help them restructure the corporate and banking sectors, establish or improve social safety nets, and alleviate the credit crunch.

8. Clear policy goals were set in each area, such as: establishing assistance centers for retrenched workers, extending protection to the informal sector, supporting investment in training, reducing school dropout rates, encouraging private sector involvement in education, creating national child health care objectives, etc.

9. These include Workmen's Compensation, Severance Pay, Voluntary Provident Fund, Employee Welfare Fund; but noticeably no unemployment insurance.

10. A review of the Unemployment Mitigation Program can be found in Pongsapich, 2002.

11. On the emerging role of civil society in Thailand, see Gough (2001), p. 174; Pongsapich (2002), pp. 243–45.

12. This is an important point and worth greater discussion for which there is little room here. A fuller exposition can be found in Blomquist, Cordoba, Verhoeven, Moser, and Bouillon (2002), p. 306.

13. The Philippines experienced improvements in key human development indicators between 1986 and 1996, particularly those related to education and health. Poverty declined from 44.2 per cent in 1985 to 31.8 per cent in 1997.

14. The government's response to the 1997 crisis was found wanting in many respects. Reduced access to basic social services was noted during the period. Findings from Reyes & Manasan (1999) echo this concern. They found that five out of six regions showed a decline in immunization coverage in 1998. Focus-group discussions noted a deterioration in the availability of drugs and medicines in local publicly run health centers. As late as September 1998, only 24 per cent of the appropriation for drugs and medicines in the Department of Health budget was covered by allotment advice. At the same time, drug prices rose by 25 to 30 per cent owing to the peso depreciation.

REFERENCES

Alderman, H., & Haque, T. (2006). Countercyclical safety nets for the poor and vulnerable. *Food Policy, 31*, 372–83.

Armstrong, J., Viossat, L.-C., & Flanagan, K. (1999). *Towards an East Asian social protection strategy*. Washington, DC: Human Development Unit: East Asia and

Pacific Region, World Bank. Retrieved from: http://siteresources.worldbank.org/SOCIALPROTECTION/Publications/20265409/SPSSPEAP.pdf.

Balisacan, A. M., Edillon, R. G., Brillantes, A. B., & Canlas, D. C. (2000). *Approaches to targeting the poor.* Quezon City: School of Economics, University of the Philippines.

Bautista, C., Angeles, L., & Dionisio, J. (2000). Philippines. In T. G. McGee & S. Scott (eds.), *The poor at risk: Surviving the economic crisis in Southeast Asia.* Final report of the Project Social Safety Net Programs in Selected Southeast Asian Countries, 1997–2000. Vancouver: Centre for Southeast Asian Research, Institute of Asian Research, University of British Columbia. Retrieved from: http://www.iar.ubc.ca/centres/csear/SSN/TOC.htm.

Blomquist, J., Cordoba, J. P., Verhoeven, M., Moser, P., & Bouillon, C. (2002). Social safety nets in response to crisis. In P. Whiteford (ed.), *Towards Asia's sustainable development: The role of social protection.* Paris: OECD. Retrieved from: http://titania.sourceoecd.org/vl=3684900/cl=29/nw=1/rpsv/cgi-bin/fulltextew.pl?prpsv=/ij/oecdthemes/99980142/v2002n4/s1/p1l.idx.

Boix, C. (2002). Globalization and the egalitarian backlash: Protectionism versus compensatory free trade. In *Workshop on "Globalization and Egalitarian Redistribution,"* Santa Fe Institute.

Bourguignon, F., & Goh, C. (2003). Trade and labor market vulnerability in Indonesia, Korea, and Thailand. In K. Krumm & H. Kharas (eds.), *East Asia integrates: A trade policy agenda for shared growth.* Washington, DC: The World Bank.

Burgoon, B. (2001). Globalization and welfare compensation: Disentangling the ties that bind. *International Organization, 55,* 509–51.

Cain, M. T., & Lieberman, S. S. (1982). *The fertility impacts of development policy in Bangladesh.* Consultants report to USAID/Dacca and the Population Section Planning Commission, Government of Bangladesh.

Coady, D., Grosh, M., & Hoddinott, J. (2004). Targeting outcomes redux. *The World Bank Research Observer, 19,* 61–85.

Cornia, G. A. (2001). Globalization and health: Results and options. *Bulletin of the World Health Organization, 79,* 834–41.

Cornia, G. A., Rosignoli, S., & Tiberti, L. (2008). *Globalisation and health: Pathways of transmission and evidence of impact.* Globalization Knowledge Network Research Papers. Ottawa: Institute of Population Health, University of Ottawa. Retrieved from: http://www.globalhealthequity.ca/electronic%20library/Globalisation%20and%20Health%20Pathways%20of%20Tranmission%20and%20Evidence%20of%20Impact.pdf.

Dev, M. (1995). India's (Maharashtra) Employment Guarantee Scheme. In J. von Braun (ed.), *Employment for poverty reduction and food security.* Washington, DC: International Food Policy Research Institute.

Echeverri-Gent, J. (1998). Guarantee employment in an Indian state: The Maharastra experience. *Asian Survey, 28*(12).

Garrett, G. (1998). Global markets and national politics: Collision course or virtuous circle? *International Organization, 52,* 782–824.

Gough, I. (2001). Globalization and regional welfare regimes: The East Asian case. *Global Social Policy, 1,* 163–89.

Gunter, B., & van der Hoeven, R. (2004). The social dimension of globalization: A review of the literature. *International Labour Review, 143,* 7–43.

Hashim, Shafruddin. (2002). Governance and social policy in Malaysia. *Towards Asia's sustainable development: The role of social protection.* Paris: OECD.

Hayes, J., Ehrlich, S., & Peinhardt, C. (2002). Globalization, the size of government, and labor market institutions: Maintaining support for openness among workers. Presented at: 2002 Annual Meeting of the Midwest Political Science Association, (unpublished).

Herring, R., & Edwards, R. (1983). Guaranteeing employment to the rural poor: Social functions and class interests in the Employment Guarantee Scheme in Western India. *World Development*, 11.

Hewison, K. (2004). Crafting Thailand's new contract. *The Pacific Review*, 17, 503–22.

———. (2006). Crafting Thailand's new contract. In H. E. Nesadurai (ed.), *Globalization and economic security in East Asia: Governance and institutions*. London: Routledge.

Holliday, I. (2000). Productivist welfare capitalism: Social policy in East Asia. *Political Studies*, 48, 706–23.

Hopkins, S. (2006). Economic stability and health status: Evidence from East Asia before and after the 1990s economic crisis. *Health Policy*, 75, 347–57.

Joo, J. (1999). Explaining social policy adoption in Korea. *Journal of Social Policy*, 28, 387–412.

Kapstein, E., & Milanovic, B. (2003). *Income and influence: Social policies in emerging market economies*. Kalamazoo, MI: Upjohn Institute.

Mansor, N., & Awang, H. (2002). The role of social safety nets in Malaysia. In P. Whiteford (ed.), *Towards Asia's sustainable development: The role of social protection* (pp. 197–214). Paris: OECD.

Norton, A., Conway, T., & Foster, M. (2001). *Social protection concepts and approaches: Implications for policy and practice in international development*. Working Papers No. 143. London: Overseas Development Institute.

Peng, I. (2004). Postindustrial pressures, political regime shifts, and social policy reforms in Japan and South Korea. *Journal of East Asian Studies*, 4.

Pongsapich, A. (2001). *Social safety nets in Thailand: Analysis and prospects*. Strengthening policies and programs on social safety nets No. 8. New York: UNESCAP.

———. (2002). Social safety nets: Programmes and projects in Thailand. In P. Whiteford (ed.), *Towards Asia's sustainable development: The role of social protection* (pp. 231–59). Paris: OECD.

Prichett, L. (2005). *A lecture on the political economy of targeted safety nets*. Social Protection Discussion Paper Series. Washington, DC: World Bank.

Puguh, B. I. (2001). *Social safety nets in Indonesia: Analysis and prospects*. Strengthening Policies and Programs on Social Safety Nets No. 8. New York: UNESCAP.

Ravallion, M. (2003). *The debate on globalization, poverty and inequality: Why measurements matter*. Policy Research Working Papers No. 3038. Washington, DC: World Bank. Retrieved from: http://www-wds.worldbank.org/servlet/WDSContentServer/WDSP/IB/2003/05/30/000094946_03051604080285/Rendered/PDF/multi0page.pdf.

Ravallion, M., Datt, G., & Chaudhuri, S. (1993). Does Maharashtra's Employment Guarantee Scheme guarantee employment? Effects of the 1988 wage increase. *Economic Development and Cultural Change*, 41, 251–71.

Reyes, C. M., & Manasan, R. G. (1999). *The social impact of the regional financial crisis in the Philippines*. MIMAP Research Paper 41. Ottawa: International Development Research Centre.

Rodrik, D. (1997). *Has globalization gone too far?* Washington, DC: Institute for International Economics.

———. (1998). *Where did all the growth go? External shocks, social conflict and growth collapses*. Discussion Papers No. DP1789. London: Centre for Economic Policy Research.

Scheve, K., & Slaughter, M. J. (2004). Economic insecurity and the globalization of production. *American Journal of Political Science*, 48, 662–74.

Smith, J., & Subbarao, K. (2003). *What role for safety net transfers in very low income countries?* Social Safety Nets Primer Series. Washington, DC: World Bank.

Torres, R. (2001). *Towards a socially sustainable world economy: An analysis of the social pillars of globalization.* Geneva: International Labour Office.

United Nations Economic and Social Commission for Asia and the Pacific, (2001). *Strengthening policies and programmes on social safety nets: Issues, recommendations and selected studies.* Social Policy Papers No. 8. Bangkok: United Nations. Retrieved from: http://www.unescap.org/esid/psis/publications/spps/08/2163.pdf.

van der Hoeven, R., & Lübker, M. (2005). Financial openness and employment: A challenge for international and national institutions. In *2006 Meeting, Global Development Network*, St. Petersburg. Geneva: International Policy Group, International Labour Office. Retrieved from: http://ctool.gdnet.org/conf_docs/Hoeven_Paper_Lunch%20Time%20Session_ILO.pdf

Van Ginneken, W. (2003). Extending social security: Policies for developing countries. *International Labour Review, 142.*

Wagstaff, A., Watanabe, N., & van Doorslaer, E. (2001). *Impoverishment, insurance, and health care payments.* Health, Nutrition, and Population Network. Washington, DC: World Bank.

Whiteford, Peter, ed. (2002). *Towards Asia's sustainable development: The role of social protection.* Paris: OECD.

World Bank, International Monetary Fund, Asian Development Bank, and Inter-American Development Bank. (2001). *Social safety nets in response to crisis: Lessons and guidelines from Asia and Latin America.* Submitted to the APEC Finance Ministers. Washington, DC: Inter-American Development Bank. Retrieved from: http://www.iadb.org/sds/POV/publication/publication_21_2744_e.htm.

World Health Organization. (2000). *The World Health Report 2000. Health Systems: Improving Performance.* World Health Report. Geneva: World Health Organization.

7 Global Financing for Health
Aid and Debt Relief

Sebastian Taylor and Michael Rowson

INTRODUCTION

Improving health equity between and within countries, as other chapters in this book discuss, requires generous social protection policies, universal forms of health system financing, and investments in social determinants of health (SDH), such as education, water/sanitation, and active labor-market policies. States need to be able to raise sufficient revenue to fund such investments, an ability that for many low-income countries has been compromised by various aspects of globalization: capital flight, declines in foreign direct investment, and substantial loss of tariff revenues as a result of import liberalization. In this chapter we address two specific forms of positive global financial flows: official development assistance (ODA), more commonly shorthanded as aid, and debt relief. While distinct, these two sets of flows are highly entwined and subject of intense international, scholarly, and civil society debates. These debates involve questions of adequacy, effectiveness, linkage, and conditionality. In addressing such questions, this chapter first discusses general trends and issues in aid, before focusing specifically on aid for health. It then turns to debt financing and debt relief, before concluding with how both aid and debt relief should be approached if global equity in health (and in access to SDH) is to be improved. It is important to note at the outset that debt is only one part of the web of inter-linking domestic and international constraints on poverty reduction; and that aid, even when reformed for greater pro-poor disbursements, is only one means of redressing some of these constraints. Changes in trade and global governance are equally essential, and the neglect of one by emphasis on another (e.g., "trade not aid") is unlikely to affect meaningful improvements in global health equity.

OFFICIAL DEVELOPMENT ASSISTANCE (ODA)

Official development assistance (ODA), or aid, predates the Second World War, predominantly in terms of colonial transactions and transfers (Führer,

1996). The modern architecture of ODA emerged at the end of World War II, with the formation of the United Nations and the Bretton Woods institutions, the World Bank and the International Monetary Fund (IMF). Underpinning the concept of ODA was the success of the Marshall Plan, which rebuilt European infrastructure destroyed during the war; the establishment of the Organization for Economic Cooperation and Development (OECD); the rise of independent postcolonial states in many parts of the developing world; and the polarities and client-state relationships of the Cold War. Those historical origins of aid help to illuminate how and why ODA, most acutely in its bilateral (nation-to-nation) form, reflects a complex geopolitical and economic interplay of interests that continues to distort aid flows today.

Contemporary ODA has a reasonably precise meaning. It is defined as grants or loans to developing countries with promotion of economic development and welfare as the main objective (Organisation for Economic Co-operation and Development [OECD], 2006). ODA includes technical cooperation, generally referring to the employ of expert consultants frequently from the donor country, but excludes financing for military ends. Much ODA is provided as straight grants. Where external finance is provided as a loan, it must include a minimum 25 percent grant element to qualify as aid.

In absolute terms aid grew strongly between 1950 and 1990 (Führer, 1996); as a proportion of donors' gross national income (GNI), the volume is less impressive. The 1969 Report on International Development recommended that donors give 0.7 percent of their gross domestic product (GDP) (now renamed GNI) as aid. That target has been met consistently only by a few Northern European countries (Norway, Sweden, Luxembourg, Netherlands, and Denmark). In 2005, total donor country assistance averaged only 0.33 percent of GNI (OECD Development Assistance Committee, 2006). As debt relief scaled up during the 1990s, ODA fell in both absolute and proportional amounts. One argument for this decline has been that other financial flows, in particular foreign direct investment (FDI), were becoming more important than aid. There is some truth in this for some parts of the world, but the relative volumes of ODA and FDI differ dramatically between global regions. In 1997, Latin America received net flows of $13 per capita in ODA and $62 per capita in FDI. For the same period, sub-Saharan Africa (SSA) received $27 per capita ODA and just $3 per capita FDI (OECD, 1998). SSA remains heavily dependent on aid; between 1991 and 2002, ODA made up over 90 percent of all financial flows into the region (Ahmed & Cleeve, 2004), generating spirited debates about the risks of aid dependency.

At the end of the 1990s, with the adoption of the Millennium Development Goals (MDGs), aid began to rise again and was projected to rise further still (Figure 7.1).

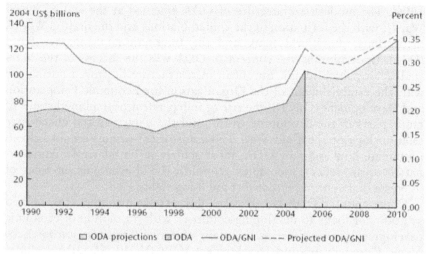

Figure 7.1   Trends in ODA, actual and projected, 1990–2010.
Source: (OECD Development Assistance Committee, 2005).

But there are three caveats:

1. The total volume of aid (compared to observable global need) remains chronically low.
2. Increasing the short-term volume of aid (the "big push" or "Africa Marshall Plan" approach) without sustained financing and coherent allocation across both social and economic sectors risks short-term gains that could easily be followed by stagnation or reversals.
3. The form that aid takes may be at least, or more, important than its volume.

AID: FORMS, USES, AND IMPACT

Aid can take multiple forms, including general budget support (GBS) paid directly to government, sector-wide support where donors create a larger combined pool within a recipient country, infrastructure investment and project financing, technical cooperation and food aid. These differing forms carry lighter or heavier conditions for use set primarily by donor institutions, and vary significantly in their impacts (Griffin & Enos, 1970; Most & Van Den Berg, 1996; Mavrotas, 2003; Rajan & Subramanian, 2006; Sundberg & Gelb, 2006; Thiele, Nunnenkamp, & Dreher, 2006).

One key distinction in form can be drawn between aid given as *special-purpose* and *non-special-purpose* grants (Independent Evaluation Office, 2006). Special-purpose grants include debt relief, technical cooperation, food and emergency aid, and the administrative costs of aid itself. Non-special-purpose grants include funding for infrastructure development, health, and education, and can be used to meet capital and recurrent costs (World Bank & International Monetary Fund, 2006). Non-special-purpose grants enhance spending in the social sectors (for example, strengthening health and education systems), and are more strongly associated with poverty reduction than are special-purpose grants; yet only 8 percent of current increases in aid qualify as non-special-purpose (Sundberg & Gelb, 2006; World Bank & International Monetary Fund, 2006). Less effective or efficient special-purpose grants made up the lion's share of aid between 2001 and 2004, at around 70 percent of the total (ActionAid International, 2005). This emphasis on special-purpose aid does not accord with the contemporary donor rhetoric about the importance of aid targeting poverty reduction; nor does the fact donor commitments rarely translate into what is actually disbursed (Michaud, 2003). In 2005 only 70 percent of pledged ODA was delivered (Afrodad Zimbabwe & 25 other nongovernmental organizations, 2005; Rajan & Subramanian, 2006).

Aid can also be split between *short- and long-run* finance, referring respectively to investments in so-called productive sectors such as agriculture and social sectors such as education and health. We say "so-called" because this dichotomy is more ideological than empirical or theoretical. Recent evidence, for example, shows that social sector investments should equally be considered productive sectors, inasmuch as economic growth is associated with improved health and literacy levels of a country's population (Commission on Macroeconomics and Health, 2001). At the same time, this raises a fundamental ethical consideration: should aid be allocated and/or evaluated primarily on the basis of its contribution to economic growth? Or should other considerations, such as meeting basic human needs, whether or not economic growth ensues, be the appropriate metric? From a global health equity vantage, some degree of economic growth is important since in many recipient countries it is a necessary, though insufficient, condition to improving the ability of governments, families, and individuals to meet basic needs. It has been argued that under the influence of the MDGs, the trend in ODA has shifted towards social sector spending at the expense of investments in infrastructure and other sectors more directly linked to economic growth. Levels of aid to agriculture, for example, have fallen perilously. Between 2000 and 2004, total US Agency for International Development (USAID) assistance to African agriculture rose modestly, from US$459 million to US$514 million, while USAID's African health budget almost doubled. Overall, between 2000 and 2003, agriculture's share of total bilateral ODA declined from 13 percent to 9 percent; during the same period, health-related aid grew by 115 percent (Howard, 2005). To the extent that agricultural assistance favors small producers and domestic food security rather than large-scale export crop production, its decline would have important negative effects on human needs and health equity. In other words, for aid to be more fully effective in supporting adequate and equitable distribution of SDH, it needs to extend beyond the formal health sector itself and incorporate strategic investments in economic growth sectors that will disproportionately benefit the poor (i.e., a pro-poor investment bias) (Maxwell, 2005; Addison, Mavrotas, & McGillivray, 2005a).

AID EFFECTIVENESS

For aid to be effective in reducing poverty it must first be disbursed for that purpose, yet after sixty years of ODA experience and evaluation, this is still not the case (Collier & Dollar, 1999). Aid continues to be directed to countries for reasons other than developmental, much less basic human, need. Geopolitical, geostrategic, trade- and security-related interests strongly influence the decisions donors make about where to send their aid, an effect originally amplified by the Cold War (Boone, 1996; Hoebink, 1997; Schraeder, Hook, & Taylor, 1998; Alesina & Dollar, 2000; Hopkins, 2000; Stiglitz, 2002; Khan, 2003). At the extreme, "developmental or humanitarian concerns, such as reduction of poverty, receive relatively little or zero weight in the [aid allocation] process" (McGillivray, 2003, p. 7). Instead, many major bilateral donors allocate in favor of former colonies (Mosley, 1981; Congressional Budget Office, 1999; Neumayer, 2003; Mazzotta, 2005; Isopi & Mavrotas, 2006); Japanese aid is influenced by historical and geopolitical sphere-of-influence considerations (Khan, 2003; Cooray, Gottschalk, & Shahiduzzaman, 2005); while US aid is positively associated with geopolitical considerations and links with trading partners. As a result of donor favoritism, less than a quarter of total ODA available in recent years actually went to the poorest countries (Acción International para la Salud & 19 other nongovernmental organizations, 2005). Over 60 percent of the total increase in ODA between 2001 and 2004 went to Afghanistan, the Democratic Republic of Congo (DRC), and Iraq—three countries of political and economic strategic interest to powerful donor countries, but accounting for less than 3 percent of the developing world's poor (World Bank & International Monetary Fund, 2006). Despite donor rhetoric on the need for good governance and good policy environments in recipient countries, the level of corruption in a potential recipient country appears to have virtually no influence over aid allocation (Isopi & Mavrotas, 2006).

Aid efficiency and effectiveness are undermined by other factors. Donors, for example, can make aid they give conditional on recipients using the money to buy donor-produced goods and services (tied aid), recouping to donors a considerable part of the aid disbursed. It has been argued that if tied aid is well designed and effectively managed it does not necessarily compromise the quality or effectiveness of aid (Sowa &

White, 1997). The OECD, however, estimates that tying aid reduced its value by $5–$7 billion in 2003 (Organisation for Economic Co-operation and Development, 2004), while the United Nations Development Program (UNDP) finds that tied aid is roughly 25 percent less effective in achieving its stated purposes than untied (United Nations Development Programme, 2003). In spite of donor commitments to reverse this practice, 40–45 percent of total bilateral aid in 2005 remained tied, raising the costs of goods and services by an estimated 15–30 percent, and 40 percent in the case of food aid (Acción International para la Salud & 19 other nongovernmental organizations, 2005).

Aid flows also rise and fall unpredictably, making coherent development planning by recipient countries difficult. Analysis suggests that the aid effectiveness is more strongly associated with the stability of the flow than with the actual amount (Lensink & White, 2000; Quartey, 2005). Aid volatility can also be directly detrimental to health.[1] Econometric analysis of child mortality across seventy-five developing countries between 1995 and 2000 found that "both low levels [of aid] and high volatility of donor funding for health explained the relatively slow progress of some countries in reducing under-five mortality" (World Bank & International Monetary Fund, 2006, p. 61).

Low levels of aid can also diminish its effectiveness. Keeping aid disbursements low is sometimes argued as necessary due to problems with aid absorption, that is, that recipient countries may not have the institutional and infrastructural capacity to absorb and usefully spend large amounts of donor finance (de Renzio, 2005). The question of absorption has been especially problematic in the case of aid to health, in that it applies linear thinking to a circular phenomenon. In order to increase the capacity of the health system in a developing country to absorb and use external finance, it is necessary to invest in strengthening that health system (Jamison, Breman, Measham, Alleyne, Claeson, Evans, Jha, Mills, & Musgrove, 2006). Evidence suggests that absorptive capacity is considerably higher in recipient country systems where assistance is targeted to both human and infrastructure development and is adequately sequenced (Attaran & Sachs, 2001; Sachs, 2004).

Some donors and aid analysts further argue for limiting aid disbursements or placing strong conditions on their use, arguing that unconditional finance, once within the recipient country's national budget, can be redirected domestically to other fiscal purposes, such as subsidizing tax relief, offsetting debt service costs, financing other public expenditure priorities, or feeding corruption. While this problem of aid leakage, or fungibility, is a genuine one, it is by no means inescapable; the degree of loss of aid impact through fungibility varies dramatically from one recipient context to another (Pack & Pack, 1993). Rather than reducing aid, or overwhelming recipients with spending conditions, the question of fungibility makes more urgent the need for a transparent framework—such as that provided by attention to SDH, and linking cross-sectoral investments with health outcomes—by which donors and recipients can verify the relationship between aid and pro-poor or proequity public expenditure (McGillivray, 2003; Amprou, Guillaumont, & Guillaumont, 2005; Thiele et al., 2006).

CHALLENGING AID'S CRITICS

In the early postwar period, aid was viewed somewhat mechanistically as a means to prompt growth through front-loading capital and capacity (Lewis, 1955; Rostow, 1960; Chenery & Stout, 1966); it was assumed that, with appropriate inputs, poor countries would "take off" and undergo accelerated development. But takeoff, in many instances, did not happen. A subsequent body of aid critiques emerged arguing that aid was either ineffective or counterproductive, distorting market function, creating inflationary pressure, increasing size of government and bureaucratic inefficiency, encouraging rent-seeking, weakening governance relationships between state and population, and financing consumption rather than investment (Friedman, 1958; Griffin & Enos, 1970; Voivodas, 1973; Mosley, 1980; Bauer, 1981; Mosley, Hudson, & Horrell, 1987, 1991; Boone, 1996; Svensson, 2000; Easterly, 2003; Quartey, 2005; Schneider, 2005; Rajan & Subramanian, 2005, 2006). Many of the early attacks on aid effectiveness, however, were analytically weakened by missing, inadequate, or poor-quality data and derived their conclusions as much from political ideologies critical of public transfers as from evidence. As well, little notice was taken of often comparable or larger financial flows from recipient to donor countries in the form of profit repatriation, capital flight, and (after circa 1980) debt service.

By the late 1990s, partly as a result of improving data, new analysis brought to light a more positive relation between ODA and growth (Burnside & Dollar, 2000; Hansen & Tarp, 2000; Hermes & Lensink, 2001; Beynon, 2001; Morrissey, 2001; McGillivray, 2003, 2004). Meta-analysis reported consistently positive associations across dozens of individual empirical studies, even in unfavorable policy environments (Cassen, 1986; Collier & Dollar, 1999; Hansen & Tarp, 2000; Gounder, 2001; Morrissey, 2002; Harms & Lutz, 2003; Clemens, Radelet, & Bhavnani, 2004; Dalgaard, Hansen, & Tharp, 2004; McGillivray, 2004; Snowdon, 2005; Addison, Mavrotas, & McGillivray, 2005c). A new controversy then developed. World Bank research suggested that aid effectiveness was conditional on the policy environment in the recipient country; that is, some countries were "good performers" in terms of macroeconomic management and should be rewarded with aid, while implicitly or explicitly "bad performers" should not (Burnside & Dollar, 2000). These research findings were quickly challenged. Easterly, Levine, and Roodman (2003) found that extending the time frame of the original study causes the positive association of ODA, policy environment, and growth to disappear. It has also been suggested that the World Bank's definition of a "good policy environment" oversimplifies complex political conditions across different countries, and favors "policy conditions" neither wholly under government control nor uniformly associated with growth (Berthélemy & Varoudakis, 1996; Lensink & White, 2000; Mosley, Hudson, & Verschoor, 2004). One synthesis concludes: "We show that even with the present allocation, aid is effective in lifting around 30 million people per annum sustainably out of absolute poverty. With a poverty-efficient allocation this would increase to around 80 million people" (Collier & Dollar, 1999, p. 2). Moreover, emphasis in many of these studies on aid and growth likely also underestimates the wide range of aid's noneconomic objectives and impacts, most obviously, finance to projects providing direct support to people in highly vulnerable conditions.

In summary, poverty is the single greatest threat to health for people in many recipient countries and aid can be effective in reducing it. That effectiveness can be severely compromised by the way aid is allocated and the form (including spending conditions) it takes. The Commission for Africa (2005, p. 58) concluded that "the system for allocating aid to African countries remains haphazard, uncoordinated, and unfocused, to a degree that should be unacceptable." For aid effectiveness to improve, there needs to be a transparent relationship between the developmental needs for which it is given and the purposes to which it is put (Acción International para la Salud & 19 other nongovernmental organizations, 2005). The dominance of political, economic, and strategic interests that still characterize much bilateral aid distorts the placement of resources to true development needs and undermines the very discussion of effectiveness.

AID FOR HEALTH

Health for centuries has been a central concern of international relations and development. However, this concern has been expressed primarily in terms of communicable disease and the threat of pandemics to national and international security and trade (Sandler & Arce, 2002). Postcolonial investment bias towards urbanization and industrialization, and cost-effectiveness emphasis on treatment rather than prevention in the 1980s and 1990s, further entrenched a highly biomedical approach (Justice, 1989; Wick & Shaw, 1998). This caveat notwithstanding, development assistance for health (DAH) can be a very effective form of aid, providing comparatively inexpensive improvements (including improvements directed at the poor), working better than other forms of external financing even in weak policy environments, and offering exceptionally high economic benefits of such improvements (Jamison et al., 2006).

DAH has also increased steadily in the last thirty-five years, growing by roughly 5.4 percent annually. Between 1990 and 2004, overall DAH rose from US$2 billion to US$11–$12 billion (Michaud, 2003; Schieber, Fleisher, & Gottret, 2006). But the total of DAH remains low relative to need. The Commission on Macroeconomics and Health (CMH) estimates that aid for health will need to rise to around US$34 per capita per annum by 2007, and to US$38–$40 per capita by 2015, in order to "deliver basic treatment and care for the major communicable diseases, early childhood, and maternal illnesses" (Commission on Macroeconomics and Health, 2001). This estimate included only limited measures to deal with the rising burden of chronic noncommunicable diseases. As Sachs (2007) shows, in many SSA countries the health ministry might be able to capture, at best, the equivalent of US $10/capita for public health expenditures. Assuming an 8 percent annual growth in GDP, no increase in costs, and improved systems of revenue capture, these countries would be over two decades away from self-financing such a basic package, and likely a half-century away from any health system adequate to the expanding needs of their population.

If DAH is to increase to levels commensurate with the harsh arithmetic of such need, however, it will also require a redirection in focus. During the 1990s much of the increase in health aid was concentrated in just three areas—immunization, HIV/AIDS, and new product development (Jamison et al., 2006). Between 2000 and 2004 allocations to HIV/AIDS, TB, and malaria took up one-fifth of total global health aid (Michaud, 2003), reflecting the health focus and financial draw of the MDGs (Jamison et al., 2006). Excluding aid allocated to HIV/AIDS (which rose approximately tenfold), remaining DAH between 1993 and 2003 actually declined as a share of ODA, from 5.4 percent to 5 percent (MacKellar, 2005). Based on their proportional contribution to the global burden of disease, measured in disability adjusted life years (DALYs), HIV/AIDS and reproductive and maternal health are internationally overfunded while injury, mental health, and nutritional disorders are underfunded (MacKellar, 2005). Between 1993 and 2003 noncommunicable disease accounted for 48.9 percent of the total burden of disease in DAH-recipient countries, but received 0 percent of directly assignable [DAH] interventions (MacKellar, 2005). When directly assignable and imputed interventions are included, noncommunicable disease still received less than a quarter of the total DAH allocation, while communicable diseases received 72.9 percent (MacKellar, 2005).

If increased aid is to be channeled to health, and it is accepted that action on health involves action across development sectors, then the evidence suggests that conceptual and structural changes will be required to make aid for health more appropriate. Investing in large-scale disease programs or focusing aid exclusively within conventional health systems and services, while immensely important in themselves, will not address the bulk of poor health in developing countries, nor the inequity in health among different groups. Aid investments in good quality health care services and in action on SDH are not alternative pathways. They are necessary and complementary.

Donor underinvestment in health-systems capacity may be related to the proliferation of new global health initiatives (GHI). GHIs can channel large amounts of health aid into development but in many cases do so outside the recipient government's core budget process. Although there are sometimes good reasons for this (see Box 7.1), such off-budget health spending can fragment national health policymaking, creating a gravitational effect towards public sector investment in parallel programs for specific diseases with diminished attention to strengthening the infrastructure of a comprehensive national health system. The World Bank estimates that as much as 50 percent of health aid runs outside domestic budgeting, with 30 percent escaping government reporting altogether (Sundberg & Gelb, 2006; World Bank & International Monetary Fund, 2006). Off-budget global and vertical health programming can result in policy that underserves pro-poor health system strengthening, and health action that does not adequately acknowledge the "structural dimensions of poverty" (Marcus, Wilkinson, & Marshall, 2002; Sobhan, 2005; Independent Evaluation Office, 2006; Wood, 2006).

But another part of the problem is that much health aid is not eligible as core funding; a recent study of fourteen recipient countries found that "a high share of today's ODA for health and education is transferred in forms that cannot be applied to core budgetary outlays" (World Bank & International Monetary Fund, 2006, p. 60) such as recurrent costs of wages or personal emoluments. This suggests that a larger proportion of DAH should be provided through relatively flexible financing instruments, such as general budget support (GBS),[2] assuming reform of the IMF requirements described in Box 7.1. The quid pro quo of the increased flexibility GBS provides is that recipients should agree to a considerably stronger form of accountability, including reporting on health equity impacts and investments in SDH.

While donors have long recognized the need to act on the structural causes of disease (or SDH), their practices in health aid remain heavily sector-specific and technocratic (Sachs, 2004). The HIV/AIDS pandemic has brought into sharp relief the socioeconomic origins of many of the drivers of infection, highlighting what has been described as the need for a *paradigm shift* in health aid to address broader development factors (Economic and Social Commission for Asia and the Pacific, 2003). Yet that paradigm shift is far from being achieved as the 2003 US President's Emergency Plan for AIDS Relief (PEPFAR) illustrates. Leaving aside the ideological origins of PEPFAR's emphasis on ABC (abstinence, fidelity, condom use), the breakdown of allocations between 2004 and 2006 (Figure 7.2) shows a preference for investment in treatment over prevention and a shift in funding away from preventive action, from over one-third in 2004 to less than a quarter two years later.

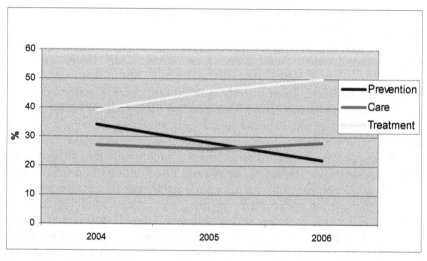

Figure 7.2   President's Emergency Plan for AIDS Relief (PEPFAR), 2004–2006.
Source: Authors' calculations.

The Millennium Development Goals (MDGs), while possibly the greatest moment in postwar commitment to international aid and with a central focus on public health (Sachs, 2004), similarly represent problems of donor overinfluence, technical overemphasis, inattention to action on underlying social, political, and economic inequities, and lack of systemic and sustained financial commitments addressing not only aid volatility but also aid implementation and equity in its distribution. The health-specific goals perpetuate a privileging of infectious diseases and encourage quick-fix investments and technical approaches (Jamison et al., 2006). Neither do the MDGs address the issue of equity. By concentrating on aggregate health as the measure of achievement, they reinforce an emphasis on health as an average outcome across an undifferentiated population. Action towards the health MDGs carries no *necessary* benefit for vulnerable groups in recipient countries, except where they are affected by progress in other goals such as those for poverty and nutrition (Gwatkin, 2005; Spinaci, Currat, Shetty, Crowell, & Kehler, 2006). Conditions of extreme vulnerability, social exclusion, and health inequity could remain entrenched even if the goals are met. There is also considerable doubt regarding whether the MDGs, even if met, can be sustained, given their simplistic focus on downstream factors and negligible action on the underlying socioeconomic, cultural, political, and environmental conditions that contextualize poor health and health inequity (Leipziger, Fay, Wodon, & Yepes, 2003; Ahmed & Cleeve, 2004; Therkildsen, 2005).

The international donor community is not unaware of these problems. The Paris Declaration on Aid Harmonization (2005) specifically highlighted the urgent need for aid to be more coordinated globally, and to be more aligned with, and supportive of, recipient countries' own national development plans. There is an already existing global mechanism for coordinating and aligning aid towards effective, recipient-owned poverty reduction—the Poverty Reduction Strategy Paper (PRSP). The PRSP protocol was launched under the Poverty Reduction Grant Facility (PRGF) as a complement to the Heavily-Indebted Poor Country (HIPC) Initiative on debt relief in 1999. To understand the strengths and limitations of the PRSP process with respect to aid, however, it is first necessary to examine the origins of, and international efforts to mitigate, developing world debt.

HISTORY OF THE DEBT CRISIS AND DEBT RELIEF INITIATIVES

The fundamental causes of the debt crisis that unfolded in the 1970s were a combination of economic slowdown and inflation in the developed world and wars in Vietnam and the Middle East. Members of the Organization of Petroleum Exporting Countries tripled the price of oil in 1973; this dramatic price rise led to a further slowdown in the rate of economic growth and rising inflation in developed nations and other oil-importing countries. The "petrodollars" created by the rise in oil prices, meanwhile, were deposited in Western banks, which then lent the money to developing countries at low interest rates. For the poorest countries, official lending from developed country governments (particularly their export credit agencies), as well as from multilateral institutions such as the IMF and World Bank, also rose. A second oil price shock in 1979 was followed by dramatic increases in interest rates in the industrialized economies, as conservative governments came to power in the United States, West Germany, and the United Kingdom on a platform of fiscal monetarism to tackle inflation. Global recession followed.

For developing countries this was a triple blow. Rising prices of oil necessitated ongoing borrowing from foreign lenders whose high-interest-rate policies worsened their burden of loan repayments. Meanwhile, less demand from the developed economies for their exports reduced the resources with which they could repay their debts. Throughout the developing world, with the recent exception of SSA, annual debt-servicing costs quickly and dramatically outstripped the annual amounts of aid funding poorer countries received, a pattern that persists today. In 1982, when the Mexican government threatened to default on its debt repayments, the world financial system was thrown into crisis. At this point, the World Bank and IMF stepped in to bail out developing countries with new loans that would ease the liquidity crisis.

The developing world was affected unevenly by what was quickly called the debt crisis. The more diversified and less exposed East Asian economies were able to withstand the worst effects. The economies of Latin America and SSA were particularly badly hit. In Latin America commercial lending dominated the debt profile. In SSA it was bilateral and multilateral lending. The debt crises in these regions thus took somewhat different paths. African economies were particularly vulnerable because they were also affected by a steep decline in the prices of their major exports, nonfuel primary commodities, due to the global recession (United Nations Conference on Trade and Development, 2004). Poor economic governance, and sometimes outright corruption on the part of both lenders and creditors, also contributed to the accumulation of debts that could not be paid back. Although also affected by deep economic crisis, the debt-distressed wealthier Latin American nations were given some relief through bailouts and rescheduling initiatives, most notably the Brady Plan of 1989, which focused on the

Table 7.1   Heavily Indebted Poor Countries Potentially Eligible to Receive Debt Relief

Completion Point[a] (23 Countries)	Decision Point[b] (10 Countries)	Predecision Point[c] (8 Countries)
Benin	Burundi	Chad
Bolivia	Chad	Comoros
Burkina Faso	Democratic Republic of Congo	Côte d'Ivoire
Cameroon	Republic of Congo	Eritrea
Ethiopia	The Gambia	Kyrgyz Republic
Ghana	Guinea	Liberia
Honduras	Haiti	Somalia
Madagascar	Burundi	Sudan
Malawi	Chad	Togo
Mali		Central African Republic
Mauritania		Nepal
Mozambique		
Nicaragua		
Niger		
Rwanda		
São Tome Principe		
Senegal		
Sierra Leone		
Tanzania		
Uganda		
Zambia		
Benin		

Source: Adapted from World Bank, 2008b.

Notes: [a]Completion point countries have gone through the initiative and should now receive the full debt cancellation available under the initiative. [b]Decision-point countries have achieved satisfactory performance under IDA/IMF programs, have a poverty reduction strategy paper (or an interim one) in place, and have a plan for clearing debts to foreign creditors. These countries are eligible for interim debt relief. [c]Predecision-point countries refer to those countries that are eligible for debt relief under HIPC but which have not met the criteria for entry into the initiative. For further details see World Bank, 2008a.

commercial debt of middle-income countries. However, a number of poorer economies, mostly in SSA, became ever more indebted, as they took on more loans to pay off older official debt and still ran up arrears. These countries became known as the Heavily Indebted Poor Countries (HIPCs) (see Table 7.1). The HIPCs have seen a massive increase in debt over the past four decades—from close to zero in 1970 to over US$200 billion in 2004—while their per capita incomes stagnated. Figures for the thirty-five of the forty HIPCs that are located in SSA underline the basic dilemma. While these countries have received US$294 billion in loans and paid back US$268 billion between 1970 and 2002, they still are left with a debt stock of US$210 billion (United Nations Conference on Trade and Development, 2004).

Debt cancellation on a small scale for these poorer countries was first initiated with the Paris Club's Toronto terms of 1988, which started to reduce their official bilateral (or Paris Club) debt but not debts to the multilateral institutions such as the World Bank and IMF (United Nations Conference on Trade and Development, 2004). The terms of bilateral debt cancellation were gradually expanded, but overall indebtedness continued to climb. Finally, in 1996 creditors proposed a more comprehensive scheme under which multilateral debt could be cancelled: the HIPC Initiative. Countries qualified if they were very poor (i.e., if they qualified for assistance from the World Bank's International Development Association program) and if their debt burden crossed certain thresholds of debt sustainability. The most important of these were measurements of the ratios of the stock of public debt to a country's exports and to the government's revenues. Countries also had to have a six-year track record of compliance with an IMF economic reform program.

The HIPC process was accelerated by a transnational civil society campaign—Jubilee 2000—that called for cancellation of the unpayable debt of the world's poorest nations by the millennium year. This led to a reformulation of eligibility criteria at the Group of Seven (G7) summit in Cologne in 1999. Qualification thresholds were adjusted downwards, interim debt relief was to be provided, and the completion point at which countries received full debt relief was no longer at the end of the full six years of IMF-mandated reform but could be adjusted to the pace of a country's economic reforms. Finally, debt cancellation was linked to debtor countries formulating Poverty Reduction Strategy Papers (PRSPs) which would show how they were going to use the proceeds from debt relief for the benefit of their populations. PRSPs are intended to organize all relevant domestic and external resources (i.e., both aid and debt relief) under the management of the recipient government, and in consultation with subnational stakeholders, to produce a comprehensive framework for budgetary allocations and programs aimed at reducing poverty. The PRSP has come to exercise a powerful influence over the fiscal choices and behavior of recipient governments. PRSPs act as a kind of gatekeeper to most major sources of international finance (World Health Organization/World Bank, 2003; Independent Evaluation Office, 2006). Failure to gain approval on a new PRSP can have a dramatic downward effect on the availability of other aid (Marcus et al., 2002). To the extent that PRSPs (and the PRGF) tend to emphasize macroeconomic stability and restraint, they can prevent increases in public sector spending such as those required for education and health system strengthening (see Box 7.1).

In 2005, the HIPC Initiative was transformed into the Multilateral Debt Relief Initiative (MDRI) announced at the G7 Summit in Gleneagles, Scotland. Major creditors now allowed 100 percent cancellation of the debts owed by HIPC nations to three multilateral institutions—the IMF, the African Development Fund (AfDF), and the International Development Association (IDA)—with the proviso that the latter two institutions receive compensatory funding from donors. One hundred percent cancellation was later agreed to by the Inter-American Development Bank, albeit on different terms (United Nations Conference on Trade and Development, 2004; International Development Association & International Monetary Fund, 2006).

Box 7.1   MTEFs and public investments for health and education.

The IMF's role as lender of last resort to developing countries is waning as many middle-income countries have paid off their outstanding loans, declared their intent to cease borrowing from the IMF, and begun developing from their foreign currency reserves regional funds to finance short-term macroeconomic instabilities without having to suffer the fund's policy imperatives. The IMF, however, retains considerable policy control over countries reliant on aid or debt relief, since it must sign off on these countries' macroeconomic strategies in order for them to qualify for such transfers. The IMF's sign-off "is also regarded as a valuable seal of approval by foreign investors" (Ooms, Van Damme, Baker, Zeitz, & Schrecker, 2008, p. 3).

A key element of IMF policy is a ceiling on the percentage of GDP going to public sector wages, even when short-term funding is available from donors. The rationales offered include avoiding future debt (if the aid flows should dry up), reducing inflation risk, and avoiding currency appreciation that would reduce the competitiveness of a country's exports. A 2007 report by the IMF's own Internal Evaluation Office corroborated earlier criticism of expenditure ceilings by civil society observers, finding that in 29 sub-Saharan countries just twenty-seven cents of every incremental dollar in development assistance was budgeted for new programs, with the balance used for paying down domestic debt and accumulating foreign exchange reserves (Independent Evaluation Office, 2007; see also Working Group on IMF Programs and Health Spending, 2007). In addition to its obvious negative consequences, this practice encourages vertical funding through global health initiatives, since these funds are not counted as part of the general government budget (Ooms et al., 2008). This weakens the ability of governments to develop more coherent public health systems, creates internal "brain drain" from public systems to shorter-term financed vertical programs, and engenders inefficiencies in organizational and reporting requirements. Further, as donors become more aware that aid funding is not being used for its intended purposes, they may become less intent on increasing aid financing (Ooms et al., 2008).

HAS HIPC DELIVERED DEBT SUSTAINABILITY?

The HIPC Initiative represented recognition by creditors that debt sustainability (meaning the ability of countries to maintain an adequate level of debt-servicing payments) was an issue, and that debtor countries' domestic needs could not be ignored (Martin, 2004). However, the initiative has proceeded exceptionally slowly, at a pace dictated by the creditors (Mandel, 2006). The choice of debt sustainability indicators itself (debt stock at or below 150 percent of export earnings; and debt stock at or below 250 percent of government revenues) was controversial from the launch of the initiative in 1996. Martin (2004, p. 17) notes that

> the amount of debt relief under HIPC was determined by eligibility thresholds which (according to public statements by Fund and Bank officials) were based on initial analysis . . . and then modified to suit political compromises amongst G7 creditors, balancing the need to include strategic G7 allies and their desire to keep costs down.

The World Bank Independent Evaluation Group's evaluation of HIPC (Independent Evaluation Group, 2006) notes that in the thirteen postcompletion-point countries the average NPV (net present value) debt-to-export ratio has declined from 310 percent to 142 percent, lower than the 150 percent target. Similarly, the five countries that eventually qualified under the revenue criterion have seen their debt-to-revenue ratio decline by more than half between decision and completion point from 445 percent to 181 percent (Independent Evaluation Group, 2006, p. 18), well below the target. Improvements in these two core indicators can in part be attributed to increased exports and revenue mobilization by the HIPCs themselves (Independent Evaluation Group, 2006) and to improvements in the terms of loans being made to HIPCs (United Nations Conference on Trade and Development, 2006), rather than to debt cancellation per se. The MDRI is predicted to result in the cancellation of 80 to 90 percent of eligible countries' debts, helping to lower their NPV of debt to exports to between 50 and 60 percent, both significant achievements. But under the terms of the MDRI, debtor countries will see future contributions from the IDA and AfDF reduced by the annual amount of debt-service relief they gain from these institutions. While countries may be able to claw some of this money back if they achieve good policy performance, the MDRI may not actually provide additional new resources to HIPCs. Moreover, while the debt burden of the HIPCs declined in absolute terms from 1995 to 2002, it has been rising again since. Worryingly, the World Bank's Independent Evaluation Group (Independent Evaluation Group, 2006) notes that in eleven of thirteen postcompletion-point countries, debt sustainability indicators are deteriorating, mainly on account of new borrowing. It is therefore questionable to what extent HIPC delivers an exit from the debt problem. This issue is being compounded by the sudden availability of Chinese loans for African governments, leading the United Kingdom (UK) government to warn that further debt problems could be building (McGreal, 2007).

While HIPC was meant to deliver comprehensive debt reduction, some commercial and bilateral creditors outside the main formal Paris Club grouping have not felt themselves bound by the initiative (Independent Evaluation Group, 2006). This is causing sustainability problems for some HIPCs and allowing some creditor countries to free ride on the debt relief given by others. HIPCs owe about US$2 billion to commercial creditors, some of whom are increasingly litigious (International Development Association & International Monetary Fund, 2006). In 2007 the activities of so-called vulture funds—private investors who buy up poor country debts at a fraction of their book value and then press claims in the courts for the full legal value of the debt—have been in the media. Politicians from across the political spectrum have condemned the actions of the vulture funds, but there is little they can do, as the transactions of the vultures are perfectly legal.

Many HIPCs further suffer from significant problems with domestic debt, a fact that is not taken into account when measuring sustainability which only deals with foreign debt. Yet, as the United Nations Conference on Trade and Development (United Nations Conference on Trade and Development, 2004, p. 40) notes, there is a link between domestic and foreign debt "as economic agents borrow to fill the private savings investment gap, the fiscal gap and/or the foreign exchange gap." HIPCs' lack of access to international capital markets also forces a greater reliance on domestic financing. As a result, interest payments on domestic debt have been absorbing larger amounts of government resources.

HAS DEBT RELIEF DELIVERED RESOURCES THAT BENEFIT SDH?

SDH are obviously wide-ranging whereas most research to date has looked only at whether debt relief has freed up money for expenditures on poverty reduction or on health and education. Although poverty-reduction-related public spending in twenty-eight decision-point HIPCs rose during the implementation of PRSPs from 6.4 percent to 8.1 percent of GDP, most of this was channeled to education (Independent Evaluation Group, 2006). Finance to health and to infrastructure such as agriculture and transport, core elements of a pro-poor SDH public spending agenda, remained steady or fell (Independent Evaluation Group, 2006), although other evidence suggests that debt relief can help to raise overall social expenditures (Thomas, 2006; United Nations Conference on Trade and Development, 2006). However, other factors, such as increased aid, may be responsible for the observed rise in poverty-reducing expenditures; and the net gains in health and SDH expenditures (apart from education) appear to be modest at best. This is likely because the new funds made available by debt relief are themselves not large. The World Bank and IMF (International Development Association & International Monetary Fund, 2006) argue that debt service payments by twenty-nine decision-point countries have been reduced by about 2 percent over the period 1999–2005, releasing new resources for poverty reduction. However, it is clear that debt reduction is not releasing anywhere near the level of resources needed to meet the MDGs (Thomas, 2006).

Importantly, the benefits of debt relief will only be apparent if they are truly additional to revenue already raised domestically and from foreign sources. There is a lack of studies on this question, although there has been a degree of speculation about debt relief's additionality to aid. Historical analyses of the relationship between debt and aid suggest that past debt relief has not been additional to aid (Bird & Milne, 2003; Arslanalp & Henry, 2006). More recent assessments of the additionality question, however, have been more upbeat. IEG (Independent Evaluation Group, 2006) notes that net annual transfers to HIPCs have increased substantially over the period of the implementation of the initiative from US$7.3 billion in 2000 to US$15.8 billion in 2004. They argue that US$4 billion of this increase is attributable to debt relief, and that the 11 percent annual increase of nondebt relief transfers over the same period suggests donors "have not . . . cut back on non-debt-relief transfers, and that debt relief was additional in the aggregate" (Independent Evaluation Group, 2006, p. 11). Nevertheless there are still a number of questions over whether additionality will last and how far HIPCs are skewing aid distributions amongst all developing countries.

UNCTAD (United Nations Conference on Trade and Development, 2006), for example, suggests that although ODA has risen to unprecedented levels in 2005—at US$106.5 billion it is 31.4 percent higher than 2004—this was primarily the result of substantial debt relief awards to Nigeria and Iraq. Since debt cancellation is generally counted as an aid contribution, allowing donors to save money by financing one against the other (Addison, Mavrotas, & McGillivray, 2005b; Arslanalp & Henry, 2006), actual new disbursements of ODA are likely to fall. Whether this will affect the HIPCs is unclear, although as of July 2008 over US$40 billion of promised new aid to Africa made at the G8 summit in 2005 has failed to be delivered (Africa Progress Panel, 2008). Furthermore, aid to HIPCs has not been additional when assessed over the whole lifetime of the initiative—that is, from 1996, rather than from 1999 to 2000.

While in aggregate aid can be seen as additional, it is clearly not where it has been used to refinance the multilateral development institutions. Martin calculates that over US$3.5 billion of OECD aid has been promised to the HIPC Trust Fund or used directly to cancel multilateral debt owed by HIPCs. There have been further contributions to the value of US$1.5 billion to the IMF's HIPC Trust; and the Inter-American Development Bank has also received funds (Martin, 2004). This trend was also reflected in the MDRI under which two of the three participating institutions are to be reimbursed for any cancellation they make. Finally, it is also unclear whether aid to non-HIPCs is rising at the same rate as aid to HIPCs. Killick (2004, p. 7) observed a redistribution of resources away from non-HIPCs since the launch of the initiative and concluded that there is "a real sense in which the poor countries outside the HIPC scheme are subsidising those who live in HIPC countries." The distribution of aid between HIPCs and very poor non-HIPCs clearly has to be monitored, and the gain of one group of countries at the expense of the other is not compatible with the values of global health equity.

Parallel to the debates on additionality, commentators have been examining an important underlying issue: is debt relief or aid better at delivering what poor countries need? Martin (2004) argues that debt relief can be more helpful than aid because:

1. It is more stable, predictable, and countercyclical than aid.
2. Tied into the PRSP framework, it increases developing country ownership.
3. It has lower transaction costs.
4. It stimulates private capital flows, aid flows, savings, and investment, whereas there is little evidence for similar dynamic effects of other flows.
5. It has encouraged antipoverty spending.
6. By generating improved fiscal management, it has also stimulated better coordinated and longer-term aid to poor countries.

Bird and Milne (2003) question some of these assertions, arguing that a restoration of sovereignty and policy autonomy would require much larger-scale debt relief than has been contemplated. They also suggest that program aid might be faster disbursing, as debt relief only becomes available to countries over an extended period (i.e., the time over which they would have repaid the debt), and also because there are very often delays in disbursement of debt relief. Furthermore, as Martin points out, 100 percent cancellation of debt relief would "exceed aid flows in only ten HIPCs and averages only 10 percent of exports. So potential gains from each percentage increase in aid, and especially from improved market access, are much greater than those from additional debt relief"(Rabnis & Stewart, 2001; Martin, 2004, p. 37).

CONCLUSION

The HIPC/MDRI debt cancellation for the poorest countries has released modest new resources to address SDH and the ambitious agenda launched by the UN Millennium Summit in 2000. For the poorest countries, substantial further resources will be needed to meet the international targets.

Given the ongoing need for low-income countries to generate capital for investment, there will inevitably be a reason for them to look for further international credit. Substantially enhanced efforts will therefore be needed over the long term to prevent a further buildup of debt. This cannot be done simply by focusing on the narrow economic sustainability indicators deployed under HIPC. Rather, the international community needs to focus on promoting "debt responsibility" (Hurley, 2007, p. 17). Five measures are needed to achieve debt responsibility:

1. Adjustment of some of the basic debt sustainability indicators used by HIPC would be important. The usefulness of the NPV debt to exports criterion has been questioned. Looking at debt-service payments as a percentage of government revenue would be a more helpful way of measuring how far debt is constraining poverty reduction spending (Martin, 2004).
2. A thorough assessment of low-income countries' vulnerability to incurring high levels of debt needs to be made, and should go beyond the revenue/exports criteria discussed earlier. There have also been calls for a focus on the price volatility of a country's key commodities, the extent of diversification of its exports, the burden of HIV/AIDS, the frequency of natural disasters, and other structural factors when assessments of debt sustainability are made (Martin, 2004; United Nations Conference on Trade and Development, 2004).
3. More transparency is needed in the loan contraction process. Government borrowers and lenders should be subject to parliamentary scrutiny (Hurley, 2007). Commercial creditors who refuse to provide debt relief when needed could be exposed. There is an urgent need to help countries facing lawsuits from commercial creditors. Martin (2004) suggests a legal assistance facility to help HIPCs in this position.
4. The delays and creditor control over the HIPC process have reinvigorated calls for a more balanced approach to debt cancellation, including reforms to the international financial architecture that would provide for independent arbitration and mediation between the claims of creditors and debtors (United Nations Conference on Trade and Development, 2006).
5. A number of commentators and reports have called for debt cancellation to be based on the resources needed for countries to meet the MDGs. Even the G8, at its meeting in Kananaskis, Canada, in 2002, said that "no country committed to poverty reduction, good governance and economic reform will be denied the chance to achieve the Millennium Goals through lack of finance" (Mandel, 2006, p. 11). Nevertheless, complete debt cancellation alone will not allow some poor countries to reach internationally agreed targets, as they will still require even higher levels of aid; and these targets themselves, as noted earlier, fail to address adequately SDH, raising questions about the sustainability of

their achievement. Some are alarmed at the prospect of such deep cancellation and suggest that it will create moral hazard, as countries are
encouraged to become even more indebted in the future. On the other
hand, UNCTAD notes "there is no greater moral hazard than the one
entailed in constant restructuring and partial debt forgiveness based on
creditors' perspectives and interests . . . " (United Nations Conference
on Trade and Development, 2004, p. 71).

6. Finally, the HIPC/MDRI initiatives only deal with countries receiving
   funds from the World Bank's International Development Association
   concessional finance facility or the IMF's Poverty Reduction and Growth
   Facility. Such funding is only made available to the poorest developing
   countries that fall below a particular income level. Most of the world's
   poor do not live in HIPC-eligible countries. To achieve meaningful and
   sustainable improvements in global health equity, debt relief should be
   offered to a broader range of debt-distressed developing countries.

In fact, a more radical interpretation of the concept of debt sustainability
is proposed by Mandel (2006). Mandel starts by using the work of Peter
Edward (2006), who argues that the international US$1-a-day poverty line
is an arbitrary cutoff point for defining absolute poverty. He argues that
US$3-a-day would be a better target; on average this level of consumption
(roughly what one would expect at the bottom end of the income scale in a
country with annual GNI/capita of around US$5,000) corresponds to a life
expectancy of between 70 and 74 years. This, he argues, would be a better
or more "moral" figure for a poverty line. Mandel suggests that we can use
this "moral poverty line" to calculate the amount of debt relief that should
be given to developing countries. Based on a sample of 136 developing countries, he argues that between 31 percent and 43 percent of all outstanding
developing-country debt—affecting ninety-three to 107 nations—needs to
be cancelled if poverty is to be reduced and the MDGs met.

Evidence and past experience similarly indicate a suite of essential
reforms to the international aid architecture, starting with recognition
that aid is important; and that it has been effective in promoting economic
growth, reducing poverty, and improving health. Currently aid does not
do this with agreed-upon or acceptable levels of regularity or reliability.
Several changes can be made to strengthen its capacity for positive impact,
both generally and on health and health equity.

1. Quantities of aid and DAH are inadequate. An achievement of the
   Commission on Macroeconomics and Health (2001) was to shift
   global thinking about aid from millions to billions. A step shift is
   required in the total quantum of aid.
2. Aid allocation should not be so tightly tied to the current form of
   policy selectivity, focusing too heavily on donor-driven assumptions of appropriate macroeconomic conditions and governance. If

selectivity is applied, it should be guided to countries demonstrating real proequity policy choices. This would include transparent monitoring of pro-poor public expenditure, including indicators of equity in both health outcomes and across a range of social determinants of health, and protected finance for health system strengthening.

3. Aid through flexible instruments such as general budget support should be increased as a proportion of the total, using the PRSP as a planning and monitoring tool for action on SDH. This perforce requires substantial change in the public expenditure ceilings imposed or recommended by the IMF; as well as reforms to the PRSP process to make it more accountable for health equity and improvements in SDH (see Box 7.2).

4. The system of aid allocation requires radical reorganization. Reversing the current trend of increasingly fragmented bilateral, multilateral, and private funding lines, a global, pooled funding system should be agreed on and established, multilaterally operated, with eligibility and allocation determined according to agreed needs and developmental objectives, and multiyear stability of donor inputs and recipient receipts.

Perhaps, more fundamentally, our conception of aid needs to change. Aid is still seen as temporary assistance, a sort of noblesse oblige on the part of wealthy countries whose riches derived, in part, from the impoverishing exploitation of many of the present aid-dependent countries. Criticisms of this aid dependency abound, both in donor countries wary of political corruption or committed to free-market "boot-strapping" ideals of growth, and in recipient countries where the conditionalities of aid are viewed as a new form of colonialism (Ooms & Hammonds, 2008). Problems of corruption, fungibility, and colonial conditionalities

---

Box 7.2 Strengthening PRSPs through a social determinants of health approach.

To date, the poverty reduction strategy process has been something of a missed opportunity. A number of actions can improve PRSP with respect to health and health equity in developing countries:

1. A more explicit emphasis on the PRSP as a process of improving national policy coherence and intersectoral actions on SDH.
2. More support from donors and national governments for funding intersectoral work on SDH.
3. More international focus on building up intersectoral action in the health field, led by WHO.
4. More support to health ministries attempting to engage with finance ministries and the IMF on the size of the health budget.
5. Assured access to flexibilities in expenditure planning (MTEF) for key recurrent costs (such as health human resources).

are real and must be confronted; but the notion that today's aid-dependent countries can, with the right macroeconomic framework and fairer trade rules, grow into fiscal independence within an ethically defensible time frame is mistaken. The pragmatic reality, then, is that aid transfers are required if those who have benefited most from the past three decades of global market integration accept any responsibility for improving health equity on a global scale.

NOTES

1. Even when the pandemic was widely acknowledged, "ODA support [for HIV/AIDS] fluctuated widely but without much upward trend" in part due to donors failing to respond to the epidemiological evidence (Attaran & Sachs, 2001).
2. Full GBS funding remains relatively rare (approximately 5 percent of total current ODA) (Daniels, 2001; Morrissey, 2002; de Renzio, 2005); although GBS makes up a little over a quarter of ODA allocated in 2004–05 by the Strategic Partnership for Africa, specific country case studies have shown considerable difficulties in implementation (Foltz, 1994; Schneider, 2005). One reason for difficulties—and corresponding hesitancy on the part of donors—is the perception of weakness in recipient countries' public expenditure management (PEM) (DAC Task Force on Donor Practices, 2001). Donor nervousness is reflected in the DAC advice regarding direct budget support (DBS). "Where commitment to social policies is not clear, donors may prefer to use NGOs or [invest in] project" (DAC Task Force on Donor Practices, 2001). In other words, if donors do not like the recipient's policy or performance, they can throw the much vaunted processes of alignment and recipient aid ownership into reverse by reducing DBS and reverting to project aid, or even circumventing the government altogether. This exposes the profound ambivalence underlying support for increased recipient authority in the aid relationship.

REFERENCES

Acción International para la Salud & 19 other nongovernmental organizations (2005). A joint NGO statement to the High Level Forum on Health MDGs. WEMOS [online]. Retrieved from: http://www.wemos.nl/Documents/hlf_letter.pdf.
ActionAid International. (2005). *Real aid: Making technical assistance work.* Johannesburg: Actionaid International.
Addison, T., Mavrotas, G., & McGillivray, M. (2005a). Aid to Africa: An unfinished agenda. *Journal of International Development,* 17, 989–1001.
———. (2005b). *Aid, debt relief and new sources of finance for meeting the Millennium Development Goals.* WIDER Research Papers No. 2005/09. Helsinki: UNU World Institute for Development Economics Research. Retrieved from: http://www.wider.unu.edu/publications/rps/rps2005/rp2005-09.pdf.
———. (2005c). Development assistance and development finance: Evidence and global policy agendas. *Journal of International Development,* 17, 819–36.
Afrodad Zimbabwe & 25 other nongovernmental organizations. (2005). NGO Statement on Aid Effectiveness. United Nations Non-Governmental Liaison

Service [online]. Retrieved from: http://www.un-ngls.org/cso/cso7/NGO-State-
ment.pdf.

Africa Progress Panel. (2008). *Africa's development: Promises and prospects—
report of the Africa Progress Panel 2008* . London: Africa Progress Panel Secretariat. Retrieved from: http://www.africaprogresspanel.org/pdf/2008%20
Report.pdf.

Ahmed, A., & Cleeve, E. (2004). Tracking the Millennium Development Goals in
sub-Saharan Africa. *International Journal of Social Economics, 31,* 12–29.

Alesina, A., & Dollar, D. (2000). Who gives foreign aid to whom and why? *Journal
of Economic Growth, 5,* 33–63.

Amprou, J., Guillaumont, P., & Guillaumont, S. (2005). *Aid selectivity according
to augmented criteria.* No. 9. Paris: Agence Française de Developpement.

Arslanalp, S., & Henry, P. B. (2006). Policy watch: Debt relief. *Journal of Economic Perspectives, 20,* 207–20.

Attaran, A., & Sachs, J. D. (2001). Defining and refining international donor support for combating the AIDS pandemic. *The Lancet, 357,* 57–61.

Bauer, P. (1981). *Equality, the Third World, and economic delusion.* Cambridge,
MA: Harvard University Press.

———. (1991). *The development frontier: Essays in applied economics.* London:
Harvester Wheatsheaf.

Berthélemy, J., & Varoudakis, A. (1996). *Policies for economic take-off.* OECD
Development Centre Policy Briefs No. 12. Paris: OCED.

Beynon, J. (2001). *Policy implications for aid allocations of recent research on aid
effectiveness and selectivity: A summary.* Joint Development Centre/DAC Experts
Seminar on Aid Effectiveness, Selectivity and Poor Performers. Paris: OECD.

Bird, G., & Milne, A. (2003). Debt relief for low income countries: Is it effective
and efficient? *The World Economy, 26,* 43–59.

Boone, P. (1996). Politics and the effectiveness of foreign aid. *European Economic
Review, 40,* 289–329.

Burnside, C., & Dollar, D. (2000). Aid, policies and growth. *The American Economic Review, 90,* 847–68.

Cassen, R. (1986). *Does aid work? Report to an intergovernmental taskforce.*
Oxford: Clarendon, for World Bank/International Monetary Fund.

Chenery, H. B., & Stout, A. (1966). Foreign assistance and economic development.
American Economic Review, 56, 679–733.

Clemens, M., Radelet, S., & Bhavnani, R. (2004). *Counting chickens when they
hatch: The short-term effect of aid on growth.* Working Paper No. 44. Washington, DC: Center for Global Development.

Collier, P., & Dollar, D. (1999). *Aid allocation and poverty reduction.* World Bank
Policy Research Working Papers No. 2041. Washington, DC: World Bank.

Commission for Africa. (2005). *Our common interest: Report of the Commission
for Africa.* London: Commission for Africa. Retrieved from: http://www.com-
missionforafrica.org/english/report/thereport/english/11–03–05_cr_report.
pdf.

Commission on Macroeconomics and Health. (2001). *Macroeconomics and health:
Investing in health for economic development.* Geneva: World Health Organization. Retrieved from: http://www.cid.harvard.edu/cidcmh/CMHReport.pdf.

Congressional Budget Office. (1999). *Making peace while staying ready for war.*
CBO Paper. Retrieved from: www.cbo.gov.

Cooray, N., Gottschalk, R., & Shahiduzzaman, M. (2005). *Will Japan increase
aid and improve its allocation to help the poorer countries achieve the Millennium Development Goals?* No. 243 Sussex: Institute of Development
Studies.

DAC Task Force on Donor Practices. (2001). *Moving to budget support*. No. DCD/ DAC/TFDP(2001)11. Paris: Development Assistance Committee, Organization for Economic Cooperation and Development.

Dalgaard, C.-J., Hansen, H., & Tharp, F. (2004). On the empirics of foreign aid and growth. *The Economic Journal*, 114, F191–F216.

Daniels, D. (2001). *A case study on the European Commission's contribution to development assistance and health (DAH)*. CMH Working Paper Series No. WG6:7. New Delhi: WHO Commission on Macroeconomics and Health.

de Renzio, P. (2005). Increased aid vs absorptive capacity: Challenges and opportunities towards 2015. *IDS Bulletin*, 36, 20–27.

Easterly, W. (2003). Can foreign aid buy growth? *Journal of Economic Perspectives*, 17(3), 23–48.

———. (2006). *Planners vs. searchers in foreign aid*. ADB Distinguished Speakers Program. Manila: Asian Development Bank. Retrieved from: http://www.adb. org/Economics/speakers_program/easterly.pdf.

Easterly, W., Levine, R., & Roodman, D. (2003). *New data, new doubts: Revisiting "aid, policies, and growth."* Working Paper No. 26, Washington: Center for Global Development.

Economic and Social Commission for Asia and the Pacific, C. o. E. S. I. (2003). *Health and development: Selected issues: Tackling HIV/AIDS as a development challenge*. Bangkok: UNESCAP.

Edward, P. (2006). The ethical poverty line: A moral quantification of absolute poverty. *Third World Quarterly*, 27, 377–93.

Foltz, A. (1994). Donor funding for health reform in Africa: Is non-project assistant the right prescription? *Health Policy and Planning*, 9, 371–84.

Friedman, M. (1958). Foreign economic aid: Means and objectives. *The Yale Review*, 47.

Führer, H. (1996). *The story of official development assistance: A history of the Development Assistance Committee and the Development Cooperation Directorate in dates, names and figures*. No. OECD/GD(94)67. Paris: OECD. Retrieved from: http://www.oecd.org/dataoecd/3/39/1896816.pdf.

Gounder, R. (2001). Aid-growth nexus: Empirical evidence from Fiji. *Applied Economics*, 33, 1009–19.

Griffin, K., & Enos, J. L. (1970). Foreign assistance: Objectives and consequences. *Economic Development and Cultural Change*, 18, 313–27.

Gwatkin, D. R. (2005). How much would poor people gain from faster progress towards the Millennium Development Goals for health? *The Lancet*, 365, 813–17.

Hansen, H., & Tarp, F. (2000). Aid effectiveness disputed. *Journal of International Development*, 12.

Harms, P., & Lutz, M. (2003). *Aid, governance, and private foreign investment: Some puzzling findings and a possible explanation*. Discussion Paper 246. Gerzensee: Hamburg Institute of International Economics.

Hermes, N., & Lensink, R. (2001). Changing the conditions for development aid: A new paradigm? *Journal of Development Studies*, 37, 1–16.

Hoebink, P. (1997). Theorizing intervention: Development theory and development cooperation in a globalizing context. In T. van Naerssen, M. Rutten, & A. Zoomers (eds.), *The diversity of development: Essays in honour of Jan Kleinpenning*. Assen, Netherlands: Van Gorcum.

Hopkins, R. (2000). Political economy of foreign assistance. In F. Tarp (ed.), *Foreign aid & development*. London: Routledge.

Howard, J. (2005). Statement to the UN ECOSOC special event on the food crisis in Africa. In *Partnership to cut hunger and poverty in Africa*. New York. Retrieved from: http://www.un.org/docs/ecosoc/meetings/2005/docs/Howard%20Speech-%20Food%20Crises-%2027%20October%202005.pdf.

Hurley, G. (2007). *Multilateral debt: One step forward, how many back?* Brussels: European Network on Debt & Development (EURODAD). Retrieved from: http://www.eurodad.org/whatsnew/reports.aspx?id=1234.

Independent Evaluation Group. (2006). *Debt relief for the poorest: An evaluation update of the HIPC Initiative.* Washington, DC: World Bank. Retrieved from: http://siteresources.worldbank.org/INTDEBTDEPT/Resources/ieghipcupdate-evaluation2006.pdf.

Independent Evaluation Office, I. M. F. (2006). *The IMF's role in the determination of the external resource envelope in sub-Saharan African countries: Issues paper for an evaluation by the Independent Evaluation Office.* Washington, DC: International Monetary Fund. Retrieved from: http://www.imf.org/External/NP/ieo/2005/ssa/eng/121305.pdf.

———. (2007). *The IMF and aid to sub-Saharan Africa.* Washington, DC: IMF. Retrieved from: http://www.imf.org/external/np/ieo/2007/ssa/eng/pdf/report.pdf.

International Development Association & International Monetary Fund. (2006). *Heavily Indebted Poor Countries (HIPC) Initiative and Multilateral Debt Relief Initiative (MDRI)—status of implementation.* Washington, DC: IDA and IMF.

Isopi, A., & Mavrotas, G. (2006). *Aid allocation and aid effectiveness: An empirical analysis.* WIDER Research Paper No. 2006/2007 Helsinki: UNU-WIDER.

Jamison, D. T, Breman, J. G, Measham, A. R, Alleyne, G., Claeson, M., Evans, D. B, Jha, P., Mills, A., & Musgrove, P., eds. (2006). *Disease control priorities in developing countries.* Washington, DC: Oxford University Press and World Bank. Retrieved from: http://www.dcp2.org/pubs/DCP.

Justice, J. (1989). Policies, plans, and people: Foreign aid and health development. *Comparative Studies of Health Systems and Medical Care, 17.*

Khan, H. A. (2003). *The future of Japanese aid to South and Southeast Asia: A comparative analysis.* CIRJE F-Series No. CIRJE-F-233. Tokyo: Faculty of Economics, University of Tokyo.

Killick, T. (2004). Politics, evidence and the new aid agenda. *Development Policy Review, 22,* 5–29.

Leipziger, D., Fay, M., Wodon, Q., & Yepes, T. (2003). *Achieving the Millennium Development Goals: The role of infrastructure.* World Bank Policy Research Working Paper 3163. Washington, DC: World Bank.

Lensink, R., & White, H. (2000). Assessing aid: A manifesto for aid in the 21st century? *Oxford Development Studies, 28,* 5–18.

Lewis, W. A. (1955). *The theory of economic growth.* London: Allen & Unwin.

MacKellar, L. (2005). Priorities in global assistance for health, AIDS, and population. *Population and Development Review, 31,* 293–312.

Mandel, S. (2006). *Debt relief as if people mattered: A rights-based approach to debt sustainability.* London: New Economics Foundation. Retrieved from: http://www.neweconomics.org/gen/z_sys_publicationdetail.aspx?pid=223.

Marcus, R., Wilkinson, J., & Marshall, J. (2002). Poverty reduction strategy papers (PRSPs): Fulfilling their potential for children in poverty? *Journal of International Development, 14,* 1117–28.

Martin, M. (2004). Assessing the HIPC Initiative: The key policy debates. In J. Teunissen & A. Akkerman (eds.), *HIPC debt relief: Myths and realities* (pp. 11–47). The Hague: Forum on Debt and Development (FONDAD). Retrieved from: www.fondad.org.

Mavrotas, G. (2003). *Which types of aid have the most impact?*, Discussion Papers No. 2003/85. Helsinki: World Institute for Development Economics Research. Retrieved from: http://www.wider.unu.edu/publications/working-papers/discussion-papers/2003/en_GB/dp2003–085/.

Maxwell, S. (2005). Exhilarating, exhausting, intriguing: The report of the Africa Commission. *Development Policy Review, 23,* 483–98.

Mazzotta, B. (2005). *Revealed preferences in United States bilateral aid 1960–2000.* Master of Arts in Law and Diplomacy Medford: Fletcher School of Law and Diplomacy, Tufts University.

McGillivray, M. (2003). *Aid effectiveness and selectivity: Integrating multiple objectives into aid allocations.* No. 2003/71. Paris: World Institute for Development Economics Research.

———. (2004). Descriptive and prescriptive analyses of aid allocation: Approaches, issues and consequences. *International Review of Economics and Finance, 13,* 275–92.

McGreal, C. (2007, February 8). Chinese aid to Africa may do more harm than good, warns Benn. *Guardian.*

Michaud, C. (2003). *Development assistance for health (DAH): Recent trends and resource allocation, prepared for Second Consultation, Commission on Macroeconomics and Health, October 29–30, 2003.* Geneva: WHO. Retrieved from: www.who.int/entity/macrohealth/events/health_for_poor/en/dah_trends_nov10.pdf.

Morrissey, O. (2001). Does aid increase growth? *Progress in Development Studies, 1,* 37–50.

———. (2002). *Aid effectiveness for growth and development.* ODI, Opinions, 2. London: ODI. Retrieved from: http://www.odi.org.uk/publications/opinions/2_aid_effectiveness.pdf.

Mosley, P. (1980). Aid, savings and growth revisited. *Bulletin of the Oxford University Institute of Economics and Statistics, 42,* 79–85.

———. (1981). Models of aid allocation process: A comment on McKinley and Little. *Political Studies, 29,* 245–53.

Mosley, P., Hudson, J., & Horrell, S. (1987). Aid, the public sector and the market in less developed countries. *Economic Journal, 97,* 616–41.

Mosley, P., Hudson, J., & Verschoor, A. (2004). Aid, poverty reduction and the "new conditionality." *Economic Journal, 114,* F217–F243.

Most, S., & Van Den Berg, H. (1996). Growth in Africa: Does the source of investment financing matter? *Applied Economics, 28,* 1427–33.

Neumayer, E. (2003). *The pattern of giving aid: The impact of good governance on development assistance* (vol. 34). London: Routledge.

Ooms, G., & Hammonds, R. (2008). Correcting globalisation in health: transnational entitlements versus the ethical imperative of reducing aid-dependency. *Public Health Ethics, 1,* 154–170.

Ooms, G., Van Damme, W., Baker, B. K., Zeitz, P., & Schrecker, T. (2008). The "diagonal" approach to Global Fund financing: a cure for the broader malaise of health systems? *Globalization and Health, 4.*

Organisation for Economic Co-operation and Development (OECD). (1998). Aid and private flows fell in 1997. University of Pennsylvania African Studies Center [online]. Retrieved from: http://www.africa.upenn.edu/Urgent_Action/apic_71998.html.

———. (2004). *Untying ODA: Progress Report 2004.* Paris: OECD.

———. (2006). *Monitoring the Paris Declaration on aid effectiveness. 5. Definitions and Guidance.* Accessed from http://www.oecd.org/dataoecd/13/29/36306366.doc. Paris: OECD. Retrieved from: http://www.oecd.org/dataoecd/13/29/36306366.doc;http://www.oecd.org/department/0,3355,en_2649_15577209_1_1_1_1_1,00.html.

Organisation for Economic Co-operation and Development (OECD) Development Assistance Committee (2006). *Final ODA Data for 2005.* Paris: OECD. Retrieved from: http://www.oecd.org/dataoecd/52/18/37790990.pdf.

Pack, H., & Pack, J. (1993). Foreign aid and the question of fungibility. *The Review of Economics and Statistics, 75,* 258–65.

Quartey, P. (2005). *Innovative ways of making aid effective in Ghana: Tied aid versus direct budgetary support.* WIDER Research Papers No. 2005/58. Helsinki: World Institute for Development Economics Research.

Rajan, R., & Subramanian, A. (2005). *Aid and growth: What does the cross-country evidence really show?* IMF Working Paper No. 05/127. Washington: IMF.

———. (2006). What undermines aid's impact on growth? In *Trade and Growth Conference, Research Department, International Monetary Fund.* Washington, DC: International Monetary Fund. Retrieved from: http://www.imf.org/external/np/res/seminars/2006/trade/pdf/rajan.pdf.

Ranis, G., & Stewart, F. (2001). *HIPC: Good news for the poor?* Helsinki: UNU-WIDER.

Rostow, W. W. (1960). *The stages of economic growth: A non-Communist manifesto.* Cambridge: University Press.

Sachs, J. D. (2004). Health in the developing world: Achieving the Millennium Development Goals. *Bulletin of the World Health Organization, 82*, 947–52.

———. (2007). Beware false tradeoffs. *Foreign Affairs* [online]. Retrieved from: http://www.foreignaffairs.org/special/global_health/sachs.

Sandler, T., & Arce, M. (2002). A conceptual framework for understanding global and transnational public goods for health. *Fiscal Studies, 23*, 195–222.

Schieber, G., Fleisher, L., & Gottret, P. (2006). Getting real on health financing. *Finance & Development, 43.*

Schneider, A. (2005). Aid and governance: Doing good and doing better. *IDS Bulletin, 36.*

Schraeder, P. J., Hook, S. W., & Taylor, B. (1998). Clarifying the foreign aid puzzle: A comparison of American, Japanese, French and Swedish aid flows. *World Politics, 50*, 294–323.

Snowdon, B. (2005). A global compact to end poverty: Jeffrey Sachs on stabilisation, transition and weapons of mass salvation. *World Economics, 6.*

Sobhan, R. (2005). Increasing aid for poverty reduction: Rethinking the policy agenda. *IDS Bulletin, 36*, 61–67.

Sowa, N. K., & White, H. (1997). *An evaluation of Netherlands co-financing of World Bank activities in Ghana, 1993–1996.* The Hague: Ministrie van Buitenlandse Zaken.

Spinaci, S., Currat, L., Shetty, P., Crowell, V., & Kehler, J. (2006). *Tough choices: Investing in health for development—experiences from national follow-up to the Commission on Macroeconomics and Health.* Geneva: World Health Organization. Retrieved from: http://www.who.int/macrohealth/documents/report_and_cover.pdf.

Stiglitz, J. (2002). Overseas aid is money well spent. *Financial Times.*

Sundberg, M. & Gelb, A. (2006). Making Aid Work. *Finance and Development, 43.*

Svensson, J. (2000). Foreign aid and rent-seeking. *Journal of International Economics, 51*, 437–61.

Therkildsen, O. (2005). Major additional funding for the MDGs: A mixed blessing for capacity development. *IDS Bulletin, 36*, 28–39.

Thiele, R., Nunnenkamp, P., & Dreher, A. (2006). *Sectoral aid priorities: Are donors really doing their best to achieve the Millennium Development Goals?* Kiel Working Papers No. 1266. Kiel, Germany: Kiel Institute for World Economics.

Thomas, A. (2006). *Do debt-service savings and grants boost social expenditures?* IMF Working Papers WP/06/180. Washington, DC: International Monetary Fund. Retrieved from: http://www.imf.org/external/pubs/ft/wp/2006/wp06180.pdf.

United Nations Conference on Trade and Development. (2004). *Economic development in Africa: Debt sustainability: Oasis or mirage?* New York and Geneva: United Nations.

———. (2006). *Trade and development report 2006: Global partnership and national policies for development.* New York and Geneva: United Nations. Retrieved from: http://www.unctad.org/Templates/Download.asp?docid=7183 &lang=1&intItemID=2068.

United Nations Development Programme. (2003). *Human development report 2003: Millennium Development Goals: A compact among nations to end human poverty.* New York: Oxford University Press.

Voivodas, C. S. (1973). Exports, foreign capital inflow and economic growth. *Journal of International Economics, 3,* 337–349.

Wick, P., & Shaw, J. (1998). The Côte D'Ivoire's troubled economy: Why World Bank intervention failed. *Cato Journal, 18.*

Wood, A. (2006). *IMF macroeconomic policies and health sector budgets.* Amsterdam: Wemos Foundation. Retrieved from: http://www.wemos.nl/Documents/wemos_synthesis_report.pdf.

Working Group on IMF Programs and Health Spending. (2007). *Does the IMF constrain health spending in poor countries? Evidence and an agenda for action.* Washington, DC: Center for Global Development. Retrieved from: http://www.cgdev.org/doc/IMF/IMF_Report.pdf.

World Bank. (2008a). *Debt relief.* HIPC Initiative, World Bank [online]. Retrieved from: http://go.worldbank.org/KNZR2IIQG0.

———. (2008b). *Heavily indebted poor countries.* HIPC Initiative, World Bank [online]. Retrieved from: http://go.worldbank.org/AJ50UJ3KI0.

World Bank & International Monetary Fund. (2006). *Global monitoring report 2006: Millennium Development Goals: Strengthening mutual accountability, aid, trade and governance.* Washington, DC: World Bank.

World Health Organization/World Bank. (2003). *High level forum on health Millennium Development Goals: Resources, aid effectiveness and harmonization.*

8   Globalization and Health Systems Change

John Lister and Ronald Labonté

A FRAGMENTED VISION: COMMON FACTORS IN HEALTH SYSTEM REFORM

INTRODUCTION

The first "global" approach to health care was marked by the overwhelming vote of the World Health Organization's (WHO) World Health Assembly to embrace the 1978 Alma-Ata Declaration and the objective of ensuring "Health for All" by 2000. Four key principles at the center of the Alma-Ata policies were simple and clear:

1. Health, defined as "a state of complete physical, mental and social well-being, and not merely the absence of disease or infirmity," was proclaimed to be "a fundamental human right" rather than being regarded more narrowly from a less effective curative focus or "medical model."
2. Universalism reflected the drive to include the whole population of every country within a protective network of health care and health services, available on the basis of need rather than the ability to pay.
3. Health systems should be based upon primary health care (PHC), defined as "essential health care based on practical, scientifically sound and socially acceptable methods and technology made universally accessible to individuals and families in the community through their full participation and at a cost that the community and country can afford." PHC should combine primary care with the availability of accessible hospital and secondary care services (World Health Organization, 1992).
4. Health systems have an important role in supporting public participation not only in the organization and delivery of health services, but also in shaping policies and actions on the social determinants of health.

The consensus around these values represented the high point of the post-war *welfarist* approach in Western Europe and most Organisation for Economic Co-operation and Development (OECD) countries, but it was already being undermined by political developments which changed the ideological paradigm of the dominant capitalist countries. This shift began in earnest with the election of Margaret Thatcher as British prime minister in 1979, Ronald Reagan as United States (US) president in 1980, and Helmut Kohl as German chancellor in 1982. Their economic policy of *monetarism* (using high interest rates to bring down inflation), accompanied by the rise of neoliberalism and its emphasis on liberalization, deregulation, and privatization, helped to shape what later came to be called the Washington Consensus (Williamson, 1990, 2000). The policy elements of this "consensus," reflecting the political agendas of the three dominant globalizing economies, were openly embraced by the leading international financial institutions, the International Monetary Fund (IMF) and the World Bank (Stiglitz, 2002).

The impact of these changes was magnified by the economic crises which befell many newly independent states in the 1980s. These states began with aspirations to establish universal, publicly funded health care systems but were forced to seek support and accept stringent conditions (Structural Adjustment Programs, or SAPs) on loans from the World Bank and IMF and as a basis to secure global credit ratings. These conditions increasingly involved the privatization of public services, opening up of markets for private providers, and tighter restrictions on government spending on welfare, including health and education. Meanwhile, donor governments in key high-income countries attempted to transfer management techniques and economic/organizational models from the private sector as a basis to reorganize and reform public services, which were portrayed as bureaucratic, monolithic, inflexible, and inefficient. The evidence-free nostrums of "New Public Management" with its core concepts of contracts and "steering rather than rowing" (Osborne & Plastrik, 1998; Denhardt & Denhardt, 2002) emerged from this same process. The consequences have been an increased focus on curative medicine rather than public health (promotion, prevention, and protection approaches), target setting based on economic and financial rather than health-related goals, and vertical programs dictated by global bodies without reference, until very recently, to the wider implications for health care provision in the recipient countries.

The World Bank, which had been little involved in health until the mid-1980s, began advocating an increasingly neoliberal package of policies. These policies not only broke from the consensus of universalism but also focused increasingly on technical solutions, cost-efficiency, and medical models, while making use of some of the language of primary health care. With its growing focus on cost recovery (user fees), private sector providers and an explicitly two-tiered system in which only a minimal package of essential care would be available to the world's poor, the Bank's policy represented a definitive break from the values of Alma-Ata and contributed to the replacement of its more comprehensive vision of health system reform with an intervention-specific approach known as "selective" primary health care (Cueto, 2004).

By contrast, the organization tasked with driving forward the principles and values of Alma-Ata, the WHO, had gone into retreat, unable to challenge the resources and the ideological weight of the bank. The bank's vast budget for projects and research has sponsored a largely one-sided line of enquiry and debate, while the WHO found its budget frozen in real terms, requiring it to seek compromising "partnership" with the bank and, increasingly, with the private sector (see Chapter 12, this volume). The WHO's relative lack of economic knowledge was one of the factors which led it to recruit World Bank health economists, resulting in the much publicized controversies surrounding the WHO's *2000 World Health Report* (*WHR*) regarding the choice of metrics by which it evaluated the effectiveness of health systems internationally (Braveman, 1998; Gadelha et al., 2001; Navarro, 2002; Brown, 2002; Landmann Swzarcwald, 2002). This report also criticized primary health care as a failure and the Alma-Ata declaration for not referring to private financing and for a time diluted the WHO's historic commitment to the concept of a basic human right to health. The 2008 *World Health Report*, however, on the topic of primary health care, is reasserting WHO commitment to this approach, and is indicative of recent retreats from the neoliberal approaches to health sector reform discussed in this chapter.

Much global discourse on health sector reform, however, persists in promoting policies that embrace free-market values, resulting in what Unger, De Paepe, Ghilbert, Soors, & Green (2006) describe as "disintegrated care." This chapter examines the global causes and consequences of this free-market embrace, concluding with a brief set of policy cautions for those concerned with building health systems based upon principles of equity, accessibility, and meeting social needs.

Driving Towards "Disintegrated Care"

The World Bank and, until very recently, the IMF became highly influential in shaping policy in low- and middle-income countries:[1] by the late 1990s the Bank was spending around US$100 million each year on research, and it has consciously fostered an image of itself as a "knowledge bank" (Pincus & Winters, 2002). However, the Bank's influence goes beyond policy and ideology. It has discretion to grant or withhold loans; by the end of the 1990s it was the largest funder of health sector activities, overtaking the WHO, and in the six years since 2000, annual Bank lending for health-related projects has averaged US$2.5 billion—13 percent of total lending through the two branches of the World Bank serving middle- and low-income countries: respectively, the International Bank for Reconstruction and Development (IBRD) and the International Development Association (IDA) (World Bank, 2005).

In 1985 the Bank published a major document arguing the case for user fees for health care (de Ferranti, 1985). This was followed by an official Bank document which combined arguments for user fees with a concerted argument for a reduced role for the state and increased reliance on market mechanisms and the private sector (World Bank 1987). But the most influential policy document shaping health policy for developing countries was the Bank's 1993 *World Development Report (WDR)* (Walt, 1994) This report effectively proposed the consolidation of a two-tiered global health system, accepting that wealthy countries would be free to spend as much as they wished but urging that public funding of hospital care in developing countries be reduced to a rudimentary minimum, with remaining services privatized in delivery, financing, or both. The same report estimated the costs of a "minimum package" of public health and essential clinical services in the poorest developing countries at US$12 per head of population (World Bank, 1993, p. 10).

Despite critical reports on the failure of the 1993 policies to deliver even the "essential package" (Colgan, 2002) and mounting evidence of the negative impact on equity and access flowing from the imposition of user fees (Creese, 1997; England, Kaddar, Nigam, & Pinto, 2001; Nanda, 2002), the Bank continued to press low- and middle-income countries in this same direction. In 2000 American non-governmental organizations persuaded Congress to threaten a withdrawal of US funding if either the IMF or World Bank continued to make user fees for health or for education a condition of loans to developing countries (Weisbrot, 2001). One result of this was the declaration in the 2004 *WDR* that the Bank no longer had a "blanket policy" on user fees (Hutton, 2004).

The accumulating negative evidence of structural adjustment policies on the health and welfare of the world's poorest—for example, a 2001 review of seventy-six articles studying the health effects of structural adjustment programs found just 8 percent recorded positive results and 45 percent were negative (Breman & Shelton, 2001)—led the bank and IMF to reform their approach to SAPs and to launch a new policy of Poverty Reduction Strategy Papers (PRSPs) (see Chapter 7, this volume). By July 2008, sixty-six countries had produced at least one PRSP, while some countries had already produced several (International Monetary Fund [IMF], 2008). However, conditionalities and the drive to privatization were still very much alive in the Bank/IMF negotiations over the cancellation of debts for the first twenty-three Heavily Indebted Poor Countries (HIPC) (Gupta, Clements, Guin-Siu, & Leruth, 2001). HIPC countries were required to make improvements in immunization and health care delivery, including steps to slow the spread of AIDS, *before* they received the promised financial reward. In Malawi, the process dragged on for years while the country also fell victim to limits on the proportion of public spending that could be used to pay public employees (Fontana, 2005) (see Chapter 7, this volume).

These policies have not gone without criticism, even by some of the Bank's and IMF's major shareholding countries. In 2006, the British government threatened to withhold its payments to the Bank unless it dropped its requirement that poor countries liberalize their economies and privatize public sector enterprises (Elliott, 2006). In 2007, the Norwegian government did withhold 25 percent of its World Bank tranche on the basis that the Bank's continuing, if now somewhat less strident, loan and grant conditionalities would effectively prevent recipient countries from emulating Norway's social democratic policies if they so chose (Bretton Woods Project, 2008).

Other Organizations Offering the Same Menu of Market Reform

The World Bank's favored package of market-style health system reforms is echoed by the regional banks like the Asian Development Bank (ADB) and the Inter-American Development Bank (IADB). Other global forces involve the donor agencies of the world's wealthiest countries. Increasingly their assistance is channeled through the World Bank and thus subject to the Bank's market-oriented reforms. When bilateral (country to country), it often reflects the more general global economic policies of the donor country. One such example of this has been the US Agency for International Development (USAID), with a budget of almost US$1.5 billion for health development projects in 2003 (Michaud, 2003). Since its establishment as a subdivision of the State Department in 1961, USAID has been explicitly tied to the US administration of the day, and to its foreign policy objectives, with a consistent bias towards privatization, economic liberalization, private sector involvement, and socially conservative policies (USAID [US Agency for International Development], 2003; Ollila, 2005; USAID, 2006). On a worldwide scale, consultancy firms such as Abt Associates, John Snow Inc., and Management Sciences for Health (frequently funded by development assistance funds from donor countries or the World Bank) also promote the drive towards more private sector and market-style policies (Lee & Goodman, 2002). So, too, do large-scale corporations involved in health care: drug companies, private insurers, and private hospital chains and corporations including Australia's Ramsay Healthcare and South Africa's Netcare, Discovery, and Life Healthcare (Fortson, 2007).

The United Kingdom (UK) and the United States, the dominant powers in the World Bank (Walt, 1994), are strikingly similar in their eagerness to use economic levers to achieve policy change, making these two countries' interventions very different from equivalent programs advanced by other countries. For example, while the UK's Department for International Development (DFID) has been strongly criticized for promoting privatization, and working in similar fashion to USAID through private consultancies in pushing this line of policy (Hilary, 2005), Australia places little emphasis on private providers (Barraclough, 2005; Australian Agency for International Development [AusAID], 2008). The Danish aid agency Danida has explicitly criticized the impact of user fees (Danida [Royal Danish Ministry of Foreign Affairs], 2005, p. 27) and the Danish definition of the "private sector" includes trade unions. Germany's GTZ/GmbH (German Agency for Technical Cooperation) also follows a markedly different agenda from USAID and DFID. In December 2005 it jointly organized a major international conference in Berlin with the International Labour Organization (ILO) and the WHO around the theme of social health insurance in developing countries, in which the concept of social insurance is clearly linked with universalism rather than restricted to providing cover for the minority of workers in formal sector employment. The German approach is thus distinct from the World Bank concept of social insurance, which tends to lead towards the kind of two-tier system that has taken shape in Colombia and some other countries, in which the provision for the poor is quite different from and inferior to that available to formal sector employees (Homedes & Ugalde, 2005; Flores, 2006). An accompanying critique from the German organizers explicitly highlighted the "considerable and negative impacts" of policies based on the Washington Consensus, while GTZ/GmbH guidelines submitted to the conference stressed principles including "universality, solidarity, and social responsibility" (Schwefel et al., 2005, p. 6).

The health system policies promoted globally by the Bank and USAID are both highly influenced by the preponderance of health policy and health economics academics based principally in US and UK universities. While by no means all health policy specialists in these academic institutions support the market-oriented policies of the Bank and USAID, many of those who do back the Bank's line tend to benefit more readily and consistently from research funding and ready avenues for publication of their findings, and exert considerable influence in both institutions and with national governments. This grouping, described by Lee and Goodman (2002, p.116) as a small, "tightly integrated network of policy-makers, technical advisors and scholars," has largely shaped and driven the policy reforms promoted by global bodies: "Analysis of [health system] policy changes over time suggests that the process of policy initiation and formulation has been largely top-down, developed and supported through the Washington and London hubs."

Stone (2001, p. 352) refers to these "hubs" as *epistemic communities*, noting also the role of a transnational network of "élite, technical and scientific cliques" in effecting change in policy and policy agendas and becoming "entrenched in bodies such as the IMF, World Trade Organization (WTO), OECD and World Bank." The WHO itself has felt the pressure of these communities in its own health systems policy development: only two of the team drafting *WHR 2000* were from health ministries in member states, while others came from the World Bank, health insurance companies, universities, the OECD, and private health organizations, as two academic critics of the epistemic community have pointed out (Ollila & Koivusalo, 2008).

However, the eventual "consensus" often convinces only the elite community of policy shapers themselves. Even the Pan American Health Organization (PAHO) has voiced criticisms of the narrow circle that has had any voice in health policy: "It is simply unacceptable for health policy to be researched and conducted in small, closed circles of consultants and policymakers . . . It is in the very definition of good governance that people have a right to a meaningful say in the decisions that govern their lives" (PAHO [Pan American Health Organization], WHO [World Health Organization], & IDRC [International Development Research Centre], 2001, Foreword).

It would be a mistake to see all such problems as simply flowing from the World Bank/IMF. Market-style policies and ideological pressures can flow also from adaptation to the global market itself and the prevailing ideas and policy frameworks elsewhere in the market system. However, since the majority of market-style policies are more expensive to implement than the more integrated systems they replace, with high bureaucratic overhead costs, they require political commitment to drive them through, whether this be external pressure from the Bank or the ideological conviction of center-right national governments. This helps explain why the policy proposals are more often talked about than implemented (Lister, 2005). Some governments, notably those of Sri Lanka, Ghana, Thailand, and Costa Rica, have withstood pressures and retained more progressive and equitable health system policies (Rannan-Eliya & Somanathan, 2005).

While policies shaping health systems in the world's poorest countries are decided to a considerable degree in multinational institutions, nongovernmental organizations (NGOs), and aid agencies elsewhere, in high-income countries a very different situation prevails. There is pressure to clamp down on spending: the European Central Bank, charged with the stability of the euro, has advocated a cap on health care spending, proposed greater private involvement in the funding of health care and the introduction of copayments (2003), and called for greater use of private finance, coupled with the use of "market forces" to move towards "efficient solutions," and the restriction of public health care to "core services" for health care and prevention, leaving individuals to provide for "non-essential health expenditure."

Policies for the thirty wealthiest countries, however, are debated and promoted through the OECD, whose researchers have become more critical of market-style reforms in the last few years. In 2004, the final chapter of a report on a four-year OECD health project, discussing "value for money in health systems," dismissed many of the stock neoliberal policies. Cost sharing, the purchaser-provider split, decentralization, payment by results (activity-based systems of payment), and competition between providers were all found wanting (OECD Health Project, 2004). A long history of universal access to health care in most OECD countries has also made it more difficult for political parties, even those favoring increased privatization and marketization, to dismantle public health systems to the extent that occurred in many low-income countries during the imposition of SAPs.

Box 8.1   The many faces of the private sector.

Public Service International, the international organization of public sector trade unions, distinguishes between a number of levels and forms of privatization:

Privatization of ownership
Privatization of responsibility
Privatization of provision
Privatization of finance
Privatization through markets—creating conditions where the private sector can compete with the public sector for government or social insurance scheme funds (PSI, 1999, p. 9).

The World Bank's report *The Business of Health in Africa* (2007), published by its affiliate, the International Finance Corporation (IFC), which makes loans to the private sector in developing countries, further points out that, within this framework, there are various different types of "private" provision in health care:

1. As well as private-for-profit provision, there are different types of private not-for-profit provision (charities, religious groups, registered nonprofits/co-ops, each of which may or may not levy user charges).
2. Private provision that is publicly financed and under varying forms of government regulation (as is the case in most OECD countries).
3. Private finance to build, manage, and operate hospitals and facilities delivering public sector services (variously referred to as the Private Finance Initiative or Public Private Partnerships).
4. Private financing for private provision in both for-profit and not-for-profit services (the latter being, for example, community insurance schemes).

By no means do all of these variants of private sector involvement necessarily have a negative impact upon equity of access and provision, although almost all private involvement carries overhead costs, and needs to deliver some form of surplus or working balance which, in turn, can result in the diversion of public funds or resources that might otherwise have been available to fund frontline services.

MARKET PRESCRIPTIONS FOR FAILURE

Market-style policies and "reforms" do not arise spontaneously at the national level in developing countries. Still less are they a direct or inevitable response to the pressures of globalization on national economies. However, as Armada & Muntaner (2004) conclude from their literature review, such policies have mostly originated as theoretical proposals lacking any serious evidence of their effectiveness. If space is to be opened for the implementation of progressive and soundly based reforms, it is necessary first to dispel illusions in the menu of measures already established as the "norm," discussed following.

A Minimum Package of Care

The World Bank's *Investing in Health* in 1993 estimated that delivery of an "essential clinical package" would cost on average about US$12 in low-income countries and US$22 per capita in middle-income countries (World

Bank, 1993, p. 116). This was then (and often is still) well above the levels of spending in many low-income countries. Even the Bank's essential "minimum package" was estimated to require a quadrupling of poorer countries' spending on public health from US$5 billion to US$20 billion a year in 1993 prices. But the Bank warned: "The case for government financing of discretionary clinical health care—services outside the essential package—is far less compelling. In fact, governments can promote both efficiency and equity by reducing—or when possible eliminating—public funding for these services" (World Bank, 1993, p. 119).

The decision that such services should not be funded publicly means that any such services could only develop in the *private* sector, levying charges which would inevitably be unaffordable to the poor. Only the wealthy few would have access to secondary- and tertiary-level care services not available to the vast majority. And because it was unaffordable, the World Bank conception of a minimum or essential package became increasingly perceived as a *target*, effectively a "maximum" for organizations such as the WHO (Laurell & Arellano, 1996) and a priority for, first, donor countries and, eventually, the proliferation of global public-private partnership funds for health.

The *WDR* framework for policies based on a "minimum package" has persisted, not least in the very limited health aspirations of the Millennium Development Goals (MDGs), and also in the narrow focus of vertical programs for immunization and AIDS treatment. Some countries have worked to introduce social health insurance schemes in which the subsidized enrolment of the poor comes with a reduced entitlement to a "minimum package" of care, as in Colombia (where it is equivalent to just 20 percent of the value of the full insurance package) and Mexico (Flores, 2006).

Imposition of User Fees

This policy is one of the most deeply ingrained in the thinking of those responsible for policy in developing countries. A recent survey of thirty African countries found twenty-seven still imposing fees (Oxfam International, 2006). Of twenty-four priority countries supported by DFID, twenty had user fees at primary care level (Witter, 2005, p. 5).

The Bank's 2004 *WDR* actually argues that "paying for services confers power," claiming that "modest co-payments can also provide an entry ticket to clinical services for poor people by reducing capture of supposedly free services by richer groups" (World Bank, 2003, p. 143). This assumes—without evidence—that the poor can afford and will pay a "modest co-payment," and that the rich will not, even though they are better able to afford it. Any illusions that patients might be "empowered" by fees should be dispelled by the revelations in recent reports of patients being forcibly detained in Burundi for failure to pay hospital bills (Human Rights Watch, 2006) and in Ghana, where newborn babies have been held in hospital in a bid to force mothers to pay maternity bills (UN Office for the Coordination of Humanitarian Affairs, 2005; Amanfo, 2006). Schieber (1997) claims that cost sharing is a means to combat "moral hazard," an economic concept referring to egregious misuse of something that is freely or easily available, while Wang'ombe optimistically suggests that the "right" people are deterred by user fees, reducing "frivolous demand" (Wang'ombe, 1997, p. 151). However, there is little actual evidence of frivolous demand in developing countries or in other contexts (Deber, 2000), and reducing demand does not necessarily reduce the need for health care.

The validity of claims that user fees can actually lead to an increase in utilization if they are accompanied by an improvement in the quality of services and availability of drugs has also been questioned by research from Nigeria which suggests that poor users excluded by the fees are replaced by wealthier sections of the population who can afford to pay—a backward step for equity (Blas, 2004, p. 19). Those most likely to be deterred from accessing health care are the poorest—and especially women. In fact, this effect is the most consistent and predictable result from any cost-recovery program (Creese & Kutzin, 1995).

Just four of the thirty-one African countries implementing user fees claimed that either "efficiency" or "equity" was an objective (Leighton & Wouters, 1995). A study in Tanzania found that the administration of the user fee program cost more than the user fees brought in (Kessler & Alexander, 2004), while in Honduras, the fees raised less than 2 percent of the Ministry of Health's income, with two-thirds of the funds collected required to administer the fee system itself (Flores, 2006). Conversely, there have been some "astounding" successes where user fees have been abolished, notably in Uganda (Hutton, 2004).

The World Bank played a crucial role in generalizing the imposition of user fees. By 1998 about 40 percent of the Bank's health, nutrition, and population projects—and almost 75 percent of those projects were in sub-Saharan Africa—included the introduction or increased application of user fees (Dunne, 2000). Few countries have been able to establish any significant system to exempt the poor from user fees: indeed, even though the Bank's position in 1993 advocated exemptions where possible, its main focus throughout remained on introducing fees at a level that would not be a barrier to the poor, and finding ways to argue that in certain circumstances fees may actually increase the use of some services (World Bank, 1993). Yet all empirical evidence appears to confirm that in practice the imposition of charges reduces the utilization of services. The scale of the reductions observed ranged from 52 percent in Kenya (Mwabu, Mwanzia, & Liambila, 1995) to 64 percent in Zambia (Kahenya & Lake, 1994). Such evidence led the United Nations (UN) Research Institute for Social Development (UNRISD) to conclude that "Of all measures proposed for raising revenue for local people, this [user fees] is probably the most ill advised" (United Nations Research

Institute for Social Development, 2000; Whitehead, Dahlgren, & Evans, 2001, p. 834).

A variant model of user fees has been the Bamako Initiative (BI), in which the fees go into community-owned "revolving funds" to be spent and controlled locally. This model is still running in Benin, Mali, and Guinea. However, "a large proportion of the poor still do not use key health services in all three countries," and Bamako Initiative health centers have become a service for the affluent (Blas, 2004). After twelve years, government subsidies to the BI system in Guinea still benefit richer groups proportionately more than they do the poorest.

It is clear, of course, that any abolition of fees would carry significant additional costs in the short and medium term, since not only would any revenue stream be lost, but also a large body of pent-up demand would be released. Experiences from Uganda, Zambia, and South Africa (Gilson & McIntyre, 2005) show that there are real dangers if the abolition of fees is not properly prepared and resourced. If there are not appropriate increases in staffing, equipment, and other supplies, the result could be the inundation of local services. Such a change of policy therefore requires practical and material/financial support rather than simply a general Bank statement that it has "no blanket policy" on user fees.

Ooms (2006) goes further and challenges the whole "illusion" of sustainability as a criterion for planning services for the poor. Sustainability of services was part of the rationale for user fees, or for community insurance schemes such as the Bamako Initiative that have been shown to produce less equitable outcomes. Ooms points out that it is impossible for the poorest countries to sustain adequate levels of health care services from their own resources, and emphasizes the need for more long-term and guaranteed assistance from the wealthiest countries. In a recent policy debate on global health system reform, Sachs makes this point even more powerfully:

> Let's recognize the iron laws of extreme poverty involved here. A typical tropical sub-Saharan African country has an annual income of perhaps $350 per person per year, of which much income is earned in kind (as food production for home use), rather than as money income. The government might be able to mobilize 15 percent of the $350 in taxes from the domestic economy. That produces a little over $50 per person per year in total government revenues (and in many countries, much less). This tiny sum must be divided among all government functions: executive, legislative, and judicial offices; police; defense; education; and so on. The health sector is lucky to claim $10 per person per year out of this, but even rudimentary health care requires roughly four times that amount. (In rich countries, public spending on health is $2,500 per person or more.) Foreign aid is therefore not a luxury for African health. It is a life-and-death necessity (2007).

Encourage Private Health Insurance

One of the reasons the World Bank and other agencies have promoted user fees has been to stimulate the emergence of insurance schemes even in the poorest countries: but even advocates of this approach have struggled to find supporting evidence. One major USAID-funded workshop in Zimbabwe analyzing "lessons learned" on health care financing concluded that "user fees are vital to the introduction of any type of insurance system" (McEuen & McGaugh, 1997). Despite this, extensive surveys by USAID-funded Data for Decision Making (DDM) could find only limited evidence of success in such health insurance schemes operating in developing countries:[2]

> DDM research . . . indicated that only small percentages of the populations studied had any kind of health insurance, and that insurance schemes currently do not contribute significant resources to total health financing. Current insurance schemes also tend to cover mainly the more wealthy income groups or the formally employed, limiting the reach of such schemes into the lower income or rural populations (McEuen & McGaugh, 1997).

The Bank has been keen to promote community-based health insurance schemes, but many have been on a very small scale. In Kenya, one scheme studied for Partnerships for Health Reform (PHR) had managed to enlist only 0.3 percent of its target population and by 1998 had only the hospital's staff as members, while other such schemes surveyed in Uganda, Tanzania, and the Democratic Republic of Congo had either targeted tiny communities (which arguably lack the resources to create a sizable risk pool) or failed to achieve any significant wider support (Musau, 2008). A DDM-sponsored study of insurance failures in a variety of developing countries found, for example, that "Zambia's local districts are receiving less funding than before the reform, and user fees may be limiting access. In most countries insurance reforms have been associated with shifting of resources from the general 'solidarity pool' to private insurance and private providers who attend wealthier patients . . ." (Berman & Bossert, 2000, p. 10). Indeed, by 1997 the Bank concluded that "Because of cost and the pronounced market failure that occurs in private health insurance, this is not a viable option for risk-pooling at the national level in low and middle income countries" (World Bank, 1997, p. 8).

The Bank's ideologically driven search for market-led policies as a means to resolve gaps in health care has led it into the contradictory position of promoting policies which research shows to be ineffective, such as social health insurance in countries with very small proportion of formal sector workers and a patchwork of small-scale insurance schemes which have also proven to be unable to draw in sufficient low-income subscribers to cover the rural and urban poor. Nonetheless, eight years later, together with its most commercial, propprivate sector wing, the International Finance Corporation (IFC), the Bank was again collaborating with leading neoliberal academics and executives from major health insurance companies and health maintenance organizations (HMOs), discussing the economics of voluntary health insurance at low-income levels (Wharton School, 2008). At the end of 2007, the IFC again took the lead in establishing a US$500 million "equity investment fund" plus another US$400–US$500 million vehicle to finance local banks lending to entrepreneurs setting up for-profit business in African health care, looking to a market projected by McKinsey's at US$21 billion a year by 2016 (*Economist*, 2007). The IFC argues that investors could expect "compelling financial returns" on their investment, and focuses strongly on for-profit private providers (International Finance Corporation, 2007).

Promote Contracts with the Private Sector or NGOs

The enthusiasm of some donors for the establishment of contracts with the private sector or NGOs in low- and middle-income countries appears to flow predominantly from the desire to transfer ideological norms and organizational paradigms—including some which would create electoral difficulties if applied in the donor countries themselves—from the developed to the developing countries, regardless of the managerial and other problems that inevitably arise.

Its link to globalization is that contracting out services ("steering rather than rowing") is part of the economic and *new public management* philosophy dominating much global policy discourse, which aims for a minimal public sector and maximum private sector involvement. Moreover, the recipients of the contracts are likely to be multinational corporations or their subsidiaries whose interests in global services provision has underpinned, in part, the European Union's push for further liberalization commitments by developing countries under the WTO General Agreement on Trade in Services (GATS). Contracts can in theory be used to regulate any part of the health system, covering not only support services, but also clinical care, again from public or private sector providers. However the contract culture that has emerged leaves a number of unresolved problems. As Ling (2000, p. 99) explains, "Contracts always have 'gaps,' performance indicators can always be manipulated or used perversely, and even worse, as 'contract culture' takes over from trust and good will, everyone looks to exploit these opportunities more forcefully."

Purchasing from Private Providers in Developing Countries

Developing countries can face pressure from global bodies and from powerful donors (notably the World Bank and USAID) which are ideologically committed to privatization and the expansion of the private sector (Akin, Birdsall, & de Ferranti, 1987; World Bank, 1993; Skaar, 1998; Mudyara-bikwa, 2000; IFC [International Finance Corporation], 2002). In 1997, for example, Peru's government opened up health services for private sector providers as a condition of IMF financial support. Most loans to Latin American and Caribbean countries from the World Bank and International Development Bank (IDB) favored private financing and provision of health systems in place of public sector provision: one 1998 loan to Nicaragua involved "modernizing" public hospitals by creating private wards for fee-paying patients (Armada & Muntaner, 2004, pp. 31–32). Among the alleged attractions of the policy in the eyes of its enthusiasts is that it facilitates "using the private sector's greater flexibility and generally better morale" and "using competition to increase effectiveness and efficiency" (Loevinsohn & Harding, 2005). Yet an extensive USAID-funded literature review has noted that "contracting health services to the private sector is a policy that is frequently recommended, but evidence of its effectiveness is lacking" (Rannan-Eliya & Somanathan, 2005, p. 9). This lack of supporting evidence has not deterred USAID, whose Private Sector Partnerships (PSP) web site notes with approval changes in Indonesia which it claims had "successfully shifted market share from predominant reliance on the public sector to reliance on the private sector. The Indonesian case study examines the policies and programs implemented to incentivize the private sector to enter the Reproductive Health/ Family Planning marketplace" (USAID, 2008).

Private provision of health care, however, often combines higher costs beyond the reach of poorer households with very low quality treatment. McPake & Mills (2000, p. 813) further find that private-for-profit providers seldom offer services "of a public health nature," even immunization. Instead they "over-prescribe in general" and tend to use excessive, unnecessary technology. Evidence from developed economies (UK) and in some developing countries such as Thailand shows that far from improving efficiency, the purchase of publicly funded care from private sector providers serves to increase costs and thus drain resources out of limited public sector budgets (Brugha & Zwi, 2002; Lister, 2008; Player & Leys, 2008).

Maximum Involvement of the Private Sector

Without drawing clear distinctions between private for-profit and nonprofit providers, both the World Bank and USAID want to promote greater collaboration with the private sector. Axelsson, Bustreo, and Harding (2003) making explicit if evidence-free presumptions of "greater cost effectiveness of the private sector compared to the public sector" and the superior "efficiency" of the for-profit private sector (Skaar, 1998). Governments would be relied upon to purchase, regulate, and, in some cases, subsidize private sector services. The Bank's commercial lending arm, the International

Finance Corporation (IFC), which clearly favors the for-profit private sector, welcomes the fact that "[t]he aim of much of recent health care reforms in several countries has been to increase the role of the private sector as the provider (rather than the financer) of care" (International Finance Corporation, 2002, p. 3).

The IFC only supports financially viable (profitable) projects. Its strategy is primarily centered in urban areas where (especially in poorer countries) the private market is "most mature" (International Finance Corporation, 2002, p. 36). It wants to "contribute to the financial protection against ill health and to the strengthening of the middle class," and evinces little interest in the health of the poorest (International Finance Corporation, 2002). It now views Africa as an expanding and potentially profitable market for health care provided on a for-profit basis (International Finance Corporation, 2007).

However, even nonprofit private provision may be no more, or even *less*, efficient than centrally funded public systems. Costa Rica, for example, has been under pressure from the Bank to privatize its health system, the most successful in Central America and one which provides comprehensive primary health care to over 90 percent of the population. However, its experiments with nonprofit provider cooperatives in the early 1990s showed them to be more expensive, less efficient, and no better in quality than the mainstream public sector services. The co-ops also had a negative impact on the efficiency and costs of the public clinics (Homedes & Ugalde, 2005).

The dismal evidentiary record of private sector involvement led to the Bank muting somewhat its enthusiasm, with the health chapter in its 2004 *World Development Report* including a number of passages highlighting market failure and the shortcomings of private sector providers. The 2004 *WDR* explicitly rejects any "one size fits all" system and places little emphasis on decentralization, competition, privatization, user fees, or market-style mechanisms that were once its health policy mainstays and which, apparently, remain so with its commercial IFC lending arm.

Privatization of Existing Public Sector Services

Privatization of services hitherto provided by publicly owned agencies may be linked with moves to decentralization or corporatization (Preker & Harding, 2000; Sein, 2001), or may flow from other aspects of New Public Management and policy reform.

Some World Bank economists see privatization as following naturally from what they term the "autonomization" and corporatization of hospitals (Preker & Harding, 2000). However, very little full-scale privatization of health care facilities and services has been carried through in more advanced economies, or even in the transition economies of the former Soviet Union and Eastern Europe. In Chile, the Pinochet regime drastically cut health care spending to 34 percent of its 1974 level by 1990. The proportion of private beds more than doubled to 25 percent between 1981 and 1992. But even under a military dictatorship and at its peak of "authoritarian neo-liberalism," Pinochet pulled back from privatizing the entire system, and left 75 percent of hospital beds in the public sector (Taylor, 2008).

Public-Private Partnerships

A different adaptation to the pressures of the market can be found in the emerging UN and WHO concept of Global Public Private Partnerships (GPPPs) (Buse & Walt, 2000). By 2001 around seventy such partnerships were identified, many of them involving drug companies and research projects (Buse & Waxman, 2001; Evans & Chen, 2002).

This stance has been controversial among NGOs and within the WHO's own structures. Critics point out that the WHO, with its global budget from all sources of US$1.7 billion per year in 2004–2005 (rising to an average US$2.4 billion per annum over the six years to 2013), with a majority coming in voluntary donations, and upwards of US$500 million a year in contributions from specific health initiatives (Director-General, 2008; WHO, 2008), is potentially vulnerable to political and economic pressure from much wealthier drug companies and private corporations, making any "partnership" profoundly unequal (Hardon, 2001). There are also fears that the privately backed campaigns may result in a reduced local capacity to produce vaccines, and a rejection of local generic products by a skeptical public convinced that the cheaper product is inferior (Hardon, 2001). Any attempt to provide developing countries with the modern medical techniques that have enabled health gains in the advanced economies would also require the additional development of modern, well-equipped hospitals and specialist staff—yet the resources and commitment to this are lacking (see Chapters 7 and 9, this volume).

Competition between Rival Service Providers

To create conditions for competition, centralized systems must be broken up and decentralized. Although competition brings with it new overheads in the form of transaction costs, the Bank has not explicitly broken from the assumption in its 1987 and 1993 policy documents that competitive, market-style policies with maximum use of the private sector are a general formula to address the reform of health care systems to all countries and circumstances, even though the possibilities for establishing genuine competition between health care providers, or even "managed competition" between rival health funds, are largely restricted to the wealthier countries.

In developing countries, where incomes are chronically low, promarket reformers fear that competition between providers would be eliminated if publicly provided services were available free of charge to all, including the wealthiest service users. This, they argue, would deter the wealthy and middle classes from either paying into private insurance schemes or pay-ing to use alternative private hospitals (Shaw & Ainsworth, 1995). Even where a degree of competition exists, it by no means guarantees a positive long-term outcome for health care services to the poor. One USAID-funded study of Tanzania notes the profoundly unequal lack of provision of com-petitive for-profit private health care in rural areas (Munishi, Yazbeck, & Lionetti, 1995).

Decentralization—Does One Size Fit All?

The call for decentralization is a theme running through most studies and reports advocating health system reform in wealthy and poor countries alike. It is "generally recognized as a major strategy for health reform" (Rannan-Eliya, van Zantern, & Yazbeck, 1996, p. 5; Valentine, 2008). In abstract, the notion of "transferring power from unconcerned and inef-ficient central bureaucrats to the people" is hard to oppose (Homedes & Ugalde, 2005). Yet as much as any element of the generic health reform prescription, decentralization needs to be geared to the specific needs and political and social realities in each country. The results of decentralization can also prove very different from those intended, as an extensive literature review for USAID-funded Partnership for Health Reform discovered:

1. Control over service provision may be captured at local level by elites who are even less responsive than central government to the needs of the poor.
2. Urban populations are often more politically influential than rural populations and therefore better placed to keep a larger share of resources.
3. Decentralization may also offer new openings for local-level corruption.
4. The new system may find itself struggling in the face of a lack of local managerial skills and expertise.
5. Decentralization may also mean smaller-scale and less well-resourced providers, which wind up delivering less training and skills for staff and lower quality care.
6. Smaller organizations also lose potential bargaining power and econ-omies of scale in negotiation with major suppliers.
7. Smaller-scale, more local structures almost inevitably offer less scope to tackle inequalities in the terms and conditions of health workers (Rannan-Eliya et al., 1996, pp. 5–6).

Granting local hospitals and health services powers to raise local funds may liberate local entrepreneurial talent in a wealthy area but condemn poorer inner-city and rural health services to permanent underfunding and second-class status (Mackintosh, 2001; Homedes & Ugalde, 2005). In Mexico, for example, an IDB report found that decentralization led to a serious decline in the quality and quantity of primary and hospital services for the poor (Homedes & Ugalde, 2005, p. 87). The results of decentralization have been "mixed, at best" (Bossert, 2000, p. 3).

Corporatization

The notion of going beyond decentralization to establish local health care providers as autonomous, free-standing corporate bodies in their own right has been gathering momentum among the advocates of market-style reforms (Preker & Harding, 2003). In the developed countries, this is not new. The British government's marketizing measures separated provider units from purchasers and led to "self-governing trusts," the first of which were launched in 1991. New Zealand's government also experimented along the same lines in the early 1990s, with profoundly mixed results (Lovelace, 2003). "Foundation Hospitals" in Spain and Sweden (and now Britain) have gone further in floating hospitals as free-standing "corporatized" enterprises with their own discretion to borrow funds and conduct deals with the private sector. This type of autonomy may prove, as with one Swedish hospital, simply a transition point to full-scale privatization (Busse, van der Grinten, & Svensson, 2002). The Swedish government later prohibited any further privatization of health services. Hospital autonomy in Brazil has not improved the quality of care (Homedes & Ugalde, 2005), while in other countries, including Argentina, Chile, Uruguay, Ecuador, and Tunisia, relatively limited experiments with hospital autonomy have yielded mixed and generally poor results (Preker & Harding, 2003).

These policies, we will argue later, are attributable to globalization forces alone. National, demographic, and technological factors, and the political preferences of elites within nations, also affect the willingness and extent of their adoption. There is one uniquely global set of pressures, however, that are affecting health systems: that of trade treaties.

Health as Commodity: The Pressure for Global Trade in Health Services

Services are assuming an increasingly important economic role in most high- and some middle-income countries. The key trade treaty covering services is the WTO's General Agreement on Trade in Services (GATS), designed specifically to increase trade in all forms of such services. There are four "modalities" of this trade (with examples from health services):

1. Cross-border delivery of services (laboratory analyses, telehealth).
2. Consumption of services abroad (health/medical tourism).
3. Commercial presence (foreign investors in private health insurance or facilities).

4. Presence of persons (special GATS visas for temporary movement of health workers from one country to another).

Of key concern is the impact of liberalization of services trade in sectors important to health: health care, education, water, and sanitation. GATS proponents argue that whether liberalization in these services produces a net public health gain or loss depends upon the domestic regulatory structures put in place to manage its impacts (Adlung & Carzaniga, 2002). This may be true. But, with respect to health services, the 2000 *WHR* cautioned, "Few countries have developed adequate strategies to regulate the private financing and provision of health services," noting that "the harm caused by market abuses is difficult to remedy after the fact" (World Health Organization, 2000).

Health and other essential public services meet basic human needs in a way that many other services do not; and commitments made under the GATS essentially lock in existing levels of commercialization with the prospect of increased liberalization in that service sector only increasing, and never decreasing, the extent of commercial involvement. Countries can elect to commit only some sectors and not others, although there is a requirement for all WTO member nations to continue negotiations to progressively liberalize all service sectors. While few developed countries have made substantial health services commitments (with some, such as Canada, emphatically declaring their intention never to do so), many developing countries have done so (Adlung & Carzaniga, 2006), often with fewer limitations than those specified by high-income countries and without a full awareness of the consequences. These consequences include the right of foreign investors or service providers to invoke trade dispute resolution processes if denied access to a country's domestic market, so denying similar opportunities to domestic actors will become politically infeasible.

Measures to increase private investment and provision in health services are often justified on the basis that they "free up" public resources for more effective and targeted provision to the poor. The weight of evidence, however, finds the opposite: commercialization in health services or insurance creates inequities in access (Barrientos & Lloyd-Sherlock, 2000; Bennett & Gilson, 2001; Cruz-Saco, 2002; Barrientos & Lloyd-Sherlock, 2003; Hutton, 2004) and also in health outcomes (Koivusalo & Mackintosh, 2005). Much of this chapter so far has refuted this claim. The experience of Thailand in cross-border health services trade offers further and more particular cautions.

Thailand has not made commitments in health services under the GATS but has actively participated in global trade in health services since the early 1990s, notably the promotion of private urban hospitals and health tourism. Facilitated through tax incentives to investment in private hospitals, this has enabled a rapid and substantial rise in the number of foreign patients being treated, most coming from high-income countries such as Japan, the United States, Taiwan, the UK, and Australia, but also increasingly from Middle Eastern oil-rich nations. In 2001, more than one million foreign patients were estimated to have been treated in both private and public facilities (though predominantly in the former). The government policy is to continue to increase the number of foreign patients.

The resources used to service one foreigner may be equivalent to those used to service four or five Thais, equivalent to three or four million Thai patients in 2001. In order to address the increased demand for health professionals created by foreign patients and the internal brain drain, the Thai government in 2004 approved a policy to increase by over 10,000 the number of doctors in the following fifteen years. This measure may address some of the future shortage of physicians, but does not address immediate needs or deal with the question of how incomes generated by medical tourism can be better harnessed to benefit the local population (Pachanee & Wibulpolprasert, 2006).

The rapid growth in medical tourism, estimated at over 30 percent annually, is not restricted to Thailand. Other countries ramping up private hospitals for private, or privately insured, overseas patients are India, Singapore, South Korea, and the Philippines. Increasingly, such hospitals are seeking ISO or other forms of certification to convey levels of quality comparable to that of hospitals in high-income countries. Together with the flow of health workers from developing to developed countries (primarily nurses, many of whom end up working in private extended-care facilities for elderly persons), we are witnessing the rapid creation of a global private health system for those who can afford it. The long-term implications for public health systems—which, unlike private systems, remain locked within national borders—are troubling, especially given the lack of adequate public health systems and health workers in many of the countries seeking to benefit from these private flows.

Governments may still want to experiment with commercialization in some components of their health systems. But until governments have demonstrated their ability to regulate private investment and provision in health services in ways that enhance health equity, they should avoid making any commitments in binding trade treaties. It is not clear that any government, anywhere in the world, has met this test. There are further political and ethical considerations associated with the GATS, underscored by the South African experience. One of the last acts of that country's apartheid regime was to commit to fully liberalize trade in health services. The postapartheid government subsequently passed national legislation guaranteeing certain health rights by requiring inter alia needs testing before service providers can set up shop in different parts of the country. Intended to improve equity in access, this provision violates its GATS commitments, leaving the country vulnerable to costly disputes (Sinclair, 2005). Such an outcome—while still only potential—leads some to call for canceling all existing GATS commitments on health services and removing health services from the scope of subsequent negotiations (Woodward, 2005).

Is Globalization the Real Driver of Health Sector Reforms?

So far this chapter has examined the prevailing pattern of change or "reform" to health systems and one common feature emerges: whether the changes have arisen from the aspiration of national leaders and policymakers to match global trends or been imposed by global bodies, none of the main menu of policies arises directly from globalization as such. Of course the predominance of neoliberalism reflects the economic and ideological domination of transnational corporations and the wealthiest OECD countries. This can also result in increased political pressure on middle- and low-income countries to comply with the line of "reform" favored by the international financial institutions and donor agencies.

But the policies that feature most prominently in the checklist of health system reforms associated with such advice are themselves not a logical or necessary response to external global pressures. The available evidence suggests that these policies do not result in leaner or more cost-effective government. They do not reduce, but *increase* costs; they do not increase, but *impede* efficiency. If the aim is to restrict government and other spending or to be more competitive, any country would do better to avoid these expensive "reforms."

Nor are the policies an appropriate response to the burden of disease and health needs. For example, all but a tiny handful of Bank documents, studies, and projects completely ignore the issue of mental health care provision, despite the appalling lack of resources for mental health (WHO, 2001; Beeharry, Whiteford, Chambers, & Baingana, 2002), and similarly ignore the rapidly growing issue of the health needs of older people (Lloyd-Sherlock, 2005). The favored menu of reforms, instead, is drawn from an ideological "one size fits all" approach, and has been applied with various degrees of commitment and conviction by national governments that have had little or no hand in devising them.

So if globalization itself is not the direct wellspring of reforms and policies to reshape health systems, how can its influence and impact on health care best be understood? Stiglitz, a latter-day Keynesian critic of the IMF and World Bank, defines globalization as "the closer integration of the countries and peoples of the world which has been brought about by the enormous reduction in costs of transportation and communication, and the breaking down of artificial barriers to the flows of goods, services, capital, knowledge and (to a lesser extent) people across borders" (Stiglitz, 2002, p. 9).

To understand what has gone wrong with globalization, Stiglitz focuses attention on "the three main institutions that govern globalization: the IMF, the World Bank and the WTO" (2002, p. 10). Stiglitz also points to the abrupt change of emphasis in the World Bank following a "purge" of its top officials in the early 1980s, to be replaced by neoliberals appointed under Ronald Reagan. An organization which had once investigated the failure of markets in developing countries and focused on government action to reduce poverty was transformed into one which saw "government as the problem"; there was a similar sea change in the IMF (Stiglitz, 2002, pp. 13–14).

These changes at the top level of two global bodies have had a major and lasting impact on the health systems of the developing countries. Following the Stiglitz approach, the effects of globalization on health systems can be most clearly identified in the low- and middle-income countries through analyzing the impact of global institutions, including the WHO and the new global donor bodies (e.g., the Bill and Melinda Gates Foundation, the Global Fund to Fight AIDS, Tuberculosis and Malaria (GFATM), the President's Emergency Plan for AIDS Relief [PEPFAR]) on financially dependent governments. By contrast, the OECD countries, whose governments generally enjoy greater scope for autonomy in decision making, within the context of well-developed health systems, but which also face generally greater political pressures arising from public expectations, have mostly charted more limited and cautious paths of reform.

Where is the Counterfactual?

A growing body of increasingly critical and independent literature has begun to question assumptions that have stood unproven at the center of World Bank/ IMF orthodoxy since the early 1980s. The most recent examples include the debunking of five common "myths" on health systems including the notion that private providers are more efficient than the public sector (Hsiao & Heller, 2007), and Wagstaff's critical review of the limitations of social health insurance (2007). However, it is less easy to find evidence to support a counterfactual analysis, since few countries have had the combination of political will and material/human resources to pursue an alternative course.

Some counterfactuals, although largely hypothetical, have been estimated on an economic basis. In Sri Lanka an estimate has been made of the economic benefit that would have accrued if a malaria eradication program had been in place over the thirty years 1947–1977: this calculates that national revenues would have increased by US$7.4 billion at a cost of just US$52 million (Sabri, 2004). We also have a good idea what many countries of sub-Saharan Africa would have aspired to in the way of health services in the absence of pressure from the World Bank and IMF SAPs, since a number of them took the opportunity immediately after achieving independence to establish publicly funded health care, free at point of use, and supported by substantial economic expansion in the 1960s and early 1970s. Most of these—such as Kenya, Uganda, Zimbabwe, and post-1979 Nicaragua—registered substantial gains in life expectancy and reductions in child mortality (Gatheru & Shaw, 1998; Birn, Zimmerman, & Garfield,

2000; Colgan, 2002). By contrast, health outcomes have fallen back in almost every country that has implemented SAPs since the 1980s, which sharply reduced state spending on health care and imposed user fees. It must be recognized, however, that this was not purely the result of health policy: the same period was also the one of sharp economic decline and the start of the HIV/AIDS epidemic, which weakened health systems were in no position to confront.

Despite poor evidence to support it, the odds have been stacked in favor of market-oriented health sector reform, not least because of the lack of coherent opposition. Yeates (2001, p. 29) notes the "marked absence" of any international institution with equivalent influence and economic power to the Bank or IMF "advancing a social democratic or redistributive agenda." The voice of the WHO can easily be ignored by governments preoccupied with the conditionalities of loans and credit ratings from the international financial institutions, or securing USAID funding for a project.

While there is absence of solid evidence to support a "counterfactual" model, the Bank itself acknowledged in its 2004 *WDR* the striking success of the Cuban government's health system, despite Cuba's very obvious rejection of every one of the Bank's main lines of health system reform. Cuba's health system has remained centralized, nationalized, and free to all at point of use (with the exception of copayments for prescriptions), is funded from state revenues, and has managed to combine an extensive and effective network of primary health care and public health together with high-technology hospital treatment. In the absence of significant economic growth, and despite over forty years of a US economic blockade and sixteen years after losing Soviet economic support, Cuba has continued to spend 6.6 percent of gross domestic product (GDP) on health care, increasing life expectancy and reducing child mortality to levels comparable to Canada, and better than those in the United States (PAHO, 2008).

The unique political context of Cuba suggests that it could not be read across as a "counterfactual" to other developing countries, few of which have had leadership willing to remain as committed for over four decades to such a radical set of policies and priorities that required economic sacrifices in other sectors. The ongoing US embargo, forcing Cuba's exclusion from the mainstream of world trade and market pressures, and its alignment with countries willing to defy US pressure, have also allowed an enlarged "policy space," permitting a very different line of policy from indebted African countries dependent on IMF loans.

However, some other governments in very different circumstances (notably Sri Lanka, Ghana, Thailand, and Costa Rica) have also withstood pressures to conform to the globalized menu of health reform and retained more progressive and equitable policies, delivering improved health outcomes for their population. While the conventional wisdom of neoliberalism has been that governments in low-income countries lack the tax base to roll out or sustain publicly funded health care, this assumption is strongly contested by Rannan-Eliya & Somanathan (2005), drawing conclusions from a systematic survey of sixteen Asian countries. They argue that user fees could be reduced or eliminated by government spending as little as 2 percent of GDP on a universal health system that would give most benefit to the poor.

Insofar as globalization—in the form of global bodies compelling dependent governments into following a line of policy, or global charities implementing vertical programs without building any wider or sustainable infrastructure of health care—can be seen as the driver of health sector "reforms," it appears to be driving them in the opposite direction to the available evidence and delivering predictably poor results. The success of policies contrary to those prescribed by the World Bank/IMF appears to be as consistent as the failure of the neoliberal reforms in improving health and delivering equitably accessible health systems (Homedes & Ugalde, 2005; Unger et al., 2006). The Bank's 2004 *WDR* is strikingly short of positive examples to illustrate the usefulness of the policies it had prescribed for over fifteen years.

By contrast, even relatively limited resources channeled along more productive (and evidence-informed) lines can improve health equity and deliver remarkable human (and economic) benefits not only to the poor but to the whole of society. In contradistinction to the nostrums that still dominate global policy discourse on health system reform, the Health Systems Knowledge Network of the WHO Commission on Social Determinants of Health in its narrative review of evidence concluded rather succinctly that the key overarching features of heath systems that generate preferential health benefits for socially disadvantaged groups, as well as general population gains, are:

1. The leadership, processes, and mechanisms that leverage intersectoral action across government departments to promote population health.
2. Organizational arrangements and practices that involve population groups and civil society organizations, and particularly those working with socially disadvantaged groups, in decisions and actions that identify, address, and allocate resources to health needs.
3. Heath care financing and provision arrangements that aim at universal coverage and offer particular benefits for socially disadvantaged groups (specifically, improved access to health care, better protection against the impoverishing costs of illness, and the redistribution of welfare between rich and poor that sustains health equity gains).
4. The revitalization of primary health care, as a strategy that reinforces and integrates the other health equity promoting features (Gilson, Doherty, Loewenson, Francis, with inputs and contributions from members of the Knowledge Network, 2007).

Needed now is a new global epistemic community, projecting a vision-ary health reform project based upon what has worked well in the past, that can expose the weaknesses of so-called reforms that have not proved themselves to be either beneficial or cost-effective, and promote an alter-native line of policy that can replace these failed and costly policies with a new approach that will enable health systems to deliver more and better treatment on a more equitable basis in the future.

NOTES

1. The IMF remains highly influential in most low-income and least developed countries which are still reliant on it to manage balance-of-payment prob-lems or currency crises; but an increasing number of South Asian and Latin American countries are pooling their own foreign currency reserves to man-age these problems without IMF assistance and intrusion (Weisbrot, 2006).
2. The workshop included participation of government representatives, health staff, academics, NGOs, and donor agencies from Botswana, Ghana, Malawi, Mozambique, South Africa, Zambia, and Zimbabwe, with addi-tional representatives from Ethiopia, Kenya, and Uganda (McEuen & McGaugh, 1997, p. xi).

REFERENCES

Adlung, R., & Carzaniga, A. (2002). Health services under the General Agreement on Trade in Services. In C. Vieira & N. Drager (eds.), *Trade in health services: Global, regional and country perspectives* (pp. 13–33). Washington, DC: Pan American Health Organization. Retrieved from: http://www.paho.org/English/HDP/HDD/06Adlu.pdf .

———. (2006). Update on GATS commitments and negotiations. In C. Blouin, N. Drager, & R. Smith (eds.), *International trade in health services and the GATS—current issues and debates* (pp. 83–100). New York: World Bank.

Akin, J., Birdsall, N., & de Ferranti, D. (1987). *Financing health services in devel-oping countries: An agenda for reform.* World Bank policy studies. Washing-ton, DC: World Bank.

Amanfo, J. (2006). Ridge hospital detains baby over c3.2m. Ghana: *Public Agenda.*

Armada, F., & Muntaner, C. (2004). The visible fist of the market: Health reforms in Latin America. In M. Singer & A. Castro (eds.), *Unhealthy health policy* (pp. 29–42). Walnut Creek, CA: Altamira Press.

Australian Agency for International Development (AusAID). (2008). *Australia's aid program.* Global Education Web site. Australian Agency for International Development (AusAID) [online]. Retrieved from: http://www.globaleducation.edna.edu.au/globaled/go/pid/24.

Axelsson, H., Bustreo, F., & Harding, A. (2003). *Private sector participation in child health: A review of World Bank projects, 1993–2002.* HNP Discussion Papers. Washington, DC: World Bank. Retrieved from: http://siteresources.world-bank.org/HEALTHNUTRITIONANDPOPULATION/Resources/281627–1095698140167/AxelssonPrivateSector-whole.pdf.

Barraclough, S. (2005). Australia's international health relations in 2003. *Australia and New Zealand Health Policy, 2.*

Barrientos, A., & Lloyd-Sherlock, P. (2000). Reforming health insurance in Argentina and Chile. *Health Policy Plan., 15*, 417–23.

———. (2003). Health insurance reforms in Latin America—cream skimming, equity and cost containment. In Louise Haagh & Camilla T. Helgo (eds.), *Social policy reform and market governance in Latin America* (pp. 183–99). London: Macmillan.

Beeharry, G., Whiteford, H., Chambers, D., & Baingana, F. (2002). *Outlining the scope for public sector involvement in mental health.* Health, nutrition and population (HNP) discussion paper. Washington, DC: World Bank. Retrieved from: http://www-wds.worldbank.org/servlet/main?menuPK=64187510&pagePK=6419 3027&piPK=64187937&theSitePK=523679&entityID=000265513_2004051714 5654.

Bennett, S., & Gilson, L. (2001). *Health financing: Designing and implementing pro-poor policy.* London: Health Systems Resource Centre. Retrieved from: http://www.dfidhealthrc.org/publications/health_sector_financing/Health_financing_pro-poor.pdf.

Berman, P., & Bossert, T. (2000). *A decade of health sector reform in developing countries: What have we learned?* DDM Report no. 81. Cambridge, MA: Harvard School of Public Health. Retrieved from: http://www.hsph.harvard.edu/ihsp/publications/pdf/closeout.PDF.

Birn, A.-E., Zimmerman, S., & Garfield, R. (2000). To decentralize or not to decentralize; is that the question? Nicaraguan health policy under structural adjustment in the 1990s. *International Journal of Health Services, 1*, 111–28.

Blas, E. (2004). The proof of the reform is in the implementation. *The International Journal of Health Planning and Management, 19*, S3–S23.

Bossert, T. J. (2000). *Decentralisation of health systems in Latin America: A comparative study of Chile, Colombia and Bolivia. Data for decision making project.* Harvard School of Public Health. Retrieved from: http://www.hsph.harvard.edu/ihsp/publications/pdf/lac/Decentralization45.PDF.

Braveman, P. (1998). *Monitoring equity in health: A policy-oriented approach in low- and middle-income countries.* Geneva: WHO. Retrieved from: http://www.gega.org.za/download/braveman.pdf.

Breman, A., & Shelton, C. (2001). *Structural adjustment and health: A literature review of the debate, its role-players and presented empirical evidence.* CMH Working Paper Series No. WG6:6. Geneva: WHO: Commission on Macroeconomics and Health.

Bretton Woods Project. (2008). Donor contributions to IDA up record amount: Norway, civil society not satisfied. *Update, 59,* 1 February.

Brown, P. (2002). WHO to revise its method for ranking health systems. *British Medical Journal, 324,* 190.

Brugha, R., & Zwi, A. (2002). Global approaches to private sector provision: Where is the evidence? In K. Lee, K. Buse, & S. Fustukian (eds.), *Health policy in a globalising world* (pp. 63–77). Cambridge: Cambridge University Press.

Buse, K., & Walt, G. (2000). Global public-private partnerships: Part I—a new development in health? *Bulletin of the World Health Organization, 78,* 549–61.

Buse, K., & Waxman, A. (2001). Public-private health partnerships: A strategy for WHO. *WHO Bulletin, 79,* 748–54.

Busse, R., van der Grinten, T., & Svensson, P. G. (2002). Regulating entrepreneurial behaviour in hospitals: Theory and practice. In R. B. Saltman, R. Busse, & E. Mossialos (eds.), *Regulating entrepreneurial behaviour in European health care systems.* Buckingham, UK: Open University Press.

Colgan, A.-L. (2002). *Hazardous to health: the World Bank and IMF in Africa.* Africa Action Position Paper. Washington, DC: Africa Action. Retrieved from: www.africaaction.org/action/sap0204.htm.

Creese, A. (1997). User fees: They don't reduce costs, and they increase inequity. *British Medical Journal,* 315, 202–3.

Creese, A., & Kutzin, J. (1995). *Lessons from cost-recovery in health. Forum on health sector reform.* Discussion Paper no.2. Geneva: WHO Division of Strengthening Health Services.

Cruz-Saco, M. A. (2002). *Global insurance companies and the privatisation of pensions and health care in Latin America—the case of Peru.* In GASPP Seminar No. 5 organized in collaboration with the ILO-SES Programme and WHO, at the University Centre (IUC), 26–28 September 2002, in Dubrovnik, Croatia. Waltham, MA: Brandeis University. Retrieved from: http://www.brandeis.edu/ibs/rosenberg_papers/cruz-saco_paper.pdf.

Cueto, M. (2004). The origins of primary health care and selective primary health care. *American Journal of Public Health,* 94, 1864–74.

Danida (Royal Danish Ministry of Foreign Affairs). (2005). *Africa—development and security: The government's priorities for Danish cooperation with Africa 2005–2009.* Copenhagen: Ministry of Foreign Affairs. Retrieved from: http://www.netpublikationer.dk/um/4888/pdf/africa_development.pdf.

Deber, R. (2000). Thinking before rethinking: Some thoughts about babies and bathwater. *Healthcare Papers,* 1, 25–32.

de Ferranti, D. M. (1985). *Paying for health services in developing countries: An overview.* World Bank Staff Working Papers No. 721. Washington, DC: World Bank. Retrieved from: http://www-wds.worldbank.org/external/default/WDS-ContentServer/WDSP/IB/2003/06/14/000178830_98101903430786/Rendered/PDF/multi0page.pdf.

Denhardt, J. V., & Denhardt, R. B. (2002). *The new public service: Serving, not steering.* New York and London: M.E. Sharpe.

Director-General, (2008). *WHO financial report 2004–2005.* No. A59/28. Geneva: World Health Organization. Retrieved from: http://www.who.int/gb/ebwha/pdf_files/WHA59/A59_28-en.pdf.

Dunne, N. (2000). Fees issue entangles US debt relief plan. *Financial Times* October 17.

Economist. (2007). Of markets and medicines. Big donors are betting on Africa's private sector to improve health. *The Economist* December 19.

Elliott, L. (2006). Britain issues World Bank £50m ultimatum. *The Guardian* September 14.

England, S., Kaddar, M., Nigam, A., & Pinto, M. (2001). *Practice and policies on user fees for immunization in developing countries.* Geneva: WHO Department of Vaccines and Biologicals. Retrieved from: http://www.who.int/vaccines-documents/DocsPDF01/www564.pdf.

Evans, T. C., & Chen, L. C. (2002). *Public-private partnerships in global health.* New York: The Rockefeller Foundation. Retrieved from: http://www.fas.harvard.edu/~acgei/Publications/Chen/LCC_PublicPrivate_Partnerships.pdf.

Flores, W. (2006). *Equity and health sector reform in Latin America and the Caribbean from 1995 to 2005: Approaches and limitations.* Toronto: International Society for Equity in Health. Retrieved from: http://www.iseqh.org/docs/HSR_equity_report2006_en.pdf.

Fontana, A. (2005). *"In limbo": Current status of some HIPC decision point countries.* Brussels: EURODAD European Network on Debt and Development. Retrieved from: http://www.eurodad.org/whatsnew/reports.aspx?id=722.

Fortson, Danny. (2007). Australian health giant Ramsay buys Capio UK. *The Independent* September 7.

Gadelha, A. J., Ugá, A., Almeida, C., Landmann Szwarcwald, C., Travassos, C., Viacava, F., et al. (2001). *Report of the workshop "Health Systems Performance—the World Health Report 2000."* Geneva: World Health Organization.

Retrieved from: http://www.who.int/health-systems-performance/docs/articles/oswaldocruz_report.pdf.

Gatheru, W., & Shaw, R., eds. (1998). *Our problems, our solutions: An economic and public policy agenda for Kenya*. Nairobi, Kenya: Institute of Economic Affairs.

Gilson, L., & McIntyre, D. (2005). Removing user fees for primary care in Africa: The need for careful action. *British Medical Journal, 331*, 762–65.

Gilson, L., Doherty, J., Loewenson, R., Francis, V., with inputs and contributions from members of the Knowledge Network. (2007). *Challenging inequity through health systems: Final report, Knowledge Network on Health Systems, WHO Commission on Social Determinants of Health*. Geneva: WHO Commission on Social Determinants of Health. Retrieved from: http://www.who.int/social_determinants/resources/csdh_media/hskn_final_2007_en.pdf.

Gupta, S., Clements, B., Guin-Siu, M. T., & Leruth, L. (2001). Debt relief and health spending in heavily indebted poor countries. *Finance and Development, 383*.

Hardon, Anita. (2001, March). Immunisation for all? A critical look at the first GAVI partners meeting. *HAI Europe, 6*(1), 1–9.

Hilary, J. (2005). DFID, UK and public services privatization: Time for change. *Global Social Policy, 5*, 134–36.

Homedes, N., & Ugalde, A. (2005). Why neoliberal health reforms have failed in Latin America. *Health Policy, 71*, 83–96.

Hsiao, W., & Heller, P. S. (2007). *What should macroeconomists know about health care policy?* IMF Working Papers No. WP/07/13. Washington, DC: International Monetary Fund. Retrieved from: http://www.imf.org/external/pubs/ft/wp/2007/wp0713.pdf.

Human Rights Watch. (2006). *A high price to pay: Detention of poor patients in Burundian hospitals*. New York: Human Rights Watch. Retrieved from: www.hrw.org; http://hrw.org/reports/2006/burundi0906/.

Hutton, G. (2004). *Charting the path to the World Bank's "no blanket policy on user fees": A look over the past 25 years at the shifting support for user fees in health and education, and reflections on the future* . London: Department for International Development Health Systems Resource Centre. Retrieved from: http://www.dfidhealthrc.org/Shared/publications/Issues_papers/04Hut01.pdf.

International Finance Corporation. (2002). *Topical briefing on health and investing in private healthcare: Strategic directions for IFC*. Washington, DC: IFC.

———. (2007). *The business of health in Africa. Partnering with the private sector to improve people's lives*. Washington, DC: International Finance Corporation World Bank Group. Retrieved from: http://www.ifc.org/ifcext/healthinafrica.nsf/AttachmentsByTitle/IFC_HealthinAfrica_Final/$FILE/IFC_HealthinAfrica_Final.pdf.

International Monetary Fund (IMF). (2008). *Poverty reduction strategy papers (PRSP) (Sorted by country)*. International Monetary Fund [online]. Retrieved from: http://www.imf.org/external/NP/prsp/prsp.asp.

Kahenya, G., & Lake, S. (1994). *User fees and their impact on utilization of key health services*. Lusaka, Zambia: UNICEF.

Kessler, T., & Alexander, N. (2004). *Assessing the risks in the private provision of essential services. Discussion paper for G-24 Technical Group* No. 31. New York and Geneva: United Nations Conference on Trade and Development. Retrieved from: http://www.unctad.org/en/docs/gdsmdpbg2420047_en.pdf; http://www.g24.org/un-kea04.pdf.

Koivusalo, M., & Mackintosh, M. (2005). Health systems and commercialisation: In Search of good sense. In M. Mackintosh & M. Koivusalo (eds.), *Commercialization of health care: Global and local dynamics and policy responses* (pp. 3–21). Basingstoke, UK: Palgrave Macmillan.

Landmann Swzarcwald, C. (2002). On the World Health Organisation's measurement of health inequalities. *Journal of Epidemiology and Community Health,* 56, 177–82.

Laurell, A. C., & Arellano, O. L. (1996). Market commodities and poor relief: The World Bank proposal for health. *International Journal of Health Services,* 26, 1–18.

Lee, K., & Goodman, H. (2002). Global policy networks: The propagation of health care financing reform since the 1980's. In K. Lee, K. Buse, & S. Fustukian (eds.), *Health policy in a globalising world* (pp. 97–119). Cambridge: Cambridge University Press.

Leighton, C., & Wouters, A. (1995). Strategies for achieving health financing reform in Africa. *World Development,* 24, 1511–25.

Ling, T. (2000). Unpacking partnership: The case of health care. In J. Clarke, S. Gerwitz, & E. McLaughlin (eds.), *New managerialism, new welfare* (pp. 82–101). London: Sage Publications, Ltd.

Lister, J. (2005). *Driving the wrong way? A critical guide to the global "health reform" industry.* London: Middlesex University Press.

———. (2008). *The NHS after 60: For patients or profits?* London: Middlesex University Press.

Lloyd-Sherlock, P. (2005). Epidemiological change and health policy for older people in developing countries: Some preliminary thoughts. *Ageing Horizons,* 2, 21–24.

Loevinsohn, B., & Harding, A. (2005). Buying results? Contracting for health service delivery in developing countries. *The Lancet,* 366, 676–81.

Lovelace, J. C. (2003). Foreword. In A. S. Preker & A. Harding (eds.), *Innovations in health service delivery: The corporatization of public hospitals.* Washington, DC: World Bank.

Mackintosh, M. (2001). Do health care systems contribute to inequalities? In D. Leon & G. Walt (eds.), *Poverty, inequality and health: An international perspective* (pp. 175–93). Oxford, UK: Oxford Medical Publications.

McEuen, M., & McGaugh, J. (1997). Initiatives in health care financing: Lessons learned. HHRAA/DDM East/Southern Africa Regional Workshop Proceedings. Data for Decision Making Project. Cambridge, MA: Harvard School for Public Health.

McPake, B., & Mills, A. (2000). What can we learn from international comparisons of health systems and health system reform? *Bulletin of the World Health Organization,* 78, 811–20.

Michaud, C. (2003). *Development assistance for health (DAH): Recent trends and resource allocation.* Prepared for Second Consultation, Commission on Macroeconomics and Health, October 29–30, 2003. Geneva: WHO. Retrieved from: www.who.int/entity/macrohealth/events/health_for_poor/en/dah_trends_nov10.pdf.

Mudyarabikwa, O. (2000). *An examination of public sector subsidies to the private health sector: A Zimbabwe case study.* Equinet Policy Series No. 8. Harare: Regional Network for Equity in Health in Southern Africa (Equinet) with University of Zimbabwe Medical School.

Munishi, G. K., Yazbeck, A. D. K., & Lionetti, D. (1995). *Private sector delivery of health care in Tanzania.* Major Applied Research Paper No. 14. Bethesda, MD: HFS, Abt Associates.

Musau, S. N. (2008). *Community-based health insurance: Experiences and lessons learned from East and Southern Africa.* Technical Report No. 34. Bethesda, MD: Partnerships for Health Reform.

Mwabu, G., Mwanzia, J., & Liambila, W. (1995). User charges in government health facilities in Kenya: Effect on attendance and revenue. *Health Policy and Planning,* 10, 164–70.

Nanda, P. (2002). Gender dimensions of user fees: Implications for women's utilization of health care. *Reproductive Health Matters,* 10, 127–34.

Navarro, V. (2002). The World Health Report 2000: Can health care systems be compared using a single measure of performance? *American Journal of Public Health,* 92, 31–34.

OECD Health Project. (2004). *Towards high-performing health systems.* Paris: OECD. Retrieved from: http://www.oecd.org/dataoecd/15/23/31737305.pdf.

Ollila, E. (2005). Global health priorities—priorities of the wealthy? *Globalization and Health,* 1.

Ollila, E., & Koivusalo, M. (2008). The World Health Report 2000: World Health Organization health policy steering off course-changed values, poor evidence, and lack of accountability. *International Journal of Health Services,* 32, 503–14.

Ooms, G. (2006). Health development versus medical relief: The illusion versus the irrelevance of sustainability. *PLoS Medicine,* 3, 1202–05.

Osborne, D., & Plastrik, P. (1998). Banishing bureaucracy. *Policy Options,* 33–38.

Oxfam International. (2006). *Zambia uses G8 debt cancellation to make health care free for the poor.* Press release. Retrieved from: http://www.oxfam.org/en/news/pressreleases2006/pr060331_zambia.

Pachanee, C. A., & Wibulpolprasert, S. (2006). Incoherent policies on universal coverage of health insurance and promotion of international trade in health services in Thailand. *Health Policy and Planning,* 21, 310–18.

PAHO (Pan American Health Organization), WHO (World Health Organization), & IDRC (International Development Research Centre). (2001). *Research on health sector reforms in Latin America and the Caribbean: Contribution to policymaking.* Paper for pre-summit of the Americas Forum. Ottawa: International Development Research Centre. Retrieved from: www.idrc.ca/lacro/docs/conferencias/paho_idrc.html.

PAHO (Pan American Health Organization). (2008). *Social protection in health schemes for mother, newborn and child populations: Lessons learned from the Latin American region.* Washington, DC: PAHO

Pincus, J. R., & Winters, J. A. (2002). *Reinventing the World Bank.* Ithaca, NY: Cornell University Press.

Player, S., & Leys, C. (2008). *Confuse and conceal: The NHS and independent sector treatment centres.* Monmouth: Merlin Press.

Preker, A. S., & Harding, A. (2000). *The economics of public and private roles in health care: Insights from institutional economics and organizational theory.* Health, Nutrition and Population. Washington: World Bank.

———. (2003). *Innovations in health service delivery: The corporatization of public hospitals.* Human Development Network Health, Nutrition and Population Series. Washington, DC: World Bank.

PSI (Public Service International). (1999). Health and Social Services briefing Notes. Paris: PSI.

Rannan-Eliya, R., & Somanathan, A. (2005). *Access of the very poor to health services in Asia: Evidence on the role of health systems from Equitap.* Workshop Paper 10. London: DFID Health Systems Resource Centre.

Rannan-Eliya, R. P., van Zantern, T. V., & Yazbeck, A. (1996). *First year literature review for applied research agenda.* Partnerships for Health Reform Applied Research Paper 1. Bethesda, MD: Abt Associates. Retrieved from: http://www.healthsystems2020.org/content/resource/detail/642/.

Sabri, B. (2004). Health and development. *Eastern Mediterranean Health Journal,* 6, 758–65.

Sachs, J. D. (2007). Beware false tradeoffs. Foreign Affairs [online]. Retrieved from: http://www.foreignaffairs.org/special/global_health/sachs.

Schieber, G. J. (1997). *Innovations in health care financing.* Proceedings of a World Bank Conference, March 10–11, 1997. World Bank Discussion Paper No. 365. Washington, DC: World Bank.

Schwefel, D., Vuckovic, M., Korte, R., Doetinchem, O., Bichmann, W., & Brandrup-Lukanow, A. (2005). *Health, development and globalisation: Guidelines and recommendations for international cooperation—executive summary.* Eachborn, Germany: GTZ(GmbH). Retrieved from: http://detlef-schwefel.de/215e%20Schwefel%20health%20and%20globalization.pdf.

Sein, T. (2001). *Health sector reform—issues and opportunities.* Regional Health Forum. Retrieved from: www.searo.who.int/en/Section1243/Section1310/Section1343/Section1344/Section1352_5256.htm.

Shaw, R. P., & Ainsworth, M., eds. (1995). *Financing health services through user fees and insurance: Case studies from sub-Saharan Africa.* Washington, DC: World Bank.

Sinclair, S. (2005). *The GATS and South Africa's National Health Act: A cautionary tale.* Ottawa: Canadian Centre for Policy Alternatives.

Skaar, C. M. (1998). *Extending coverage of priority health care services through collaboration with the private sector: Selected experiences of USAID cooperating agencies.* Major Applied Research No. 4 Working Paper 1. Bethesda, MD: Abt Associates.

Stiglitz, J. (2002). *Globalisation and its discontents.* London: Penguin.

Stone, D. (2001). Think tanks, global lesson-drawing and networking social policy ideas. *Global Social Policy, 1,* 338–60.

Taylor, M. (2008). The reformulation of social policy in Chile 1973–2001: Questioning a neoliberal model. *Global Social Policy, 3,* 21–44.

UN Office for the Coordination of Humanitarian Affairs. (2005, September 16). Ghana: Despite new health scheme, newborn babies detained in hospital pending payment. *IRIN News.*

Unger, J.-P., De Paepe, P., Ghilbert, P., Soors, W., & Green, A. (2006). Disintegrated care: The Achilles' heel of international health policies in low and middle-income countries. *International Journal of Integrated Care, 6,* e14.

United Nations Research Institute for Social Development. (2000). *Visible hands: Taking responsibility for social development.* Geneva: UNRISD. Retrieved from: http://www.unrisd.org/unrisd/website/document.nsf/0/FE9C9439D82B525480256B670065EFA1?OpenDocument.

USAID (United States Agency for International Development). (2003). This is USAID. USAID [online]. Retrieved from: http://www.usaid.gov/about_usaid/.

———. (2003). USAID history. USAID [online]. Retrieved from: http://www.usaid.gov/about_usaid/usaidhist.html.

———. (2006). Users' guide to USAID/Washington health programs. Washington, DC: USAID [online]. Retrieved from: http://pdf.usaid.gov/pdf_docs/PNADG713.pdf; http://www.usaid.gov/our_work/global_health.

———. (2008). PSP-One Policy. Private sector partnerships for better health. Private Sector Partnerships-One [online]. Retrieved from: http://www.psp-one.com/section/technicalareas/policy.

Valentine, W. (2008). WHO spearheads multi-country study of decentralisation and health system change. *The Bridge (WHO-Europe),* Spring.

Wagstaff, A. (2007). *Social health insurance reexamined.* World Bank Policy Research Working Papers No. WPS 4111. Washington, DC: World Bank. Retrieved from: http://www-wds.worldbank.org/external/default/WDSContentServer/IW3P/IB/2007/01/09/000016406_20070109161148/Rendered/PDF/wps4111.pdf.

Walt, G. (1994). *Health policy: An introduction to process and power.* London: Witwatersrand University Press/Zed Books.

Wang'ombe, J. K. (1997). Cost recovery strategies in sub-Saharan Africa. In G. J. Schieber (ed.), *Innovations in health care financing: Proceedings of a World Bank conference, March 10–11, 1997* (pp. 155–61). Washington, DC: World Bank.

Weisbrot, M. (2001). *The "Washington Consensus" and development economics.* Draft paper prepared for the discussion at the UNRISD meeting on the need to rethink development economics, 7–8 September, 2001, Cape Town, South Africa. Geneva: United Nations Research Institute for Social Development (UNRISD) . Retrieved from: http://www.unrisd.org/80256B3C005BCCF9/htt pNetITFramePDF?ReadForm&parentunid=3AD5D5F2520B7436C1256BC90 04C3D2C&parentdoctype=paper&netitpath=80256B3C005BCCF9/(httpAux Pages)/3AD5D5F2520B7436C1256BC9004C3D2C/$file/weisbrot.pdf.

———. (2006). *Latin America: The end of an era.* Washington, DC: Center for Policy and Economic Research. Retrieved from: http://www.cepr.net/documents/publications/end_of_era_2006_12.pdf.

Wharton School. (2008). *Wharton impact conference. Voluntary health insurance in developing countries.* March 15–16, 2005. Philadelphia: Wharton School of the University of Pennsylvania. Retrieved from: http://hc.wharton.upenn.edu/ImpactConference/agenda.html.

Whitehead, M., Dahlgren, G., & Evans, T. (2001). Equity and health sector reforms: Can low-income countries escape the medical poverty trap? *The Lancet, 358,* 833–36.

Williamson, J. (1990). What Washington means by policy reform. In J. Williamson (ed.), *Latin American adjustment: How much has happened?* (pp. 7–38). Washington, DC: Institute for International Economics.

Williamson, J. (2000). What should the World Bank think about the Washington Consensus? *The World Bank Research Observer, 15,* 251–64.

Witter, S. (2005). *An unnecessary evil? User fees for healthcare in low-income countries.* London: Save the Children. Retrieved from: http://www.savethechildren.org.uk/en/docs/An_Unnecessary_Evil.pdf.

Woodward, D. (2005). The GATS and trade in health services: Implications for health care in developing countries. *Review of International Political Economy, 12,* 511–34.

World Bank. (1993). *World development report 1993: Investing in health.* New York: Oxford University Press.

———. (1997). *Health, nutrition, and population sector strategy.* Washington, DC: International Bank for Reconstruction and Development/World Bank. Retrieved from: http://docserver.ingentaconnect.com/deliver/connect/wb/9780821340400/v1n1/s1.pdf?expires=1217538022&id=45335559&titleid=7750&accname=University+of+Ottawa&checksum=3E84A1667EE7F507463E60C7A133AD0E.

———. (2003). *World development report 2004: Making services work for poor people.* New York: Oxford University Press.

———. (2005). *The World Bank annual report 2005. Year in review.* Washington, DC: The International Bank for Reconstruction and Development/The World Bank. Retrieved from: http://siteresources.worldbank.org/INTANNREP2K5/Resources/51563_English.pdf.

WHO (World Health Organization). (1992). *Basic Documents* (39th ed.). Geneva: WHO.

———. (2000). *The world health report 2000. Health systems: Improving performance.* World Health Report. Geneva: World Health Organization.

———. (2001). *The world health report 2001. Mental health: New understanding, new hope.* Geneva: WHO. Retrieved from: http://www.who.int/entity/whr/2001/en/whr01_en.pdf.

———. (2008). *Medium-term strategic plan 2008–2013.* Geneva: World Health Organization. Retrieved from: http://www.who.int/gb/ebwha/pdf_files/AMTSP-PPB/a-mtsp_2en.pdf.

Yeates, N. (2001). *Globalization and social policy.* London: Sage.

9 Globalization and the Cross-Border Flow of Health Workers

Corinne Packer, Ronald Labonté, and Vivien Runnels

INTRODUCTION

Recent decades have seen an increase in cross-border flows of health professionals. Of greatest health equity concern are flows from poorer countries which have existing and severe shortages of health human resources (HHR) and high burdens of disease to richer countries with shortages (but much less severe) and comparatively lower burdens of disease. Operating simultaneously, "push" and "pull" factors serve to create human capital flight or "brain drain" where workers with high levels of training or technical skills emigrate in search of a job and a better life for themselves and their families. While not a new phenomenon, such migration has been accelerated by the past three decades of globalization. The deteriorating economic and broader social and environmental conditions in many so-called "source" countries, for example, are at least partly attributable to liberalization or other forms of global market integration, directly and negatively affecting working conditions, availability of jobs and career development, and thus serving to "push" health workers out of their countries (Marchal & Kegels, 2003). Conditionalities associated with loans or debt relief from the international financial institutions (IFIs) that constrain governments' abilities to pay adequate salaries or to provide incentives for health workers to remain exacerbate the situation. Globalization also makes it easier for rich countries to "pull" or attract health professionals. Border barriers in high-income countries are being actively lowered for professional, technical, and skilled immigrants, even as they are (frequently) raised for semi- or lesser-skilled individuals. High-income countries, such as the United States (US), Australia, New Zealand, Canada, and, until very recently, the United Kingdom (UK), have come to rely on the immigration of foreign-trained health workers to fill their own HHR vacancies. Although there have been attempts to frame the flows of health professionals as a continuous "brain circulation" rather than a brain drain, evidence demonstrates that HHR flow overwhelmingly and increasingly from poorer to richer countries, with the poorest countries unable to replace or attract new workers. For these countries, the inevitable result is diminished health care access and services, both critical barriers to improving global health equity. Other factors associated with globalization foster HHR migration, notably the internationalization of professional credentials and, in some instances, notably the European Union (EU), of citizenship. Professional credentials in health as in other fields are increasingly recognized across borders, particularly where free trade areas have been formed. Eased migration and mobility (including, for instance, through cheaper, faster, and easier travel, multilingualism, postcolonial ties, and common academic curricula) have contributed to a veritable sense of "global citizenship" worldwide with professional credentials serving as passports. Finally, regional and global trade agreements, key tools of modern globalization, can facilitate international labor mobility.

In exploring these issues, this chapter begins by describing some of the known empirics of HHR density and flows. It then examines in more depth how these flows relate to globalization, and what their impacts have been, notably on lower-income source countries. (We accept as given that receiving countries benefit both health-wise and economically by these flows.) The chapter concludes by reviewing critically the feasibility and desirability of various policy options to manage health-professional migration.

THE GLOBAL PICTURE

Most analysts have found strong evidence indicative of major and enduring global shortages in nurses and doctors over the next decades (Bach, 2003; Joint Learning Initiative, 2004; Liese & Dussault, 2004). While workforce prediction is imprecise, recent surges in HHR out-migration from a number of poor countries to a small handful of rich countries instantiates a trend likely to continue, in some cases risking a virtual collapse in source nations (Pond & McPake, 2006). As in many facets of globalization discussed in this book, the effects to date of the global HHR flow have been highly asymmetrical, with the main receiving countries being high-income, largely (though not exclusively) Anglophone countries. According to a 2008 Organisation for Economic Co-operation and Development (OECD) report, New Zealand has the highest proportion of migrant doctors among OECD countries, and one of the highest for nurses (Zurn & Dumont, 2008). The World Health Organization's (WHO) *World Health Report* 2006 indicates the United States received the highest number of foreign-trained doctors and nurses, followed by the UK. As one simple metric of this asymmetry: doctors trained in sub-Saharan African countries (SSA), largely at public expense, who now work in OECD countries represent close to one-quarter of the current total physician workforce in those SSA source countries.

Table 9.1 Doctors and Nurses Trained Abroad Working in OECD Countries

OECD country	Doctors from Abroad		Nurses from Abroad	
	Number	% of Total	Number	% of Total
Australia	11,122	21	—	—
Canada	13,620	23	19,061	6
Finland	1,003	9	140	0
France	11,269	6	—	—
Germany	17,318	6	26,284	3
Ireland	—	—	8,758	14
New Zealand	2,832	34	10,616	21
Portugal	1,258	4	—	—
United Kingdom	69,813	33	65,000	10
United States	213,331	27	99,456	5

Source: World Health Organization (2006), p. 98. Note: Only a portion of foreign-trained physicians and nurses come from underserved low-income countries.

While the literature on health worker migration is typically limited to physicians and nurses, other health workers, such as ophthalmologists and radiologists, are also part of the phenomenon of brain drain. A snapshot of pharmacists, for instance, shows a situation of global shortage, with wealthy OECD countries suffering mild but increasing shortages of pharmacists and developing countries experiencing extreme shortages (International Pharmaceutical Federation [FIP], 2006). This has obvious implications for the dispensing of antiretroviral drugs, or treatments for malaria, tuberculosis (TB), other infectious diseases, and the increasing burden of chronic disease in all developing countries. Specifically, pharmacist shortages in many SSA nations are cited as one constraint on more rapid roll-out of antiretroviral (ARV) treatments (Attaran & Walker, 2008).

The Joint Learning Initiative on Human Resources for Health (JLI), a two-year global study of the impact of HHR on health performance, aptly describes health workers as the "glue of the health system," without which technologies, drugs, infrastructure, knowledge, and information cannot be applied (Joint Learning Initiative, 2004). The situation is so severe that the JLI concluded that the fate of global health and development in the twenty-first century lies largely in the management of the HHR crisis (Joint Learning Initiative, 2004). It also documented the severe shortages currently experienced by many low-income countries. While imperfect, vacancy rates are in many instances the best available measure we have of such shortages. Ghana's Health Service, as one of the more extreme examples, had 2,002 vacancy rates of nearly 50 percent for doctors and 57 percent for nurses. A memo issued that year by the director-general of the Ghana Health Service indicated that more Ghanaian doctors worked outside the country than within (Mensah, Mackintosh, & Henry, 2005). While vacancies are not singularly a result of out-migration, as we shall discuss later, they are affected by it. Additionally, countries with relatively small workforces and inflows, such as Malawi, can be hugely affected by even numerically small outward flows (Gerein, Green, & Pearson, 2006a).

REGIONAL FEATURES

While globalization is enabling the creation of a global labor market in health professionals, its form (that is, the direction and ease of such flows) has distinctive regional features.

Europe

Some countries in Europe face specific HHR challenges. As Dubois et al. (2006) explain, states of the former Union of Soviet Socialist Republics (USSR) that became independent in the early 1990s (such as Armenia, Russia, and Ukraine) and the countries of Central and Eastern Europe (CEE) had "inherited a workforce that was especially ill-suited to the demands facing modern health care systems. Large numbers of physicians were trained but many received limited and often narrowly specialized training . . . [while] [t]heir inherited nursing workforces had low levels of skills and were ill-equipped to take on the roles adopted by their equivalents in Western Europe". Once these earlier problems were overcome, these same countries began to face the challenge of increased international mobility of professionals (Nicholas, 2007). With the enlarged European Union (EU), health professionals in CEE countries, such as Lithuania and Poland, are increasingly attracted by better-paying jobs in other EU countries (Buchan, Jobanputra, Gough, & Hutt, 2006). Slovenia, as one case, is already experiencing a significant deficit of physicians due to out-migration (Nicholas, 2007).

Some wealthier countries in Europe are experiencing challenges at a different end of the spectrum. Spain and France, for instance, presently have an oversupply of physicians and nurses (judged so by the lack of available positions for all those actively seeking employment); the lack of jobs is drawing these professionals to seek work elsewhere, which could eventually precipitate a rebound shortage in both countries. In contradistinction, other wealthy European countries, such as Ireland (where over half of newly registered nurses in 2000 were foreign-trained), the Netherlands, Norway, and the UK are or have been experiencing severe HHR deficits. The immediate impact of shortages in these countries is long waiting lists for patient treatment and surgery (Tjadens, 2002). These nations draw in physicians and nurses not only from other European countries but also from India, the Philippines, Pakistan, the Caribbean, and South Africa, as well as from rich countries such as Canada and Australia (Buchan et al., 2006). The aging populations of Western

Europe, creating more complex and HHR-demanding health problems, suggest ongoing or increasing HHR flows, particularly of nurses or other health workers capable of providing live-in care (World Health Organization, 2006).

North America, Australia, and New Zealand

Australia, New Zealand, Canada, and the United States have all experienced minor to significant shortages in domestically trained physicians and nurses (Hawthorne, 2001; Bourassa, Forcier, Simoens, & Giuffrida, 2004; Mullan, 2005). At present, all depend heavily on foreign-trained health professionals to fill important gaps in their HHR supply. If all foreign-trained physicians were to leave these countries today, one-fifth to one-third of all posts would become vacant. Certain regions within these developed countries would suffer even greater impacts. For instance, in Canada more foreign-trained physicians fill posts in rural and underserved regions than do domestically trained physicians (Canadian Institute for Health Information, 2006). The Canadian province of Saskatchewan has nearly 55 percent foreign-trained physicians, this figure rising even higher in the smaller towns and urban centers of the province (Labonté, Packer, & Klassen, 2006). Certain areas of practice, such as family medicine (general practice), would also suffer acute shortages in the absence of foreign-trained physicians (Canadian Institute for Health Information, 2005). Canada's experience is broadly generalizable: stated simply, foreign-trained physicians take jobs that domestically trained physicians do not want.

Latin America and the Caribbean

There is little literature on health worker migration from Latin America. Within the region, migration tends to be from poorer countries (e.g., Ecuador and Peru) to wealthier ones (notably Chile, where increasing numbers of public sector physicians have migrated to the private sector) (Bach, 2006). In the Caribbean, the loss of health workers has become a significant concern. At a Commonwealth Secretariat-sponsored Caribbean conference on the "managed migration" of nurses, participants estimated that the Caribbean is losing a minimum of 400 nurses annually through migration to the United States, Canada, and the UK (Public Services International, 2006). In Trinidad and Tobago it has been estimated that each year about one-third of nursing graduates resign from their duties in the public sector to take up positions abroad (Public Services International, 2006). Approximately 35 percent of posts in the region for registered nurses are vacant. As a result, some countries in the region are now actively recruiting nurses, pharmacists, and physicians from the Philippines, Cuba, Nigeria, and Guyana in order to satisfy severe staff shortages (Public Services International, 2006). Cuba singularly stands out as a considerable overproducer and intentional exporter of physicians, both for the contractual earnings repatriated by émigré health workers and as stated acts of solidarity with other developing countries. Unlike other countries with deliberate HHR export policies discussed following (India, the Philippines), Cuba does not have a domestic HHR shortage, provides health care access to all its citizens, and posts high-income country health outcomes despite being a low-income nation (Evans, 2008).

Asia and the Persian Gulf

With a quarter of the world's population, the Southeast Asia region has only 12 percent of the global health workforce. Numerous Asian countries have characteristics that foster professional mobility to key English-speaking receiving countries. They tend to be less developed than Western countries, have large and well-trained labor pools, and have the potential to supply English-speaking professionals in many different fields. India, the Philippines, and Sri Lanka are prime examples in the health care field (Khadria, 2006).

India is a principal source of physicians in the four main OECD receiving countries. It ranks number one in both the UK (10.9 percent of the total physicians workforce) and the United States (4.9 percent), supplies the second greatest number of foreign-trained physicians to Australia (4.0 percent), and the third greatest number to Canada (2.1 percent) (Mullan, 2005). The country provides the largest absolute number of physicians to recipient countries worldwide (Mullan, 2005). Developed and prosperous countries alike have also discovered India as a new source country for recruiting well-trained English-speaking nurses to meet their own shortages. In India nurses qualifying with a bachelor of science in nursing are educated and trained to international standards of "registered nurses," making it very easy for them to move abroad and work (Khadria, 2006). Private recruitment agencies have sprung up in India specifically with the aim of sending trained nurses to key Western English-speaking and Gulf countries. Around four million Indian migrants are working in Gulf countries, of whom an estimated 40,000 to 60,000 are nurses (Percot, 2006).

The Indian government in turn has established its own exporting department as a means of facilitating international migration of nurses and to safeguard them against exploitation. Yet India has amongst the lowest nurse-to-population ratios of all source countries, far behind South Africa and the Philippines, with a high number of unfilled positions, particularly in rural areas. Some of the best hospitals in the country are reportedly experiencing mass resignation and exodus of nurses to hospitals abroad (Khadria, 2006).

In the Philippines in 2002, nearly 13,000 health workers left the country to work abroad, 93 percent of whom were nurses. In December 2004, the government-administered professional licensure examination for Filipino nurses counted at least 18,000 test takers (Anon., 2006). This means that the country experienced a loss of nurses that was the equivalent of approximately two-thirds of the numbers taking the licensure exams. Like India, and for a longer period of time, the Philippines has been deliberately training nurses for export; yet, also like India, but unlike Cuba, it experiences very low nurse-to-population ratios, particularly in rural areas, and high levels of nurse vacancies (Khadria, 2006).

Evidence from Sri Lanka shows a similarly dramatic loss of physicians through internal and external migration, ranging from 15 percent to 85 percent, depending on the region. Unfortunately, the study does not provide information on the years covered by these estimates (Aluwihare, 2005). There are only around 800 specialists in Sri Lanka to serve a population of eighteen million people. Each year around sixty doctors head to the UK, Australia, and other nations in the developing world to complete their year's compulsory training to become a consultant. However, only half return, exacerbating a growing crisis in health provision (Burke, 2005). The economy of Sri Lanka, like many other professional-exporting nations, depends heavily on remittances sent home by their émigré workers. Remittances contributed 8.1 percent to Sri Lanka's gross domestic product (GDP) in 2004–2005—57 percent of the amount coming from workers in the Middle East (Central Bank of Sri Lanka, 2005).

It has been noted at international meetings on health worker migration that, while there is little hard data on health worker migration to the Persian Gulf, these states are considerable importers of health workers. Some estimate that 80 percent of health workers in the Gulf states are foreign-trained. The absence of representation from states such as Kuwait, the United Arab Emirates, Bahrain, and Saudi Arabia at international meetings on health worker migration has been noted as a concern. Although Sudan and Saudi Arabia have entered a bilateral agreement on the managed migration of Sudanese physicians to Saudi Arabia, Sudanese physicians are still being recruited through the back door.[1] The ability to circumvent provisions appears to be a weakness common to all such agreements.

Sub-Saharan Africa

African health care systems suffer severely from migration of health professionals. Physicians and nurses based in rural and poor areas move to cities for better working conditions and environments. Urban-based physicians and nurses move from the critically underequipped and underfunded public sector to the private sector (Gerein, Green, & Pearson, 2006b). There are frequently noted, though less studied, flows from the public sector to nongovernmental health organizations or other structures administering the growing number of disease-specific global health initiatives (see Chapter 8, this volume). Finally, health professionals in both private and public sectors leave to work in more developed countries to obtain higher pay, better working conditions, an overall better quality of life, and improved opportunities for them and their families.

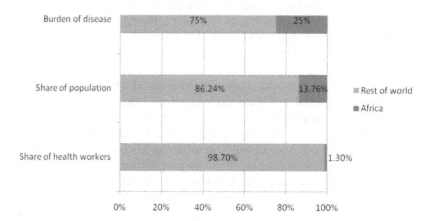

Figure 9.1 Burden of disease, share of population, and share of health workers, Africa and rest of world.

Source: Figure adapted from Our Common Interest: Report of the Commission for Africa, 2005, p. 184. Available at: http://www.cfr.org/publication/8292/our_common_interest.html.

The need for medical professionals is arguably greatest in sub-Saharan Africa (SSA) (Dovlo, 2005a; see Figure 9.1), and yet significant numbers of African-trained health workers migrate to developed countries to work each year. Six of the twenty countries with the highest physician emigration factors (arrived at by measuring the loss of physicians from a country as a proportion of the physicians remaining to do the work of health care) are in sub-Saharan Africa (Mullan, 2005). There are at least 11,000 SSA-trained physicians known to be licensed and practicing in the UK, the United States, and Canada alone (Hagopian et al., 2005). According to one report, SSA is approximately 700,000 physicians and 700,000 nurses short of staffing requirement necessary to meet the Millennium Development Goals (MDGs) (Bueno de Mesquita & Gordon, 2005).

GLOBALIZATION'S DRIVERS OF HHR MIGRATION

At the Macro Level

There are various ways to understand how globalization is influencing the global HHR flows. Framed broadly, HHR migration, as with all forms of migration, defines one aspect of globalization and the relationship between the two becomes somewhat tautological. To the extent that increased trade and investment liberalization, defining qualities of contemporary globalization, lead to higher per capita gross domestic product (GDP) and in theory enhancing the funds available for health systems, they can reduce a source country's push factors. Most low-income economies from which significant numbers of health workers are migrating, however, despite in some instances recently recording high levels of growth due to dramatic rises in world prices for their export commodities, still lack sufficient capital to develop their health systems adequately (Bundred, Martineau, & Kitchiner, 2004).

In narrower and more evidence-informed terms, there are multiple ways in which different aspects of globalization are leading to increased HHR flows from poorer to richer countries. Some of the more important of these include:

1. Deteriorating economic or broader social and environmental conditions at least partly attributable in some regions (notably Latin America and Africa) to rapid and ill-timed market liberalization required as structural adjustment conditions on grants and loans by the IFIs (the International Monetary Fund [IMF], World Bank, and regional development banks) during the 1980s and 1990s.
2. Continuing conditionalities associated with grants, loans, or debt relief from the IFIs that limit governments' spending in the public sector and therefore their abilities to employ and retain HHR through adequate salaries and incentive mechanisms (see Chapter 7, this volume).
3. Eased migration restrictions on the flows of HHR from low- to high-income countries with perceived HHR deficits. In health labor markets under conditions of global shortage, a person's professional skills become a valuable commodity; the result is out-migration of those with internationally accredited qualifications (Bundred et al., 2004).
4. Specific policies to overproduce and export HHR in order to achieve a better balance of payments via remittances, in part to create domestic conditions more favorable to foreign investors or lenders, or to improve debt-servicing capacity (though again emphasizing the stark differences between countries such as India, the Philippines, and Cuba).

Finally, because increased health inequities arise from lack of workers in poorer countries with high burdens of disease, HHR migration can also be seen as a problem requiring global policy intervention. In this framing of the HHR crisis, the empirical relationship of globalization drivers to HHR migration is less a concern than is the international *obligation* or *duty* of all nations to manage flows in a way that does not compromise their legal or normative commitments to other countries under human rights treaties or the internationally agreed upon Millennium Development Goals (see Packer, Labonté, and Spitzer, 2007, for more detailed discussion).

At the Micro Level

Individuals are motivated to migrate for different reasons (Crush, 2002; Bundred et al., 2004) that can be country-specific; at the same time, there

Table 9.2 Summary of Push and Pull Factors of HHR Migration

Push Factors	Pull Factors
Job Security	
• No jobs available • Lack of promotions • Risk of losing jobs due to lack of funds	• Jobs available • Colleagues, friends, and recruiters telling them about opportunities • Fairness in granting promotions
Working Conditions	
• Deteriorating work environment/ facilities • Inadequate medicine and equipment • Inability to treat patients appropriately • For nurses, unhappiness with prevalent social attitudes towards the profession • Significant stress, overtime, and generally poor conditions of service resulting in fatigue and burnout • Impossible patient-health care provider ratios making quality care difficult	• Satisfaction of practicing medicine and nursing as trained and capable of doing • Reasonable workload and conditions of work
Economic Considerations	
• Disarray in severely economically depressed countries • Low salaries • Inability to accrue savings • Nonpayment of salaries, housing allowance, pension	• Higher pay (and opportunities for remittances) • Reasonable remuneration—able to save money • Recruiters actively sourcing workers internationally with promise of high income and good benefits
Political Considerations	
• Political, racial, ethnic upheaval • Gender discrimination • Government training health workers for international export	• OECD countries wealthy, stable, and democratic • Absence of corruption
Physical Security	
• Criminality • Gender-based violence • Exposure to HIV—risk of infection through treatment of patients	• Safe country • Safe working environment • Appropriate medical equipment to prevent HIV infection
Quality of Life	
• Poor accommodation • Lack of transport to go to work • Inability to live a decent life	• Multiethnic and tolerant of diversity • Good quality of life
Education	
• Diminishing quality of education for children	• Greater opportunities for children—good education and ability for them to earn a decent living

Compiled from: McDonald & Crush, 2002; Bundred et al., 2004; Thomas, Hosein, & Yan, 2005; World Health Organization, 2006.

are well-established, evidence-based "push" and "pull" factors summarized in Table 9.2. There is also a well-developed culture of medical migration. Hagopian et al. explain how this culture has become firmly rooted in many source and receiving countries: it not only fails to discourage medical migration but actively encourages it. Medical school faculty in source countries are often role models of, or advocates for, the benefits of migration, and are proud of their students who successfully emigrate to higher-income countries affording greater professional opportunities (Hagopian et al., 2005).

There is little evidence that significant numbers of doctors and nurses return to their source country to practice their profession, ostensibly because the conditions which led to their departure remain unchanged. HHR shortages in the key receiving countries are merely fuelling a fire that was already started. In this light, one word, admittedly oversimplifying the situation, describes the most important and yet most complicated step towards resolving the HHR migration crisis: *retention.* For retention efforts to take root and be truly successful, the fundamental labor, economic, and social conditions that drive health workers to leave in the first place must be improved. This will require enormous adjustments in public health systems (e.g., improvements in procurement and safety procedures, in telemedicine, in the balance of skills of health workers, etc.) and increases in funds. It might be argued that remittances from émigré HHR could partly provide such funding, but remittances are private transfers not structured to finance public health services, although there is some evidence that poorer families receiving remittances often use them to purchase health care when quality publicly funded services are not available.

THE IMPACTS OF MIGRATION ON SOURCE-COUNTRY HEALTH SYSTEMS

While health care is not the only determinant of population health, it is certainly an important one. Human resources are a prerequisite for effective, quality health care, with most medical interventions requiring the services of physicians, nurses, or other types of trained health workers. A poorly resourced health workforce inevitably affects negatively the health of populations (Dussault & Dubois, 2003; Marchal & Kegels, 2003). In their correlational study of HHR and health outcomes, Anand and Bärnighausen (2007) found that human resources for health in aggregate terms (specifically physicians, nurses, and midwives) matter significantly in health outcome measures of maternal, infant, and under-five mortality rates, even after controlling for other variables that are typically used to explain health outcomes.

Shortages in HHR in poor countries can be devastating to health care and thus equity in health outcomes (Table 9.3). Significant shortages exist

Table 9.3   Selected Impacts of Inadequate HHR

Too few hospital beds causing refused or delayed treatment
Too few treatment facilities reducing level of care
Reduced emergency care
Increased wait time, reduced patient care time, and poorer infection control
Overwork in public sector pushes HHR into private sector, creating more overwork conditions in public sector caring for the poor
Increased health worker absenteeism due to overwork, stress, and emotional exhaustion, creating more overwork conditions
Care provided, of necessity, by insufficiently trained staff, particularly in rural areas

Compiled from: Aluwihare, 2005; Bach, 2006; Gerein et al., 2006a.

in certain specialties, such as anesthesiology, radiology, and pathology. Physicians with such training are in high demand in richer receiving countries and are already few in numbers in developing source countries. As physicians with specialized training take longer and cost more to train, their out-migration deals a particularly severe blow to the source country. As an example, a regional spinal injuries unit in South Africa serving a population of three million was closed in 2004 when two key doctors were recruited to open a similar unit in a Canadian city with a population of 700,000 (Bundred et al., 2004). Undergraduate and postgraduate medical education also suffers as a result of migration, affecting the next generation of HHR in some source countries (Paton, 2006). Specialized health professionals who emigrate are often among the few active or published researchers in low-income source countries. Emigration of such individuals stifles innovation and invention in dealing with persistent local public health problems, for example, HIV/AIDS, tuberculosis, and malaria (Kirigia, Gbary, Muthuri, Nyoni, & Seddoh, 2006). Finally, loss of educated health-professional pools through migration has broader impacts for societies. Physicians and their families constitute an educated sector of the population of a country and the migration of physicians depletes this pool. Physicians' spouses are also often health care professionals and children are often steered into the health profession. As such, the recruitment of one doctor overseas potentially depletes a much larger educated pool of actual and potential health professionals.

THE IMPACTS OF TRADE AGREEMENTS

A defining characteristic of contemporary globalization is the growth in the number of bilateral, regional, and multilateral trade liberalization agreements (see Chapter 5 and Chapter 8, this volume). The sheer number of bilateral agreements makes any assessment of their provisions on the movement of HHR beyond the scope of this chapter's analysis. As one recent example, however, Japan and the Philippines concluded a bilateral agreement in September 2006 that allows for up to 500 Filipino nurses or caregivers to enter Japan each year for work, professional education, or language training. This number is expected to rise as the population of elderly Japanese increases (Anon., 2006).

A number of regional trade treaties and mobility policies have incorporated specific measures designed to encourage the free movement of labor within their defined geopolitical areas.

EU

The EU has established an inclusive model of mutual recognition of qualifications in which, for example, registered nurses or midwives are free to work in any other member state. As a result, the barriers to mobility have less to do with recognition of qualification and more to do with linguistic and other barriers (Buchan, Parkin, & Sochalski, 2003).

NAFTA

The North American Free Trade Agreement (NAFTA) enables some, but not all, Canadian, Mexican, and American citizens to work temporarily in each other's countries, and provides a framework for mutual recognition of professional competency. In practice, NAFTA has encouraged movement primarily between Canada and the United States. Medical students in both countries receive a similar education. Canadian medical graduates therefore can apply for a US residency-training program and subsequent to that become licensed to practice in the United States; and vice versa (Biviano & Makarehchi, 2003). NAFTA-approved migrants do not require visas. Health workers from NAFTA countries need only a letter of employment to present at the port of entry (Ouaked, 2002).

ASEAN

The Association of Southeast Asian Nations (ASEAN) is a participant in the global trade liberalization process through the establishment of the ASEAN Free Trade Area (AFTA), which, in turn, has started to develop the ASEAN Economic Community (AEC). The AEC by 2020 will turn ASEAN into a single market with over five hundred million consumers and free flows of goods, capital, services, and skilled labor. The health services sector has been set as one of eleven priority sectors to be accelerated and fully liberalized by 2010. At present, negotiations are in the advanced stages for specific health commitments. These would include the mutual recognition arrangements for freer movements of health professionals such as physicians, nurses, and other allied health practitioners (Kovindha, 2006).

MERCOSUR

The Southern Common Market Agreement (known by its Spanish acronym, MERCOSUR) is a regional free-trade agreement between ten South American countries. It adopted provisions for trade in health services identical to those found in the General Agreement on Trade in Services (GATS) of the World Trade Organization (WTO) next discussed.

WTO

Aside from regional free-trade agreements, WTO rules have attracted the most attention in terms of implications for health worker migration. Of specific concern are the negotiations around the General Agreement on Trade in Services (GATS), a set of multilateral, legally enforceable rules designed to encourage the liberalization of trade in services (OECD, 2002). The most forceful GATS provisions are bottom-up, applying only to those sectors and measures that governments specifically agree to cover. In making commitments to these rules, governments can specify how they apply to particular services and government measures. Commitments can be unbound (applying only to current government measures) or bound (covering current and any future government measures). They can include limitations on the range of services and measures covered, or they can be without limitations. Commitments can be limited to certain ways of providing services, or they can cover all possible ways of providing the service. However, this formal flexibility is diminished by intense negotiating pressure to extend the reach of GATS rules with full, bound commitments and minimal limitations (see Chapter 5, this volume).

It is GATS Mode 4 (presence of natural persons) which most directly relates to the provision of health services by individuals in another country on a temporary basis (Bach, 2003). If a country allows the entry of foreign doctors and nurses as service providers, GATS requires that it must make its licensing requirements transparent and freely available, and must administer tests in a reasonable and impartial manner. At the same time, countries committed to allowing the entry of foreign health workers have the right to verify foreigners' credentials to ensure they are consistent with national credential rules. There are no specific limits on the cost, duration, or standards of this testing (Martin, 2003). In theory, Mode 4 has made international labor mobility for health workers easier. In practice, however, none of the high-recipient countries for foreign-trained HHR (Canada, the United States, the UK/EU, and Australia) has made commitments that would directly facilitate the movement of physicians, nurses, or other health professionals, although some are acting to ease accreditation and to establish global standards for competencies (Blouin, 2005; Broten, 2008). The possibility nonetheless remains that future commitments made under GATS Mode 4 could increase the flow of HHR from developing to developed countries.

POLICY OPTIONS TO MANAGE HEALTH-PROFESSIONAL MIGRATION

We discuss next a number of policy options that have been advanced as means to manage the migration of health workers such that global health equity does not suffer. While migration is a global phenomenon, many of these options have more to do with improving domestic supply and retention.

Reduced Reliance by Source Countries

Countries should commit to becoming self-sufficient in the development of their own domestic supply of HHR by a given target date. This would apply particularly to those OECD countries that remain heavily reliant on foreign-trained health professionals, and would eventually reduce pull factors (available positions). Recently, for example, the UK National Health Service began to explicitly prioritize hiring of locally trained over foreign-trained health workers in filling vacancies. As explained by Debbie Mellor, director of workforce development for the UK Ministry of Health, at a March 2007 International Organization for Migration (IOM)/WHO meeting on HHR migration, the UK's overall goal is to reduce reliance on non-European internationally educated nurses to between 25 percent and 30 percent of the total roster—which nonetheless remains a sizable number. Targeting a maximum reliance on HHR from developing countries, however, at least establishes an accountable baseline.

Several source countries are either actively or planning to begin training auxiliary (mid-level or substitute) health workers whose skills are presently less marketable globally. Examples are Tanzania, Zambia, South Africa, and Malawi, where, for example, health care workers (not nurses) are being trained to administer vaccinations and other limited treatments. There is no evidence that, with an adequate training curriculum, higher skilled backup and good supervision, the expanded deployment of such workers leads to a "second-class health system," as is sometimes claimed by medical and nursing organizations in both source and receiving countries.

Rural Incentive Schemes

Rural areas in both source and destination countries are critically short of health workers and are the first to lose in the global flow of HHR. One solution to this problem attempted by many countries is the offer of extra pay or other incentives to health workers who take posts in rural or other underserved areas. One study observed, however, that wage differentials for those accepting posts in these regions have to be significant to be effective in attracting physicians and nurses (Vujicic, Zurn, Diallo, Adams, & Dal Poz, 2004). Incentives are not only financial but have included subsidized housing, deferred or reduced student loan schemes, better access to

228 Corinne Packer, Ronald Labonté, and Vivien Runnels

promotions, and specialized training for those willing to go to rural areas (Physicians for Human Rights, 2004). A community service requirement that encourages health professionals to practice for a fixed period in rural and other underserved areas has also been tried in such countries as South Africa and Nigeria (Physicians for Human Rights, 2004). Another strategy that has been advanced is a requirement of internship rotation where nursing and medical school students in their final year work in both rural and urban areas (Serneels, Lindelow, Garcia-Montalvo, & Barr, 2005).

Reduced Wastage of In-Country Health Workers

Wastage of trained HHR occurs in both receiving and source (Dovlo, 2005b) countries. This occurs when a country develops or gains health professionals through in-migration but fails to employ them. As an example of a receiving country, in one province of Canada alone there are reportedly 3,000 to 4,000 skilled foreign-trained physicians who have not obtained Canadian certification and are therefore underutilized (College of Physicians and Surgeons of Ontario, 2004). While their training may not be comparable to or reach the standards Canadian licensing bodies require, it would arguably cost Canada less to bring these already knowledgeable individuals' skills up to par than to train new professionals from scratch.

At the same time, there is a considerable number of source countries with significant numbers of health professionals unemployed even when there are significant numbers of vacancies. For instance, between 1996 and 2001 there were 32,000 vacancies in nursing in the South African public sector and yet 25,000 registered nurses who were inactive or unemployed within the country, pointing to problems other than migration affecting the health sector (Gent & Skeldon, 2006). A similar situation is reportedly the case in Kenya as well (McVeigh, 2006). Globalization, for example, in the form of IMF-recommended or -required ceilings on the public sector wage bill, might play a role in this ironic situation; but it also attests to other underlying problems in HHR planning, management, and funding that account for crisis in undersupply.

Restrictions on International Mobility

Restrictions can be applied on both the exit of individuals from source countries and on their entry into destination countries. The first has generally taken the form of temporary bonding, which requires that individuals trained at public expense work for a period within country essentially to repay that cost. While intuitively appealing, there have been numerous documented problems with bonding (Chikanda, 2005; Mensah et al., 2005; Serneels et al., 2005); for example, it fails to deal with the root causes of out-migration, can increase health workers' dissatisfaction, creating an additional incentive to leave or reluctance to return home after spending years abroad, is prone to corruption and favoritism, and, when accompanied by fines, has proven easy to "buy out."

Bonding has also sometimes been criticized for potentially violating peoples' right to seek migration. If bonding is in the form of a contract for repayment of publicly subsidized education, there is no apparent violation of this right. But human rights issues do cut across many of these policy options.

Receiving countries can also place restrictions on international mobility. The South African government, for instance, does not condone the recruitment of health professionals from any Southern African Development Community (SADC) country for ethical reasons, since these neighboring countries also suffer acute HHR shortages. The South African–SADC HHR agreement includes nonretention of foreign (SADC) students who have completed their studies in South Africa.

Return of Migrants to their Source Countries

Current evidence indicates that schemes to promote the return of migrants have so far proved costly and largely unsuccessful, particularly where root factors which caused the out-migration in the first place have not been addressed. Any reduction of global health inequities through investments based on this strategy must be weighed against the opportunity costs of investing in stronger evidence-informed options. It is important, however, to distinguish health professionals who migrate primarily for purposes of advancing training that may be unavailable in their own countries. A recent Canadian study of foreign-trained physicians who eventually left Canada found that roughly half returned to their home, or neighboring, country within three years of completing their Canadian postgraduate residencies, indicative that migration for this group serves primarily as a training strategy (Watanabe, Comeau, & Buske, 2008). At the same time, the proportion of all foreign-trained physicians in Canada who left was low (around 9 percent) and those from poorer countries were least likely to return home and most likely to move from Canada to the United States— hardly convincing evidence of return migration by HHR from countries most in need.

Restitution for Loss of Human Capital

The premise of restitution is that receiving countries or émigré health professionals compensate source countries for, at minimum, the loss of training cost investment and, at maximum, estimated economic welfare losses to the country over the foregone life span of active professional service. Most source and destination countries appear to be in considerable opposition on this option. Source countries frequently argue that the scale of the "perverse subsidy" represented by such HHR flows from poor to rich, particularly in light of international commitments such as the MDGs, demands restitution. Destination countries generally counter that individuals migrate by free volition, as is their right. Yet the grounds for restitution lie precisely in other human rights treaty obligations (notably Article 12 of the International Covenant on Economic, Social and Cultural Rights, known colloquially as "the right to health"), which requires nations to avoid acting in ways that do interfere with other nations' abilities to fulfill their obligations under this right (Bueno de Mesquita & Gordon, 2005). A compromise strategy embodied in the World Health Assembly's Resolution 59.23 (May 2006), and less dramatic than calling for "restitution," emphasizes the importance of dramatically increasing training for health workers in source countries, with increased financial and nonfinancial support from "receiving developed countries." Such support could be based on some calculi of net costs and benefits to source/receiving countries (improbable), much more generous health aid transfers from receiving (donor) to source (recipient) countries (more likely, but see Chapter 7, this volume, on the need first for substantive aid reform), or transfers based on systems of global taxation on all flows of goods, capital, and people (possible, but not for some time in the future).

CONCLUSION

Migration is an inescapable feature of humankind. People always have migrated and will continue to pursue what they feel are better opportunities. But the extent to which health workers, in particular physicians and nurses, are leaving poor countries to work in rich ones is beyond simple migration. It is a symptom, not a cause, of failing health systems.

The key element in both source and receiving countries which will stem the HHR migration crisis is retention. The central component of any retention scheme is the improvement of pay and living and working conditions to encourage health workers to remain. In very straightforward terms, money will resolve this crisis, bolstered by other strategies to improve working environment and conditions and, in many source countries, the overall economic and social health of the country. This will require specific actions, as suggested in the policy options described in this chapter, from both source and destination countries as well as the international institutions (Kapur & McHale, 2005).

The impact of trade and cross-border mobility agreements on HHR flows continues to be a concern. While such agreements generally are not the cause of, nor as yet a major factor in, the outward flow of HHR, their potential to become so exists and may be on the rise. Experience with health sector liberalization has shown that inequities tend to follow in access, largely a result of internal drains from the rural public to the urban private health systems (Packer, Labonté, & Spitzer, 2007).

Various policy options to manage the migration of health workers, both proposed and in practice, have been outlined in this chapter. The best scenario would be for *both* source and receiving countries to adopt such strategies and, where relevant, enter into bilateral agreements to manage flows in a manner suitable to both countries. But as all of the chapters in this book have argued, and the evidence in terms of "push" and "pull" in the global HHR labor market substantiates, only policies that are based on redistribution, rights, and regulation are likely to lead to a sustained resolution of the ongoing crisis of "brain drain."

NOTES

1. Reported verbally by participants at the conference "A Call to Action: Ensuring Global Human Resources for Health," March 22–23, 2007, Geneva. Agenda available at: http://www.hret.org/hret/publications/ihwm.html.

REFERENCES

Aluwihare, A. P. R. (2005). Physician migration: Donor country impact. *Journal of Continuing Education in the Health Professions, 25,* 15–21.

Anand, S., & Bärnighausen, T. (2007). Health workers and vaccination coverage in developing countries: An econometric analysis. *The Lancet, 369,* 1277–85.

Anonymous. (2006). *Philippines health care paralyzed by nurses' exodus.* Retrieved from: www.healthypages.co.uk.

Attaran, A., & Walker, R. B. (2008). Shoppers drug mart or poachers drug mart? *Canadian Medical Association Journal, 178,* 265–66.

Bach, S. (2003). *International migration of health workers: Labour and social issues.* Geneva: ILO. Retrieved from: http://www.medact.org/content/health/documents/brain_drain/Bach%20Health%20worker%20Migration%20WP%20209.pdf.

———. (2006). *International mobility of health professionals: Brain drain or brain exchange?* Research Papers No. 2006/82. Helsinki: Wider World Institute for Development Economics Research. Retrieved from: http://www.wider.unu.edu/publications/rps/rps2006/rp2006–82.pdf.

Biviano, M., & Makarehchi, F. (2003). *Globalization and the physician workforce in the United States.* Sixth International Medical Workforce Conference. Ottawa, Canada. Retrieved from: www.bhpr.hrsa.gov/healthworkforce/reports/gpw.htm.

Blouin, C. (2005). The impact of trade agreements on the mobility of health workers. Background paper prepared for Canadian research study (Labonté et al. 2003–2005) on the flow of HHR from sub-Saharan Africa to Canada. Unpublished manuscript. Available from Professor Ronald Labonté: rlabonte@uottawa.ca.

Bourassa, Forcier, M., Simoens, S., & Giuffrida, A. (2004). Impact, regulation and health policy implications of physician migration in OECD countries. *Human Resources for Health, 2,* 1–11.

Broten, L. (2008). *Report on removing barriers for international medical doctors.* Toronto: Government of Ontario.

Buchan, J., Parkin, T., & Sochalski, J. (2003). *International nurse mobility: Trends and policy implications.* London: Royal College of Nursing. Retrieved from: http://www.rcn.org.uk/downloads/InternationalNurseMobility-April162003.doc.

Buchan, J., Jobanputra, R., Gough, P., & Hutt, R. (2006). Internationally recruited nurses in London: A survey of career paths and plans. *Human Resources for Health,* 4.

Bueno de Mesquita, J., & Gordon, M. (2005). *The international migration of health workers: A human rights analysis.* London: Medact. Retrieved from: www.medact.org.

Bundred, P., Martineau, T., & Kitchiner, D. (2004). Factors affecting the global migration of health professionals. *Harvard Health Policy Review,* 5, 77–87.

Burke, J. (2005, 13 February). Sri Lanka accuses NHS of luring away its medical staff. *Guardian Newspapers Ltd.*

Canadian Institute for Health Information (2005). *Canada's health care providers: 2005 chartbook.* Ottawa: Canadian Institute for Health Information. Retrieved from: http://secure.cihi.ca/cihiweb/products/HCP_Chartbook05_e.pdf.

———. (2006). *Geographic distribution of physicians: Beyond How many and where.* Ottawa: Canadian Institute for Health Information. Retrieved from: http://secure.cihi.ca/cihiweb/products/Geographic_Distribution_of_Physicians_FINAL_e.pdf.

Central Bank of Sri Lanka. (2005). *Annual report 2005.* Sri Lanka.

Chikanda, A. (2005). *Medical leave: The exodus of health professionals from Zimbabwe.* Southern Africa Migration Project. Cape Town: IDASA. Retrieved from: http://www.sahims.net/doclibrary/Sahims_Documents/Acrobat34.pdf.

College of Physicians and Surgeons of Ontario. (2004). *Tackling the doctor shortage.* The College of Physicians and Surgeons of Ontario.

Crush, J. (2002). The global raiders: Nationalism, globalization and the South African brain drain. *Journal of International Affairs,* 56, 148–72.

Dovlo, D. (2005a). Migration and the health system: Influences on reaching the MDGs in Africa (and other LDCs). In *International migration and the millennium development goals* (pp. 67–79). New York: UNFPA.

———. (2005b). Wastage in the health workforce: Some perspectives from African countries. *Human Resources for Health,* 3, 1–9.

Dubois, C. A., McKee, M., & Nolte, E., eds. (2006). *Human resources for health in Europe.* Maidenhead, UK: Open University Press. Retrieved from: http://www.euro.who.int/Document/E87923.pdf.

Dussault, G., & Dubois, C.-A. (2003). Human resources for health policies: A critical component in health policies. *Human Resources for Health,* 1.

Evans, R. G. (2008). Thomas McKeown, Meet Fidel Castro: Physicians, population health and the Cuban paradox. *Healthcare Policy,* 3, 21–31.

Gent, S., & Skeldon, R. (2006). *Skilled migration: Healthcare policy options.* Brighton, UK: Development Research Centre on Migration, Globalisation and Policy. Retrieved from: http://www.migrationdrc.org/publications/briefing_papers/BP6.pdf.

Gerein, N., Green, A., & Pearson, S. (2006a). The implications of shortages of health professionals for maternal health in sub-Saharan Africa. *Reproductive Health Matters,* 14, 40–50.

———. (2006b). The implications of shortages of health professionals for maternal health in sub-Saharan Africa. *Reproductive Health Matters,* 14, 40–50.

Hagopian, A., Ofosu, A., Fatusi, A., Biritwum, R., Esel, A., Hart, L. G., et al. (2005). The flight of physicians from West Africa: Views of African physicians and implications for policy. *Social Science and Medicine,* 61, 1750–60.

Hawthorne, L. (2001). The globalisation of the nursing workforce: Barriers confronting overseas qualified nurses in Australia. *Nursing Inquiry,* 8, 213–29.

International Pharmaceutical Federation (FIP). (2006). *Global pharmacy workforce and migration report*. The Hague, Netherlands: FIP. Retrieved from: http://www.fip.org/files/fip/HR/FIP%20Global%20Pharmacy%20and%20 Migration%20report%2007042006.PDF.

Joint Learning Initiative. (2004). *Human resources for health: Overcoming the crisis*. Cambridge, MA: Global Equity Initiative, Harvard University. Retrieved from:http://www.globalhealthtrust.org/report/Human_Resources_for_Health. pdf.

Kapur, D., & McHale, J. (2005). *Give us your best and brightest. The global hunt for talent and its impact on the developing world*. Washington, DC: Brookings Institution Press.

Khadria, B. (2006). International recruitment of nurses in India: Implications of stakeholder perspectives on overseas labour markets, migration and return. *Health Services Research*, 42 (3p2), 1429–36.

Kirigia, J., Gbary, A., Muthuri, L., Nyoni, J., & Seddoh, A. (2006). The cost of health professionals' brain drain in Kenya. *BMC Health Services Research*, 6, 89.

Kovindha, O. (2006, October 16). The right to freedom of health professional movement and the right to health care in ASEAN countries: Lecture presented at 13th Canadian Conference on International Health (CCIH), Ottawa, Canada.

Labonté, R., Packer, C., & Klassen, N. (2006). Managing health professional migration from sub-Saharan Africa to Canada: A stakeholder inquiry into policy options. *Human Resources for Health*, 4, 22.

Liese, B., & Dussault, G. (2004). *The state of the health workforce in sub-Saharan Africa: Evidence of crisis and analysis of contributing factors*. Africa region, World Bank. Retrieved from: http://siteresources.worldbank.org/AFRICAEXT/ Resources/No_75.pdf http://www-wds.worldbank.org/external/default/WDS-ContentServer/WDSP/IB/2005/07/05/000090341_20050705112206/Rendered/PDF/328040Health0workforce0AFHD0No175.pdf.

Marchal, B., & Kegels, G. (2003). Health workforce imbalances in times of globalization: Brain drain or professional mobility? *International Journal of Health Planning and Management*, 18, S89–S101.

Martin, P. (2003). *Highly skilled labour migration: Sharing the benefits*. Geneva: International Labour Organization. Retrieved from: http://www-ilo-mirror. cornell.edu/public/english/bureau/inst/download/migration2.pdf.

McDonald, D. A., & Crush, J. (2002). *Destinations unknown: Perspectives on the brain drain in Southern Africa*. Pretoria: African Insitute of South Africa.

McVeigh, T. (2006, May 21). Nurse exodus leaves Kenya in crisis. *The Observer*.

Mensah, K., Mackintosh, M., & Henry, L. (2005). *The "skills drain" of health professionals from the developing world: A framework for policy formulation*. London: Medact. Retrieved from: www.medact.org.

Mullan, F. (2005). The metrics of the physician brain drain. *New England Journal of Medicine*, 353, 1810–18.

Nicholas, S. (2007). Movement of health professionals: Trends and enlargement. *Eurohealth*, 8, 11–12.

OECD. (2002). *GATS: The case for open services markets*. Paris: OECD.

Ouaked, S. (2002). Transatlantic roundtable on high-skilled migration and sending countries issues. *International Migration*, 40, 153–66.

Packer, C., Labonté, R., & Spitzer, D. (2007). *Globalization and health worker crisis*. Globalization and Health Knowledge Network: Research Papers. Ottawa: Institute of Population Health, University of Ottawa.

Paton, Carol. (2006, April 14). Doctors—terminally ill. *Financial Mail SA*.

Percot, M. (2006). Indian nurses in the Gulf: Two generations of female migration. *South Asia Research*, 26, 41–62.

Physicians for Human Rights. (2004). *An action plan to prevent brain drain: Building equitable health systems in Africa.* PHR's Health Action AIDS Campaign. Boston: Physicians for Human Rights. Retrieved from: www.phrusa.org.

Pond, B., & McPake, B. (2006). The health migration crisis: The role of four Organisation for Economic Cooperation and Development countries. *Lancet,* 367, 1448–55.

Serneels, P., Lindelow, M., Garcia-Montalvo, J., & Barr, A. (2005). *For public service or money: Understanding geographical imbalances in the health workforce.* World Bank Policy Research Working Paper No. 3686. Geneva: World Bank. Retrieved from: http://ideas.repec.org/p/wbk/wbrwps/3686.html.

Thomas, C., Hosein, R, Yan, J. (2005). Assessing the export of nursing services as a diversification option for CARICOM economics: Report prepared for the Caribbean Commission on Health and Development, May 2005. Washington, DC: PAHO and Caribbean Commission on Health and Development.

Tjadens, F. (2002). Health care shortages: Where globalisation, nurses and migration meet. *Eurohealth,* 8, 33–35.

Vujicic, M., Zurn, P., Diallo, K., Adams, O., & Dal Poz, M. (2004). The role of wages in the migration of health care professionals from developing countries. *Human Resources for Health,* 2.

Watanabe, M., Comeau, M., & Buske, L. (2008). Analysis of international migration patterns affecting physician supply in Canada. *Healthcare Policy,* 3, e129–e138.

World Health Organization. (2006). *The world health report 2006: Working together for health.* Geneva: WHO.

Zurn, P., & Dumont, J.-C. (2008). *Health workforce and international migration: Can New Zealand compete?* Paris: Organisation for Economic Co-operation and Development.

10 Globalization, Trade, and the Nutrition Transition

Corinna Hawkes, Mickey Chopra, and Sharon Friel

INTRODUCTION

The world is characterized by huge nutritional inequities. Undernutrition, especially among children, persists at unacceptably high levels, leading to poor health in the poorest and most vulnerable communities around the world. At the same time, a "nutrition transition" to energy-dense, poor-quality diets is occurring, leading to obesity and diet-related chronic diseases (DRCD) among poor populations in middle- and high-income countries (or developed and transitioning countries).

This chapter begins with an overview of the double burden of malnutrition. It then identifies and analyzes the role of processes of globalization within the food system that are linked to the increase of poor-quality diets: the rise of transnational food corporations (TFCs), international food trade, and the use of global food advertising and promotion. It also examines how these processes are changing diets through their interaction with changes in the social system such as household livelihood and income, shifting global demographics, and increasing levels of urbanization.

THE DOUBLE BURDEN OF MALNUTRITION

Since the 1980s, the proportion of undernourished children and adults in the world has declined. The rate of decline, however, was slow; the numbers remain high; and in Africa, the actual number of undernourished people rose (Tables 10.1, 10.2, and 10.3). The Food and Agricultural Organization of the United Nations (FAO) estimates that between 2001 and 2003, 854 million people worldwide were undernourished: 820 million in developing countries, 25 million in transition countries, and 9 million in industrialized countries (FAO, 2006). In developing countries, this represents a decline of just 3 million people since 1990–92 (Table 10.1); between 2000 and 2003 there was an actual *increase* of 23 million, offsetting a decline of 26 million between 1990 and 1997. By far the largest number of undernourished people live in Asia (mainly South Asia), but it is only in Africa that the number of undernourished people has increased since 1990 (FAO, 2006). The proportion and number of stunted[1] and underweight[2] children in developing countries declined between 1980 and 2005, but in Africa, while the proportion declined, the number of stunted children increased, as did both the proportion and number of underweight (Tables 10.2 and 10.3). There were an estimated 165 million stunted and 138 million underweight children in developing countries in 2005.

Table 10.1   Number and Proportion of Undernourished People in Developing Countries, 1990–1992 and 2001–2003

Region	Number of Undernourished People (million)		Proportion of Undernourished People (%)	
	1990–1992	2001–2003	1990–1992	2001–2003
Sub-Saharan Africa	169.0	206.2	36	32
Near East & North Africa	25.0	37.6	8	9
Asia	569.7	524.0	20	6
Latin America/Caribbean	59.6	52.4	13	10
DEVELOPING WORLD	823.1	820.2	20	17

Source: Adapted from United Nations Food and Agriculture Organization, 2006, p. 32.

Table 10.2   Estimated Prevalence and Number of Stunted Children in Developing Countries, 1980 (actual) and 2005 (forecasted)

UN Region	Prevalence of Stunting (%)		Number Stunted (million)	
	1980 (actual)	2005 (forecasted)	1980 (actual)	2005 (forecasted)
Developing countries	47.1	29.0	221.35	164.70
Africa	40.5	33.8	34.78	49.40
Asia	52.2	29.9	173.37	110.19
Latin America/Caribbean	25.6	9.3	13.19	5.11

Source: Adapted from United Nations System Sub-Committee on Nutrition, 2000.

Table 10.3   Estimated Prevalence and Number of Underweight Children in Developing Countries, 1980 (actual) and 2005 (forecasted)

UN Region	Prevalence of Underweight (%)		Number Underweight (million)	
	1980 (actual)	2005 (forecasted)	1980 (actual)	2005 (forecasted)
Developing countries	37.4	24.3	175.74	137.95
Africa	26.2	29.1	22.47	42.45
Asia	43.9	25.3	145.95	93.16
Latin America/Caribbean	14.2	4.3	7.32	2.35

Source: Adapted from United Nations System Sub-Committee on Nutrition, 2000.

By numbers, micronutrient deficiency is an even larger problem. Iron deficiency and anemia affect at least 3.5 billion people in the developing world; more than 740 million people are affected by goiter (a result of iodine deficiency), and 2 billion are at risk for dietary iodine deficiency; between 78 and 254 million people are estimated to suffer from vitamin A deficiency; large numbers also suffer from zinc deficiency (United Nations System Sub-Committee on Nutrition, 2000).

Against this background, it is ironic that the proportion and number of adults and children who are overweight or obese is increasing, particularly in the developed or high-income countries of the world. According to the World Health Organization (WHO), in 2005 approximately 1.6 billion adults (age fifteen and over) worldwide were overweight, at least 400 million of whom were obese (World Health Organization, 2006). In addition, at least 20 million children under the age of five years were overweight. WHO further projects that by 2015, approximately 2.3 billion adults will be overweight and more than 700 million will be obese.

Obesity has become an important global public health concern because it is a core risk factor for the development of DRCDs such as cardiovascular diseases (CVDs), diabetes, and some cancers, as well as the associated risk factors of high blood pressure and cholesterol. Although CVDs have been the leading causes of death in developed countries for decades, CVD is now projected to be the leading cause of mortality in developing countries as well, and 80 percent of all deaths from chronic diseases occur in developing countries (World Health Organization, 2005). Worldwide, the number of individuals with diabetes is estimated to rise from 171 million (2.8 percent of the world's population) in 2000, to 366 million (6.5 percent) in 2030, 298 million of whom will live in developing countries (Wild, Roglic, Green, Sicree, & King, 2004).

Likewise, the number of people who are overweight and obese is growing particularly rapidly in developing countries, from Brazil to Morocco, India to China, Saudi Arabia to Thailand (World Health Organization, 2000; Popkin & Gordon-Larsen, 2004; Prentice, 2006). As shown in Figure 10.1, the prevalence of overweight is considerably higher in urban areas in the developing world, but in Latin America, the Middle East, and South Africa, overweight is also higher than underweight in rural areas. Moreover, the situation found in high-income countries, where prevalence of obesity and related diseases is disproportionately high among groups of lower socioeconomic status (SES), is beginning to repeat in middle-income countries. A recent review of the evidence concluded that as developing country gross national product (GNP) increases, the burden of obesity shifts towards lower SES groups. After countries cross a GNP threshold of about US$2,500 per capita, women of low SES have proportionally higher rates of obesity (Monteiro, Moura, Conde, & Popkin, 2004). In other words, in both developed and developing countries, obesity starts out as a problem among groups of higher SES but as national economies grow, the

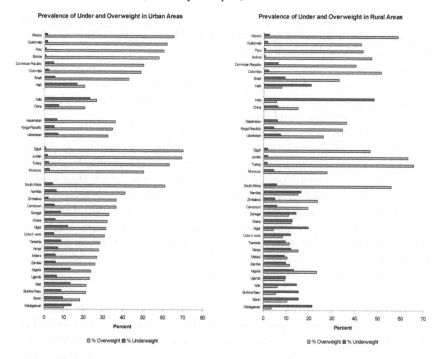

Figure 10.1 Prevalence of overweight and underweight in urban and rural areas of developing countries.

Source: Adapted from Mendez & Popkin, 2004.

risk moves towards groups of lower SES.[3] In Mexico, for example, a recent study showed that overweight and obesity doubled over a six year period in young women living in a poor community (Neufeld, Hernández-Cordero, Fernald, & Ramakrishnan, 2008). In these lower income communities, obesity has been found to coexist with undernutrition within the same household, typically consisting of an overweight mother with a stunted child (Doak, Adair, Monteiro, & Popkin, 2000; Garrett & Ruel, 2005).

These changes in nutritional status can be linked in part to changing diets. In what is often termed the nutrition transition, people are consuming more fats, sweeteners, energy-dense foods, and highly processed foods compared to traditional diets characterized by higher intake of cereals. In industrialized countries, the transition to diets higher in fats, sweeteners, and highly processed foods has been ongoing since the Industrial Revolution (Grigg, 1995). For example, in England, it is estimated that the per person consumption of fat and refined carbohydrates increased five to tenfold over the past two centuries, while the consumption of fiber-rich grains declined substantially (Uusitalo, Pietinen, & Puska, 2002). Today, this shift is taking place in middle- and low-income countries, but at a much faster rate

(Popkin, 2002). The shift typically begins with major increases in domestic production and imports of oilseeds and vegetable oils (Drewnowski & Popkin, 1997). Consumption then increases of animal-source foods (meat, milk) and processed foods such as snacks, soft drinks, breakfast cereals, and processed dairy products. The transition is also characterized by increased consumption of foods away from home, such as street foods and fast foods. As a result of these changes, people who do not consume sufficient energy to assuage hunger face nutrition insecurity through an inadequate supply of micronutrients, while those who do consume sufficient energy also face nutrition insecurity through an intake of unhealthy levels of saturated fat and free sugars.

GLOBALIZATION AND DIET: A QUESTION OF CHANGING FOOD AND SOCIAL SYSTEMS

It is widely postulated that the nutrition transition towards poor quality, energy-dense diets and the increasing prevalence of chronic disease is deeply rooted in the processes of globalization. Two plausible pathways can be identified. First, globalization-driven changes in the social system, including income growth, urbanization, and employment, can drive dietary changes. Second, globalization-related changes in the food system can alter the amount and quality of food available for consumption. Changes in both the social and food system are important in and of themselves but are of course interconnected, making it difficult to attribute exactly the influence of specific components.

CHANGES IN THE SOCIAL SYSTEM

While this chapter focuses mainly on the food system, some contextual understanding of the possible influence of globalization on the social system is necessary, particularly if we are to understand the unequal distribution observed in overnutrition (Friel, Chopra, & Satcher, 2007). Ecological studies suggest that increasing national income and urbanization are associated with changes in diet and prevalence of obesity. Countries with higher GNPs and more urbanized populations consume greater amounts of energy from fats, sweeteners, and protein (Popkin, 1999; Dixon et al., 2007). It has also been estimated that body mass index (BMI), along with systolic blood pressure and total cholesterol, increases with national income until about I$5,000 (international dollars)[4] and then levels off. BMI increases continuously with greater urbanization (Ezzati et al., 2005). Thus, to the degree that globalization has helped to generate higher national incomes and encouraged more urbanization, it is associated with the nutrition transition through changes in ways of living and associated food demands.

240 *Corinna Hawkes, Mickey Chopra, and Sharon Friel*

But it should be noted that the relationship among globalization, income, urbanization, employment, and nutrition is not straightforward. Many have disputed whether globalization really does lead to higher household incomes for all (see Chapters 2 and 13, this volume). It has already been shown that in some countries, people of lower SES consume more obesogenic diets, indicating that even if there is a relationship between rising incomes and obesity at the level of national populations, it may not operate at the individual or household level. Moreover, the nutrition transition among people of lower SES is occurring faster in today's developing countries than earlier transitions in industrialized countries. The nature of urbanization and the resulting built environment appears to have a greater adverse impact on low-income households that are more constrained by lack of transportation and lack of healthful food purchasing choices in lower-income neighborhoods (Dixon et al., 2007). Globalization-induced changes in employment conditions have possible ramifications

---

Box 10.1 Implications for diet: Changes in the Indian social system.

India's emergence as one of today's most rapidly growing economic forces arises partly because of a shift in the late 1980s away from its historical commitment to nonalignment and self-reliance, to greater international trade liberalization, liberalization of foreign direct investment, fewer restrictions on large enterprises, and liberalization of the financial sector. However, like many transitioning countries, the nature of India's integration into the globalization process and accompanying structural adjustment programs appears to have been characterized by cuts in some areas of welfare spending, low employment generation, greater income inequality, and persistence of poverty (Gupte, Ramachandran, & Mutatkar, 2001).

Since 1997, the Indian economy has grown on average by 5.4 percent each year, resulting in a burgeoning urban middle class that is roughly the same size as the whole of the United States. Juxtaposed with national wealth are the persistently high rates of poverty, which, while declining, remain a very serious problem in rural and urban slum areas. Notably, over the course of the 1990s, much of the push in urban areas was towards informal, unprotected labor. With wages not indexed to inflation, this growing group is disproportionately affected by rising food prices (Ghosh, 2002).

Both economic growth and workforce changes were enjoyed most acutely by the urban middle-class professionals and skilled workers, and helped to fuel increases in market demand for high-value foods such as meat, fruit, vegetables, and edible oils, which were highly import intensive, and have created a boom in certain consumer goods (Ghosh, 2002). Through globalization of the economy the middle-class, Indian dietary habits have converged with those of the Western world, that is, high in saturated fat and refined sugars.

Even though India experienced continued economic growth, employment, which grew by 2.5 percent per annum between 1987 and 1988, and 1993 and 1994, slowed down to 1.1 percent between 1993 and 1994, and between 1999 and 2000. During this period of globalization, work in the agriculture sector stagnated (Papola, 2005). The reduction in state subsidies supporting domestic produce, the depression of domestic prices due to cheaper imports, and technological and infrastructural factors have affected both the nature of the national food supply and employment and working conditions for those in the agricultural sector.

for nutrition security, although the evidence remains sparse. Time pressures and strain associated with precarious employment conditions make fast access to energy-dense foods more attractive. More fundamentally, changing labor market conditions mean reduced job security and limited access to benefits such as paid family leave that undermine those financial and psychosocial resources necessary for individuals and communities to make healthy living choices (Friel et al., 2007). An example of how globalization has affected diets through these changes in the social system is given in Box 10.1.

CHANGES IN THE FOOD SYSTEM

Globalization is also influencing diets by radically altering the nature of the food system. As stated by Kennedy, Nantel, and Shetty:

> [G]lobalization is having a major impact on food systems around the world . . . [which] affect availability and access to food through changes to food production, procurement and distribution and the food trade environment . . . in turn bringing about a gradual shift in food culture, with consequent changes in dietary consumption patterns and nutritional status that vary with the socio-economic strata. (2004, p. 1)

The evidence suggests that diets have been influenced by three important changes in the food system: the growth of TFCs, including transnational supermarkets; liberalization of international food trade and foreign direct investment (FDI); and global food advertising and promotion (Table 10.4). All three are fundamental to the process of globalization, and can be conceptualized as affecting diet by altering the availability, prices, and desirability of food.

Table 10.4   Globalization Processes Linked With the Nutrition Transition

Globalization Process	Dietary Implication
Growth of TFCs, including supermarkets	Increases **availability** of processed foods (fast foods, snacks, soft drinks) through growth of fast-food outlets, supermarkets, and food advertising/promotion; driven by trade and FDI. Growth of transnational supermarkets changes food **availability** (increases diversity of available products), **accessibility, price,** and way food is marketed
Liberalization of international food trade and foreign direct investment (FDI)	Imports change **availability** of foods and/or their **price;** investment changes type of foods **available,** their **price,** and the way they are sold and marketed
Global food advertising and promotion	Shapes food preferences by affecting **desirability** of different foods

The Growth of Transnational Food Processors, Fast-Food Companies, and Supermarkets

TFCs now increasingly organize food production, distribution, and marketing on a global scale. Globalization has provided powerful incentives for the formation of these transnational companies (Box 10.2). TFCs grow through FDI, often acquiring partial or complete ownership of a local company. This allows companies to buy, sell, and invest in other companies in other countries, one of the processes through which vertical integration of the global food chain is taking place.

The market power of TFCs throughout the food supply chain has grown considerably with globalization. Globally traded agricultural commodities, from bananas to sugar to coffee, are now controlled by a relatively small number of processors and retailers (Vorley, 2003). Meat producers and processors have become increasingly concentrated (Table 10.5), while the largest food processors and retailers have spread their global reach and increased sales (Table 10.6) (Hendrickson & Heffernan, 2005).

Box 10.2   How globalization has encouraged the growth of TFCs.

- FDI in the food industry as the key process by which TFCs form and grow.
- The commercialization and privatization of state food monopolies, further opening opportunities for investment by the domestic and foreign private sector.
- FDI in the service sector, the streamlining of dispute settlement mechanisms under the World Trade Organization, and stronger and broader intellectual property rights (see Chapter 11, this volume) facilitate the ability of TFCs to conduct business and increase access to capital and technology, encouraging further investment by TFCs.
- More liberalized cross-border trade and FDI facilitates "global vertical integration" by which TFCs and their buying and contracting companies and services become involved in all aspects of the production, processing, distribution, and sale of a particular food, bringing the entire food supply chain under TFC control.
- Greater liberalization of cross-border trade also facilitates "global sourcing," when a company searches for inputs, production sites, and outputs where costs are lower and regulatory, political, and social regimes favorable. Both vertical integration and global sourcing enable TFCs to cut costs and create safeguards against the uncertainty of commodity production and product sales, stimulating further growth of TFCs.

Table 10.5   Concentration Ratio (CR)[a] of Selected Food Sectors in the United States

Sector	Historical CR (date)	CR in 2003
Beef packers	72% (1990)	84%
Broilers	44% (1990)	56%
Pork packers	40% (1990)	49%
Food retailers	24% (1997)	46%

Source: Adapted from Hendrickson and Heffernan, 2005.
Note: [a]CR is the concentration (relative to 100%) of the top four firms in that specific food sector.

Table 10.6   Sales From the Largest TFCs in Food Processing and Retail, mid-2000s

Sector	TFC (country-base)	Sales US$ Billions (year)
Food processors	Kraft Foods Inc. (US)	21.9 (2003)
	Tyson Foods Inc. (US)	21.9 (2003)
	Pepsico Inc. (US)	18.3 (2003)
Food retailers	Wal-Mart (US)	244.5 (2004)
	Carrefour (France)	64.7 (2004)
	Royal Ahold (Netherlands)	59.2 (2004)

Source: Adapted from Hendrickson and Heffernan, 2005.

The most dramatic increase in power has been among food retailers, which have emerged as dominant players in the food system (Murphy, 2006). In Europe, merely 110 retail buying desks served 160 million consumers and 3.2 million farmers and producers in 2003 (Vorley, 2003). European and US-based grocery retailers are expanding transnationally: in 2002, 49 percent of French-based Carrefour's sales came from the foreign market, as did 85 percent of Dutch-based Royal Ahold's sales (Vorley, 2003). In just the ten years since Wal-Mart first started to sell food, it has emerged as the world's largest grocery chain, with 45 percent of total sales coming from groceries (Murphy, 2006). In 2004, Wal-Mart was estimated to have 6.1 percent of the global grocery market, with Carrefour at 2.3 percent. In 2003 the top thirty retailers had 19 percent of the market in Asia and Oceania and 29 percent of the market in Latin America, and in all continents mergers and acquisitions are ongoing. Supermarkets now control 50 to 60 percent of the food retail sector in Latin America. The effect of these trends is similar everywhere: supermarket chains are replacing local food shops, bringing in capital and know-how to deliver a variety of food to consumers in one place (Murphy, 2006).

TFCs have altered the food supply by increasing the availability of processed and fast foods through the growth in food-processing companies and large transnational supermarkets and fast-food outlets, and by making them more desirable through advertising and promotion (McMichael, Shetty, & McPherson, 1997; Lang, 1999; Chopra, Galbraith, & Darnton-Hill, 2002; Chopra, 2002; Hawkes, 2002, 2006; Chopra & Darnton-Hill, 2004; Kennedy et al., 2004; Kinabo, 2004; Sawaya, Martins, & Martins, 2004).

The largest foreign affiliates of TFCs in developing countries are often food companies specializing in producing some type of processed foods (Table 10.7). FDI has played a particularly important role in shaping the growing global market for such foods (Connor, 1994; Vepa, 2004; Hawkes, 2005, 2006). Food processing is now the most important recipient of FDI relative to other parts of the food system, and FDI is more important in the global processed-foods market than trade. US FDI into foreign food processing companies grew from US$9 billion in 1980 to US$36 billion in

2000. Sales by these companies increased from US$39.2 billion in 1982 to US$150 billion in 2000; trade, by contrast, generated a relatively small US$30 billion in processed food sales in 2000. While a high proportion of this FDI is still targeted at high-income countries, an increasing proportion is entering developing and transition markets, notably Latin America, Asia, and Central and Eastern Europe. The evidence also shows that as FDI into food processing companies has risen, the allocation of investment has shifted away from products for export to the home market towards foods for sale in the host market. In 1998, 74 percent of the sales of affiliates of US food companies remained in the host market.

A second trend has been the shift of FDI away from primary to highly processed foods. For instance, Central and Eastern Europe and the Baltic states attracted soaring rates of FDI in the food sector in the 1990s, concentrated on soft drinks and confectionery. The confectionery sector in Poland attracted FDI of US$963 million between 1990 and 1999, more than the FDI in meat, fish, flour, pasta, bread, sugar, potato products, fruits, vegetables, vegetable oils, and fats put together. On a global scale, this trend has led to the dominance of foreign investors in the highly processed-food sector. In China, there are numerous national and local food companies, some of which have successfully outcompeted foreign companies. But in packaged foods, such as instant noodles, soft drinks, snacks, sweet biscuits, and fast foods, foreign investors dominate. Further evidence comes from Mexico, as described in Box 10.3 (Hawkes, 2006).

This is not to underestimate the importance of domestic investment in the processed-foods industry, as shown by evidence from India. In India the consumer-food industry remains relatively small but has been growing since 1990, notably in packaged bread and biscuits. Consumption of these products has increased. Yet a relatively small proportion of this growth came from foreign relative to domestic investment: of the US$156 billion of investment in the Indian processed-foods industry between 1991 and 2002, just US$2 billion was from FDI (Vepa, 2004).

The second key aspect of the growth of TFCs has involved transnational supermarkets. Supermarkets have fast become the new locus of power in the food system and now provide an increasing amount of the world's food to consumers (Tables 10.5 and 10.6). FDI from US-based supermarket chains grew to nearly US$13 billion in 1999, up from around US$4 billion in 1990. European-based supermarkets have transnationalized to an even greater extent: Carrefour (France), Tesco (UK), and Metro (Germany) are the second, third, and fourth largest supermarkets worldwide, after Wal-Mart, the world leader (Hendrickson & Heffernan, 2007).

The growing importance of supermarkets has two important related dietary implications: shifting demand for home-produced foods or foods purchased in open ("wet") markets to increased dependence on store-bought foods supplied by TFCs; and expanding available food choices, especially of processed foods (Lang, 1999; Chopra, 2002; Cwiertka &

Box 10.3   Foreign direct investment, supermarkets, and processed foods in Mexico.

In 1994, Mexico, the United States, and Canada signed the North American Free Trade Agreement (NAFTA). The agreement contained key provisions designed to facilitate foreign investment, and stimulated a rapid acceleration of FDI from the United States into Mexican food processing. Between 1983 and 1993, US FDI into the Mexican food-processing industry increased from US$210 million to US$2.3 billion. Five years after NAFTA was signed, FDI into the Mexican food industry from the United States had risen to US$5.3 billion, nearly three-quarters of which went into the production of processed foods.

The passage of NAFTA also had a profound effect on the food retailing sector in Mexico. The number of chain supermarkets, discounters, and convenience stores grew from less than 700 in 1993 to 3,850 in 1997 and 5,729 in 2004 (Hawkes, 2006). Growth occurred largely though major investments by foreign-based retailers. Modern retailers, notably supermarkets and convenience stores, now account for 55 percent of all food retail in the country. US-based Wal-Mart de Mexico (known as Walmex) has been particularly successful; it is now the nation's leading retailer. In 2004, there were 663 million customer transactions at 420 Walmex supermarkets and discount stores and 290 Walmex restaurants in seventy-nine cities; in 2004, sales increased by 11 percent to reach a record high of US$12.4 billion. The company also employs more people (109,075) than any other company in Mexico

Large supermarkets in Mexico, like Walmex, stock a far wider range of processed foods than the small, traditional family-owned *tiendas*. During the time period of the rise of supermarkets, sales of processed foods (e.g., soft drinks, snacks, baked goods, and dairy products) expanded rapidly relative to other food groups, at a rate of 5–10 percent per year (between 1995 and 2003). Importantly, thousands of *tiendas* also sell (almost exclusively) soft drinks and snacks.

Walraven, 2002; Fajardo, 2004; Kennedy et al., 2004; Kinabo, 2004; Pingali & Khwaja, 2004; Sawaya et al., 2004; Schmidhuber & Prakash, 2004; Hawkes, 2006; Popkin, 2006; Dixon et al., 2007). The entry of supermarkets into developing countries is marked initially by specialization in the sale of processed foods; after establishment, supermarkets diversify into products like frozen meat and fruits and vegetables (Kennedy et al., 2004; Schmidhuber & Prakash, 2004; Popkin, 2006). This focus on processed foods occurs because supermarkets are better able to make available a far wider range of such foods than are small stores, to take the risks inherent in introducing new foods, and to sell them at lower prices (Hawkes, 2006). The case of Mexico again presents an illustrative example of the effect of the growth of supermarkets (Box 10.3).

Fast-food companies have grown along with supermarkets. Figure 10.2 shows that, while the number of McDonald's outlets in the United States increased rapidly between 1991 and 2001, the proportion of outlets outside the United States increased at an even faster rate. Other data show that even in countries like Tanzania, where the number of fast-food outlets remains quite small, their presence and popularity are fast rising, propelled by advertising and promotion (Kinabo, 2004).

246 *Corinna Hawkes, Mickey Chopra, and Sharon Friel*

Table 10.7 Examples of Low- and Middle-Income Countries in Which Food
Companies are Among the Three Largest Foreign Affiliates in the
Industrial or Tertiary Sector

Country	Sector (rank 1–3 by sales)	Company Name (country base)	Sales (US$ millions)[a]
Africa			
Algeria	Food, dairy (1)	Laiterie Djurdjura (France)	29.8
Cape Verde	Beverages, beer/soft drinks (1)	Ceris-Soc CV Cerveja Ref (Luxembourg)	1.8
Kenya	Food, packaged (3)	Unilever Kenya (UK)	141.0
Morocco	Food, packaged (3)	Nestlé Maroc (Switzerland)	88.4
Rwanda	Beverages, beer/soft drinks (1)	Brasseries et Limonaderies (Netherlands)	28.6
Zimbabwe	Food, meat (1)	Meat Importers (UK)	25.0
Asia / Pacific			
Cambodia	Beverages, soft (2)	Cambodia Beverage Company (Coca-Cola) (Singapore)	Not known
Samoa	Beverages, beer/soft drinks (2)	Samoa Breweries (Japan)	Not known
Central& Eastern Europe			
Albania	Beverages, soft (2)	Coca-Cola Bottling Enterprises (USA)	Not known
Bosnia-Herzegovina	Beverages, soft (3)	Coca-Cola (USA)	Not known
Croatia	Beverages, beer (1)	Zagrebacka Pivovara DD (Belgium)	49.4
Estonia	Food, meat processing (3)	Rakvere Lihakombinaat AS (Finland)	72.8
Kazakhstan	Diversified, including food (1)	Procter & Gamble (USA)	150.0
Moldova	Food, dairy (2)	Alba (USA)	Not known
Romania	Retail, including food (1)	Metro Cash and Carry SRI (Germany)	359.8
Ukraine	Beverages, soft (3)	Coca-Cola Beverages Ukraine Ltd. Co. (USA)	42.0
Latin America			
Brazil	Retail, including food (2)	Carrefour Comercio E Industria (France)	4412.0
Costa Rica	Food, fruit production (3)	Standard Fruit Company de Costa Rica (USA)	173.0
Ecuador	Food, packaged (2)	Nestlé Ecuador (Switzerland)	102.0
Mexico	Retail, including food (1)	Wal-Mart de Mexico (USA)	9607.0

Source: Hawkes, 2005. Reprinted with permission.
Note: [a]Data are taken from 1999, 2000, 2001, or 2002.

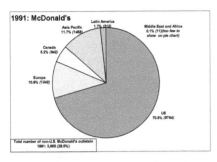 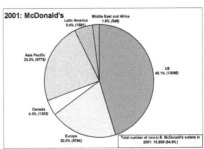

Figure 10.2 Worldwide number of McDonald's outlets, by region, 1991 and 2001 (proportion and number).

Source: Hawkes, 2002. Reprinted with permission.

TFCs and Changing Dietary Patterns

There can be no question that processed foods now loom larger in the global diet. Between 2000 and 2005, sales of packaged foods increased from US$1.095 billion to US$1.455 billion (Euromonitor, 2006). Globally, the fastest growth was in snack bars, followed by ready meals. The number of transactions at fast-food chains is also increasing in countries all over the world (Figure 10.3). Sales of processed foods in developing countries are lower than in developed countries (one-quarter or less of all food expenditures, compared with almost half), and sales of primary processed foods (e.g., fats and oils) relative to highly processed foods are greater. Yet annual sales growth of all processed foods is around 29 percent in low- to middle-income countries compared with 7 percent in high- to middle-income countries. For example, in Brazil, growth in real volume sales of hamburgers, biscuits, ready-to-eat desserts, yogurts, and flavored milk amounted to an average 27 percent between 1993 and 1997, compared with 5 percent for vegetable oils, margarines, beef, poultry, and pork meat. Sales of breakfast cereals are registering double- and triple-digit growth in many developing countries, while sales growth of ready-to-eat meals has been dramatic in Eastern Europe and Latin America. Soft-drink sales are growing rapidly in Eastern Europe, Asia, and Latin America. Vietnam, China, and Indonesia are expected to be the fastest-growing markets for packaged food retail sales over the coming years, with growth rates forecast at 11, 10, and 8 percent, respectively. Korea, Thailand, India, and the Philippines rank among the top ten growing markets, with total packaged food retail sales expected to grow by 5 to 7 percent annually.

Direct evidence on changes in the amounts of processed foods manufactured by TFCs, however, is lacking. One study (Adair & Popkin, 2005) actually suggests these foods contribute relatively few calories to diets among youth in developing countries. The study examined changes in consumption of fast foods, snacks, and soft drinks among youth in China,

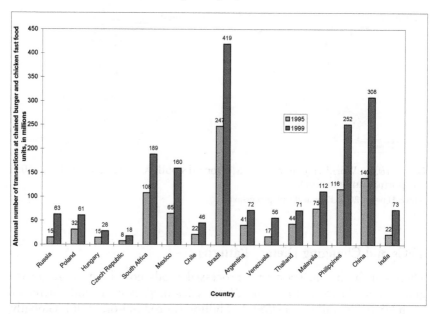

Figure 10.3   Number of transactions at chained burger and chicken outlets in selected countries, 1995 and 1999.

Source: Hawkes, 2002. Reprinted with permission.

Russia, the Philippines (Cebu in metropolitan Manila), and the United States, finding that in the United States, intake of these foods doubled from 10.5 percent to 21.2 percent of total energy intake between 1977 and 1996. The contribution of these foods to caloric intake in the other countries was much smaller. In Chinese youth, modern snacks, fast foods, and soft drinks made up less than 0.1 percent of caloric intake in both 1991 and 2000. In Russian youth, percent calories from modern snacks rose from 0.9 to 1.4 percent between 1994 and 2003, fast food remained the same at 0.2 percent, and soft drinks rose from 0.2 to 0.5 percent. In Cebu youth, percent calories from modern snacks declined from 2.6 percent to 0.6 percent between 1994 and 2002, fast food remained the same at 0.7 percent, and soft drinks rose from 1.6 percent to 3 percent. The evidence thus shows that, relative to the United States, the presence of fast foods, snacks, and soft drinks in the diets of youth remains relatively small, although these products are beginning to have more dietary significance in these countries.

There is also little direct evidence on how the growth of large supermarkets has influenced dietary patterns. It is clear that consumers are purchasing more foods at supermarkets relative to other stores, and supermarkets sell a wider range of processed foods, but the dietary impacts of this shift has not been subject to rigorous investigation.

In practice, direct measurements of consumption of foods produced by TFCs may not be the best source of evidence of dietary impact. This is because TFCs also have important indirect effects (Hawkes, 2006). TFCs have a reverberating impact on food-system change by introducing new ways to sell and promote foods and stimulating new forms of competition, thereby affecting the availability, accessibility, price, and desirability of foods not just from TFCs but from all actors in the food market

INTERNATIONAL FOOD TRADE

The Growth of International Food Trade

The rise of international food trade, especially imports, is widely perceived as an important determinant of the nutrition transition. In some countries, trade liberalization was initially adopted as a domestic, unilateral strategy. In others, eliminating quotas, lowering tariffs, and privatizing state trading agencies were undertaken as part of structural adjustment programs (SAPs) in many developing countries starting in the 1980s. The pace of reform accelerated in the 1990s as many countries liberalized food trade via global, regional, and bilateral agreements. The 1994 Agreement on Agriculture represented the first time food had been specifically addressed in the General Agreement on Tariffs and Trade (GATT). The GATT was superseded by the World Trade Organization (WTO), which continues to be the major global negotiating mechanism for the reduction of tariffs, export subsidies, and domestic agricultural support. WTO disciplines are now complemented by a proliferation of regional and bilateral agreements including the North America Free Trade Agreement (NAFTA), the Mercado Común Sudamericano (MERCOSUR), the Association of Southeast Asian Nations (ASEAN), and the Central American Free Trade Agreement (CAFTA). The result has been a more liberal regime for international food trade, although it cannot yet be described as "open," since high levels of protection still exist in various forms.

The global value of food trade grew from US$224 billion in 1972 to US$438 billion in 1998, a 95 percent increase that greatly exceeded world population growth of 53 percent during the same time period. Food now accounts for 11 percent of global trade, a proportion higher than that of fuel (Pinstrup-Andersen & Babinard, 2001; Chopra et al., 2002). In developing countries, food-import bills as a share of gross domestic product (GDP) more than doubled between 1974 and 2004, and the amount of trade made up of processed agricultural products rose much faster than primary agricultural products (FAO, 2004).

International Trade and Changing Dietary Patterns

An increase in food imports can have nutritional implications by altering food availability and/or prices, thus helping to shape preferences (Chopra et al., 2002; Chopra, 2002). But the evidence on whether food imports have actually *changed* the nature of the food supply, rather than just substituting for foods previously produced domestically, is rather thin. For example, evidence from the Philippines shows that imports (as of 1999) contributed to over 50 percent of the total supply of milk and milk products, but it is not clear whether this represents an addition to the existing milk supply or a substitution for domestically produced milk (Pedro, Barba, & Candelaria, 2004). Likewise, evidence from Colombia shows that the proportion of calories from imported foods has risen over time, but not whether this has contributed to increased energy availability (Fajardo, 2004).

More compelling evidence comes from India, where market liberalization in the mid-1990s stimulated a rapid increase in imports of low-priced vegetable oils (Hawkes, 2006), which corresponded with a simultaneous increase in consumption (Table 10.8). It also stimulated a switch in the type of oils consumed, away from traditional peanut, rapeseed, and cottonseed oils, and towards imported palm and soybean oils. This is a good example of how the nutrition transition typically begins with major increases in imports of oilseeds and vegetable oils, as shown by Drewnowski and Popkin (1997). A similar process occurred in China. During the 1990s, China implemented new tax and import regulations to encourage soybean imports. Subsequently, imports of soybeans and soybean oil increased and the amount of calories from vegetable oils available for consumption in China increased relative to what would have been produced domestically (Table 10.8). Household survey data also suggest that vegetable oil consumption has increased significantly throughout China in the past fifteen years. Still, it remains unclear whether the increase in vegetable oil imports is driving increased consumption, or whether increased consumer demand is driving increased imports.

The strongest body of evidence on the role played by trade in the nutrition transition comes from the Pacific Islands. Four different studies show that imported foods have altered the "traditional" diet, particularly by increasing fat consumption (Evans, Sinclair, Fusimalohi, & Liava'a, 2001; Schultz, 2004; Hughes & Lawrence, 2005; Cassels, 2006). Many of these changes actually preceded the modern era of economic globalization. Before 1945, each Pacific island was essentially food self-sufficient, with nutritionally adequate diets comprising locally produced staples, fish, and fruits. After 1945, Europeans colonized the islands (a different form of globalization) and foods began to be imported. This marked a specific change in the foods available on the islands: people began to consume increasing amounts of imported foods, and to change their source of calories. Increases of imports continue to this day. In Fiji, total energy supply

Table 10.8 Imports and Consumption of Vegetable Oils in India and China, 1989–1991 and 2000–2002

	1989–1991[a]	2000–2002[a]
INDIA		
Imports of soybeans (mT)	102	432
Imports of soybean oil (mT)	25,944	1,055,083
Calories available from soybean oil/cap/day	11	48
Imports of palm oil (mT)	353,790	3,317,333
Calories available from palm oil/cap/day	7	66
Calories available from peanut, cottonseed, and rapeseed oils/cap/day	107	76
Calories available from all vegetable oils/cap/day	158	231
Soybean oil as percentage of calories available from all vegetable oils (%)	7	21
Palm oil as percentage of calories available from all vegetable oils (%)	4	28
CHINA		
Imports of soybeans (mT)	1,961,944	14,368,805
Imports of soybean oil (mT)	435,735	736,254
Calories available from soybean oil/cap/day	27	78
Calories available from all vegetable oils/cap/day	141	213
Soybean oil as percentage of calories available from all vegetable oils (%)	19	37

Source: Hawkes, 2006. Reprinted with permission.
Notes: [a]The numbers are three-year averages around 1990 and 2001.

derived from imported foods rose from 43 percent to 60 percent between 1985 and 1996 (Schultz, 2004). There is evidence that Pacific Island countries are experiencing "dumping" of high-fat meat cuts, particularly cheap mutton flaps from Australia and New Zealand and turkey tails from the United States (Gittlesohn, Haberle, Vastine, Dyckman, & Palafox, 2003; Gewertz & Errington, 2007).

The availability of imported foods appears to have stimulated a change from "healthy" locally sourced foods (preimports) to "unhealthy" fatty foods (postimports). In Tonga, meat imports rose from 3,389 to 5,559 tons between 1989 and 1999, mainly high-fat chicken parts (Evans et al., 2001). Given that the population of the island increased from 96,000 to 100,000 during the time period (Populstat, 2007), this represents an increase of availability from 0.035 to 0.056 tons per capita (35 to 56 kilograms), an increase of 57 percent. In seven of the islands between 1963 and 2000, the total fat supply increased by between 5 percent and 80 percent, the largest increases in the most economically advanced islands (80 percent in French Polynesia, 65 percent in Fiji) (Hughes & Lawrence, 2005). This is because imported fats and oils have *added* to existing sources of fats, such as coconut oil. Individual imported foods providing fat include vegetable oils, margarine, butter, meat and chickens, canned meat, and canned fish. A survey on the island country of Vanuatu conducted in 1998 showed that the proportion of energy as fat consumed from imported foods was 44.8 percent for urban populations compared with 8.4 percent for rural and semirural populations. People who consumed fats from imported foods rather than traditional fats were 2.2 times more likely to be obese and 2.4 times more likely to be diabetic.

A further study provides some limited evidence of the role of food imports in the Federated States of Micronesia (Cassels, 2006). There, the initial massive dietary changes started in the 1960s and 1970s when the United States began to provide subsidies to the islands. Imported foods became more accessible and available, and a US-subsidized school feeding program encouraged the consumption of tinned foods and rice. Overweight and obesity rates rose on the islands during the same time period. A particularly important policy change occurred in 1981 with the sale of local fishing rights to the Japanese. After this, consumption of local tuna declined and consumption of tinned fish increased.

It has been argued by some, however, that changing diets have a greater influence on trade than trade has on diets. In other words, trade (in the form of increased food imports) simply meets increased demand for specific foods rather than creating demand itself. For example, Regmi, Ballenger, and Putnam (2004) examined trends in food consumption patterns worldwide, finding that consumption of products associated with a "Mediterranean diet" is increasing (i.e., olive oil, pasta, and cheese), a process the study attributes to growing incomes, GDP, and urbanization. The study presents evidence that this demand is being met by increased trade in these products, although trade continues to be hampered by high tariff barriers and transportation costs. Whether or not increased food trade creates or follows demand (or, most probably, does both), less doubt exists that food advertising and promotion are playing an important role in the globalization of diets and the subsequent nutrition transition.

FOOD ADVERTISING AND PROMOTION

The Growth of Global Food Advertising and Promotion

Advertising and promotion have been a fundamental process of globalization. From the 1980s onwards, advertising agencies transnationalized through FDI, mergers, and acquisitions and grew into vertically integrated global corporations (Hawkes, 2006). Today the global advertising and promotion market is controlled by just a handful of communications networks, mainly headquartered in the United States, Europe, or Japan. An important outcome of this global consolidation has been that agencies previously concerned solely with advertising now have additional expertise in nonmedia advertising, market research, and communications services, enabling them to supply clients with coordinated and comprehensive promotional campaigns.

The growth of transnational advertising and communications companies has deepened the role of food advertising and promotion by speeding the flow of food products into the global marketplace (Hawkes, 2006). Advertising and promotion works by attracting attention to new products, creating perceived differences between similar products, and improving the apparent value and desirability of products. In so doing, marketing encourages more consumers to consume the products and more producers to produce them, thus advancing the cycle of global market exchange and integration.

Global food advertising expenditure is high and is increasing steadily in developing countries. Total global advertising expenditure rose from US$216 billion to US$512 billion between 1980 and 2004 (World Watch, cited in Hawkes, 2006). In the United States, the food industry is estimated to spend around US$11.26 billion on advertising, more than any other industry (McGinnis, Gootman, & Kraak, 2006), and evidence suggests that the food industry is increasing its advertising expenditure in developing countries. Figure 10.4 shows that expenditure by two leading US-based brands declined in the United States in the 1990s, but increased outside the United States; Table 10.9 shows that, while the Coca-Cola Company is not among the top ten largest spenders in the United States or Western European countries, it is in developing and transitional countries. In other words, spending is greatest where companies are attempting to significantly grow their "new" (or at least newer) markets.

Evidence from Western countries shows that a significant proportion of food advertising and promotion is targeted at children and youth, and much of it is for high-calorie, nutrient-poor foods (Hastings et al., 2003; McGinnis et al., 2006). Available studies from developing countries show the same pattern. A recent systematic review of the literature from developing countries revealed that there is a great deal of food promotion to children in countries for which data is available, particularly in the form of television advertising, and that advertising is typically for highly processed, energy-dense foods (Hastings et al., 2003). In Brazil, close to 60 percent of all food advertisements in 2002 were for foods high in fats and sweeteners (Sawaya et al., 2004). In Asia food makes up a significant proportion of advertising targeted at children, ranging from 25 percent in South Korea, to 40 to 50 percent in India, 50 to 75 percent in Pakistan and the Philippines, and 70 percent in Malaysia (Escalante de Cruz, Phillips, Visch, & Bulan Saunders, 2004).

As described in Box 10.4, companies use a wide range of techniques to deliberately encourage children and youth to adopt regular and frequent consumption of these products in developing countries (Hawkes, 2002). In

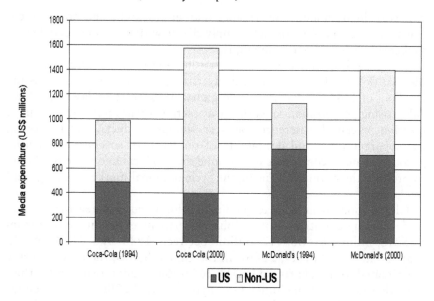

Figure 10.4 US/non-US media spending by the Coca-Cola Company and McDonald's, 1994–2000. Source: Hawkes, 2002. Reprinted with permission.

Table 10.9 Countries in Which the Coca-Cola Company was Among the Top 10 Media Spenders, 1997–2000

Country	Media Expenditure (US$ million per year)	Country	Media Expenditure (US$ million per year)
Mexico	68.8	Ukraine	3.8
Chile	54.5	Croatia	2.9
Colombia	41.2	Kazakhstan	2.7
Turkey	27.2	Indonesia	1.9
India	22.7	Vietnam	1.7
South Africa	21	Serbia	1.4
Venezuela	16.4	Lebanon	1.0
China	15.3	Kenya	0.9
Russia	13.5	Azerbaijan	0.8
Peru	12.6	Jordan	0.6
Hungary	11.7	Macedonia	0.5
Romania	5.1	Uganda	0.3
Slovakia	4.1	Bulgaria	0.3

Source: Hawkes, 2002. Reprinted with permission.

Latin America, for example, soft-drinks companies took steps in the late 1990s to "increase consumption in schools" by selling products in schools in "attractive combo" packages in Mexico and Colombia, and in Costa Rica "creat[ed] new points of sale in strategic areas of each institution."

These strategies were said to boost sales to schoolchildren by 50 percent. In India, a leading soft-drinks company used celebrity advertising as a means of "making sure people are made to want to drink more of our drinks." In China, the popularity of fast food with children was encouraged by the provision of facilities for birthday parties, play areas, and educational activities. This latter finding is supported by anthropological evidence from Asia that advertising and promotion are used to create a cultural identification with new, Western foods (Watson, 1997). In all of these developing markets, promotional activity is destined to grow given the expansion of media communications, the liberalization of rules on international advertising services, and the increasing number of children's television channels.

Food Advertising and Promotion, and Changing Diets

There is clear evidence that food advertising and promotion affect food consumption patterns. Two major systematic reviews have now concluded that food advertising targeted at children and youth does influence food choices (Hastings et al., 2003; McGinnis et al., 2006). The review by Hastings et al. (2003) was updated in 2006 and came to the same conclusions (Hastings, McDermott, Angus, Stead, & Thomson, 2007). The implications from both reviews are clear: food promotion has a significant influence on children's food behavior and diet *independent* of other factors. Although these studies focused on North America and Europe, a second review by Hastings et al. (2007) also found that children in developing countries recall, enjoy, and engage with food advertising.

The example of Thailand suggests that greater investment in advertising helps stimulate greater consumption of processed foods. The advertising and promotions industry in Thailand is among the most developed and dynamic in Asia: from 1987 to 1996, advertising expenditures grew nearly 800 percent and advertising revenues have grown at double-digit figures in recent years. Foreign ownership of advertising/marketing agencies is not restricted and, while advertising is regulated to some degree, campaigns are not subject to restrictions like maximum foreign content requirements. This relatively open market has encouraged TFCs to enter Thailand and to use the network of global marketing and communications agencies to develop highly sophisticated marketing campaigns using a wide variety of promotional techniques.

Evidence from a US-based company, Frito-Lay (a division of PepsiCo), shows that advertising does appear to increase sales, in this case, of snacks (Figure 10.5). When Frito-Lay first consolidated its presence in Thailand in 1999/2000, per capita snack consumption was still relatively low (1 kg per person per year in 1999 compared with 3 kg in Mexico and 10 kg in the United States). The company developed an aggressive strategy to increase consumption and more than doubled its promotional spending between 1999 and 2003. Frito-Lay's share of the total snack market subsequently

---

Box 10.4   Strategies used by TFCs to encourage consumption of high-calorie, nutrient-poor foods among children worldwide.

TFCs use many different strategies to promote consumption of their products, which are often termed the "5 Ps" of marketing: price, package, product, promotions, and public relations.

PRICE AND PACKAGE: Processed-foods products are often priced out of the reach of the mass market. To expand their consumer base, TFCs use a joint price/package marketing strategy of selling smaller and cheaper drinks in newer/poorer/rural markets. To expand volume, they size up portions and packages in more affluent urban areas.

PRODUCT: TFCs adapt their products to provide products preferred by local people and develop menu items specifically to appeal to children and youth.

PROMOTION: To advertise their products, TFCs utilize a huge range of techniques including signage, television advertising, sales promotions, and Web sites.
  - *Television advertisements* are designed to encourage consumers to emotionally bond with the product, via association with a special or magical moment, strong family values, fun and excitement, or local traditions. Commercials purvey glamour, and often feature young children, good-looking teens and young adults, celebrities, and animation.
  - *Premium, prize, and discount sales promotions* target children and youth. Notable examples include free/discounted toys with meals, and gifts available to collectors of product packaging. In some countries, TFCs have set up kids' clubs enabling children to access more sales promotions.
  - *Web sites* provide information about promotional campaigns and feature interactive promotions, games, and downloadable goods.

PUBLIC RELATIONS: Includes service-related marketing, TV and movie tie-ins, sports sponsorship, music, events, product sponsorship, educational competitions, and philanthropy.
  - *Service-related marketing* by fast-food companies includes the provision of services to attract children (such as play areas and birthday parties) and teens (such as Internet access and computer games).
  - *Sports sponsorship* is a major promotional vehicle for TFCs, ranging from the global scale (such as the World Cup and Olympic games) to the grassroots level (such as community sports training programs). The sports sponsored are those most popular in specific countries and those popular with youth.
  - *Sponsorship of children's and youth television shows and movies.*
  - *Sponsorship of music, events, and products* as a means of attracting teens, expanding product availability and signage, and identifying the brand with local culture. They also run a range of educational competitions, including environmental awareness campaigns and youth achievement awards.
  - *Philanthropy* extends marketing by identifying the brand with good deeds and local concerns. TFCs operate on a large scale via foundations and links with international organizations, as well as at a local level, focusing on causes such as children, education, and health.

---

grew from the low single digits in the mid-1990s to 30 percent by 2003. More importantly from a dietary perspective, the entry of Frito-Lay into the market also had the effect of stimulating total snack sales. Snack sales grew particularly rapidly from 1999 to 2004, the period of most intensive

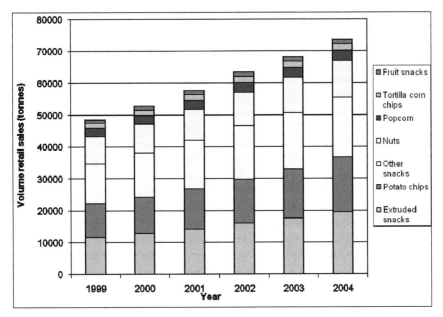

Figure 10.5 Retail sales of sweet and savory snacks in Thailand, 1999–2004.
Source: Hawkes, 2006. Reprinted with permission.

marketing, and sales volumes of the most heavily promoted products (chips and extruded snacks) increased by the largest amount (Figure 10.5). This indicates—though does not prove—that advertising and promotion played an important role in encouraging sales and consumption of snacks.

CONCLUSION

Linking the nutritional transition directly with globalization is a difficult task. Changes in diet and nutritional outcomes can be caused by a number of phenomena within social systems that are linked to globalization such as urbanization, agrarian reform, social welfare policy, and changes in relative income. Here we have concentrated mainly upon changes in the food system linked with globalization and summarized the evidence of how this can plausibly be linked to changes in diet and nutritional outcomes especially with regards to overweight and obesity.

Globalization has been strongly associated with a significant increase in the concentration of corporate ownership across the whole food-supply chain from production, processing, supply, and retailing. This is occurring across all regions of the world albeit at different rates, with Latin America and large parts of Asia experiencing the most rapid changes. Overall there is convincing evidence that globalization has magnified key supply-side drivers shaping diets. The growth of large TFCs, including supermarkets, along with increasing FDI is leading to dramatic increases in the supply, availability, advertising, and promotion of high-calorie, nutrient-poor foods (especially processed food) in middle-income countries. Although individual country case studies suggest that changes in the food supply have been very important in shaping diets, studies of individuals are too few to provide strong empirical evidence.

The pathways by which the recent changes in the food system are being experienced in different segments of the population, especially in low- and middle-income countries, are still relatively underresearched. But our review indicates that processes driving globalization exacerbate existing inequities. The diversifying nature of globalization processes has positive implications, but also raises the policy concern that these processes may encourage the uneven development of new dietary habits between rich and poor. As high-income groups in developing countries accrue the benefits of a more dynamic marketplace, lower-income groups may either continue to face inadequate access to food or to experience convergence towards poor-quality obesogenic diets, as has been observed in Western countries. People of low socioeconomic status (albeit not the poorest of the poor) are more likely to be influenced, over the long term, by the converging trends of the global marketplace, while the more affluent and educated move onto the more expensive, "healthy market" niches.

The specific impacts of globalization processes and policies also depend on other contextual factors, such as the terms of trade (ratio of the price of an export commodity to the price of an import commodity), the specifics of the trade agreement, the foodstuff, and the domestic policies and cultural traditions. Thus, the implications of globalization for the nutrition transition should always be examined in the context in which it is affecting people's everyday lives.

NOTES

1. Measure of height-for-age, which reflects cumulative effects of inadequate nutrition.
2. Measure of weight-for-age, which is a composite of stunting and wasting (weight-for-height, reflecting severe and acute weight loss).
3. This relationship is particularly strong for women and is not always the case for men.
4. Hypothetical unit of currency that has the same purchasing power that the US dollar had in the United States at a given point in time.

REFERENCES

Adair, L. S., & Popkin, B. M. (2005). Are child eating patterns being transformed globally? *Obesity Research, 13,* 1281–99.

Cassels, S. (2006). Overweight in the Pacific: Links between foreign dependence, global food trade, and obesity in the Federated States of Micronesia. *Globalization and Health, 2.*

Chopra, M. (2002). *Globalization and food: Implications for the promotion of "healthy" diets.* Geneva: World Health Organization.

Chopra, M., & Darnton-Hill, I. (2004). Tobacco and obesity epidemics: Not so different after all? *British Medical Journal, 328,* 1558–60.

Chopra, M., Galbraith, S., & Darnton-Hill, I. (2002). A global response to a global problem: The epidemic of overnutrition. *Bulletin of the World Health Organization, 80,* 952–58.

Connor, J. M. (1994). North-America as a precursor of changes in Western-European food-purchasing patterns. *European Review of Agricultural Economics, 21,* 155–73.

Cwiertka, K., & Walraven, B. (2002). *Asian food: The global and the local.* Richmond, UK: Curzon Press Ltd.

Dixon, J., Omwega, A., Friel, S., Burns, C., Donati, K., & Carlisle, R. (2007). The health equity dimensions of urban food systems. *Journal of Urban Health, 84,* 118–29.

Doak, C. M., Adair, L. S., Monteiro, C., & Popkin, B. M. (2000). Overweight and underweight coexist within households in Brazil, China and Russia. *Journal of Nutrition, 130,* 2965–71.

Drewnowski, A., & Popkin, B. M. (1997). The nutrition transition: New trends in the global diet. *Nutrition Reviews, 55,* 31–43.

Escalante de Cruz, A., Phillips, S, Visch, M., & Bulan Saunders, D. (2004). *The junk food generation: A multi-country survey of the influence of television advertisements on children.* Kuala Lumpur, Malaysia: Consumers International, Asia Pacific Office.

Euromonitor. (2006). *Packaged Food-World.* London: Euromonitor.

Evans, M., Sinclair, R. C., Fusimalohi, C., & Liava'a, V. (2001). Globalization, diet and health: An example from Tonga. *Bulletin of the World Health Organization, 79,* 856–62.

Ezzati, M., Vander Hoorn, S., Lawes, C. M., Leach, R., James, W. P., Lopez, A. D., et al. (2005). Rethinking the "diseases of affluence" paradigm: Global patterns of nutritional risks in relation to economic development. *Public Library of Science Medicine, 2,* 404–12.

Fajardo, L. (2004). *Impact of globalization on food consumption, health and nutrition in urban areas of Colombia.* No. 83. Rome: Food and Agriculture Organization of the United Nations. Retrieved from: ftp://ftp.fao.org/docrep/fao/007/y5736e/y5736e00.pdf.

FAO (Food and Agriculture Organization of the United Nations). (2004). *Globalization of food systems in developing countries: Impact on food security and nutrition.* FAO Food and Nutrition Paper 83. Rome: FAO.

———. (2006). *The state of food insecurity in the world 2006.* Rome: FAO. Retrieved from: ftp://ftp.fao.org/docrep/fao/009/a0750e/a0750e00.pdf

Friel, S., Chopra, M., & Satcher, D. (2007). Unequal weight: Equitable policy responses to the global obesity epidemic. *British Medical Journal, 335,* 1241–43.

Garrett, J. L., & Ruel, M. T. (2005). Stunted child–overweight mother pairs: Prevalence and association with economic development and urbanization. *Food and Nutrition Bulletin, 26,* 209–21.

Gewertz, D., & Errington, F. (2007). The alimentary forms of the global life: The Pacific Island trade in lamb and mutton flaps. *American Anthropologist, 109,* 496–508.

Ghosh, J. (2002). *Social policy in Indian development.* Geneva: United Nations Research Institute for Social Development (UNRISD). Retrieved from: http://

260   *Corinna Hawkes, Mickey Chopra, and Sharon Friel*

unrisd.org/unrisd/website/document.nsf/ab82a6805797760f80256b4f005da1a
b/7ee221555523155dc1256c77003cfaed/$FILE/ghoslong.pdf.

Gittelsohn, J., Haberle, H., Vastine, A. E., Dyckman, W., & Palafox, N. A. (2003).
Macro- and microlevel processes affect food choice and nutritional status in the
Republic of the Marshall Islands. *American Society for Nutritional Sciences,*
133, 310S–313S.

Grigg, D. (1995). The nutritional transition in Western Europe. *Journal of Historical Geography,* 22, 247–61.

Gupte, M. D., Ramachandran, V., & Mutatkar, R. K. (2001). Epidemiological
profile of India: Historical and contemporary perspectives. *Journal of Biosci-
ences,* 24, 437–64.

Hastings, G., McDermott, L., Angus, K., Stead, M., & Thomson, S. (2007). *The
extent, nature and effects of food promotion to children: A review of the evidence.* Geneva: World Health Organization.

Hastings, G., Stead, M., McDermott, L., Forsyth, A., MacKintosh, A. M., Rayner,
M., et al. (2003). *Does food promotion influence children? A systematic review
of the evidence.* London: Food Standards Agency.

Hawkes, C. (2002). Marketing activities of global soft drink and fast food companies in emerging markets: A review. In *Globalization, Diets and Noncommunicable Diseases.* Geneva: World Health Organization.

———. (2005). The role of foreign direct investment in the nutrition transition.
Public Health Nutrition, 8, 357–65.

———. (2006). Uneven dietary development: Linking the policies and processes
of globalization with the nutrition transition, obesity and diet-related chronic
diseases. *Globalization and Health,* 2.

Hendrickson, M., & Heffernan, W. (2005). Concentration of agricultural markets:
February 2005 [online]. Retrieved from: http://www.nfu.org/issues/economic-
policy/resources/heffernan-report/.

———. (2007). *Concentration of agricultural markets: April 2007.* http://www.
nfu.org/issues/economic-policy/resources/heffernan-report/ [online]. Retrieved
from: http://www.nfu.org/wp-content/2007-heffernanreport.pdf.

Hughes, R. G., & Lawrence, M. A. (2005). Globalization, food and health in Pacific
Island countries. *Asia Pacific Journal of Clinical Nutrition,* 14, 298–306.

Kennedy, G., Nantel, G., & Shetty, P. (2004). *Globalization of food systems in
developing countries: A synthesis of country case studies.* FAO Food and Nutrition Paper No. 83. Rome: Food and Agriculture Organization of the United
Nations. Retrieved from: ftp://ftp.fao.org/docrep/fao/007/y5736e/y5736e00.
pdf.

Kinabo, J. (2004). *Impact of globalization on food consumption, health and nutrition in urban areas: A case study of Dar es Salaam, United Republic of Tanzania.* No. 83. Rome: Food and Agriculture Organization of the United Nations.
Retrieved from: ftp://ftp.fao.org/docrep/fao/007/y5736e/y5736e00.pdf.

Lang, T. (1999). Diet, health and globalization: Five key questions. *Proceedings of
the Nutrition Society,* 58, 335–42.

McGinnis, J. M., Gootman, J. A., & Kraak, V. I. (2006). *Food marketing to children and youth: Threat or opportunity?* Washington, DC: National Academies
Press.

McMichael, A. J., Shetty, P. S., & McPherson, K., eds. (1997). *The public health
impact of globalisation of food trade.* Chichester, UK: John Wiley & Sons.

Mendez, M., & Popkin, B. (2004). Globalization, urbanization and nutritional
change in the developing world. In *Globalization of food systems in developing
countries: Impact on food security and nutrition* (pp. 55–80). FAO Food and
Nutrition Paper 83. Rome: Food and Agriculture Organization of the United
Nations. Retrieved from: ftp://ftp.fao.org/docrep/fao/007/y5736e/y5736e00.pdf.

Monteiro, C. A., Moura, E. C., Conde, W. L., & Popkin, B. M. (2004). Socioeconomic status and obesity in adult populations of developing countries: A review. *Bulletin of the World Health Organization, 82*, 940–46.

Murphy, S. (2006). *Concentrated market power and agricultural trade.* ECOFAIR Trade Dialogue Discussion Papers No. 1 Heinrich Böll . Retrieved from: http://www.tradeobservatory.org/library.cfm?refid=89014.

Neufeld, L. M., Hernández-Cordero, S., Fernald, L. C., & Ramakrishnan, U. (2008). Overweight and obesity doubled over a 6-year period in young women living in poverty in Mexico. *Obesity, 16*, 714–17.

Papola, T. S. (2005). *Workers in a globalising world: Some perspectives from India, Globalisation and Labour Mobility in India and China 2005.* Melbourne: ABERU.

Pedro, M. R. A., Barba, C. V. C., & Candelaria, L. V. (2004). Globalization, food consumption, health and nutrition in urban areas: A case study from the Philippines. *FAO Food and Nutrition Paper, 231–52.*

Pingali, P., & Khwaja, Y. (2004). *Globalization of Indian diets and the transformation of food supply system.s* No. 04–05. Rome: Agricultural and Development Economics Division, Food and Agriculture Organization of the United Nations. Retrieved from: http://www.fao.org/docrep/007/ae060e/ae060e00.htm.

Pinstrup-Andersen, P., & Babinard, J. (2001). Globalization and human nutrition: Opportunities and risks for the poor in developing countries. *African Journal of Food and Nutritional Sciences, 1*, 9–18.

Popkin, B. M. (1999). Urbanization, lifestyle changes and the nutrition transition. *World Development, 27*, 1905–16.

———. (2002). The shift in stages of the nutrition transition in the developing world differs from past experiences! *Public Health Nutrition, 5*, 205–14.

———. (2006). Technology, transport, globalization and the nutrition transition food policy. *Food Policy, 31*, 554–69.

Popkin, B. M., & Gordon-Larsen, P. (2004). The nutrition transition: Worldwide obesity dynamics and their determinants. *International Journal of Obesity, 28*, S2–S9.

Populstat. (2007). TONGA: historical demographical data of the whole country. Retrieved from: http://www.populstat.info/Oceania/tongac.htm.

Prentice, A. M. (2006). The emerging epidemic of obesity in developing countries. *International Journal of Epidemiology, 35.*

Regmi, A., Ballenger, N., & Putnam, J. (2004). Globalisation and income growth promote the Mediterranean diet. *Public Health Nutrition, 7*, 977–83.

Sawaya, A. L., Martins, P. A., & Martins, V. J. B. (2004). *Impact of globalization on food consumption, health and nutrition in urban areas: A case study of Brazil.* No. 83. Rome: Food and Agriculture Organization of the United Nations. Retrieved from: ftp://ftp.fao.org/docrep/fao/007/y5736e/y5736e00.pdf.

Schmidhuber, J., & Prakash, S. (2004). Nutrition transition, obesity & noncommunicable diseases: Drivers, outlook and concerns. *SCN News, 29*, 13–19.

Schultz, J. (2004). *Globalization, urbanization and nutrition transition in a developing island country: A case study in Fiji.* No. 83. Rome: Food and Agriculture Organization of the United Nations. Retrieved from: ftp://ftp.fao.org/docrep/fao/007/y5736e/y5736e00.pdf.

United Nations System Sub-Committee on Nutrition. (2000). *4th report on the world nutrition situation: Nutrition throughout the life cycle.* Geneva: ACC/SCN in collaboration with International Food Policy Research Institute. Retrieved from: http://www.unsystem.org/scn/Publications/4RWNS/4rwns.pdf.

Uusitalo, U., Pietinen, P., & Puska, P. (2002). Dietary transition in developing countries: Challenges for chronic disease prevention. In *Globalization, Diets and Noncommunicable Diseases.* Geneva: World Health Organization.

Vepa, S. S. (2004). *Impact of globalization on the food consumption of urban India*. No. 83. Rome: Food and Agriculture Organization of the United Nations (FAO).

Vorley, B. (2003). *Food, Inc. corporate concentration from farm to consumer*. London: IIED.

Watson, J. L., ed. (1997). *Golden Arches East: McDonald's in East Asia*. Stanford, CA: Stanford University Press.

Wild, S., Roglic, G., Green A., Sicree, R., & King, H. (2004). Global prevalence of diabetes: Estimates for 2000 and projections for 2030. *Diabetes Care, 27*, 1047–53.

World Health Organization. (2000). *Obesity: Preventing and managing the global epidemic—report of a WHO consultation*. Geneva: WHO. Retrieved from: http://whqlibdoc.who.int/trs/WHO_TRS_894.pdf.

———. (2005). *Preventing chronic diseases: A vital investment*. Geneva: WHO. Retrieved from: http://www.who.int/chp/chronic_disease_report/contents/en/index.html.

———. (2006). *Obesity and overweight*. WHO Fact Sheets No. 311. Geneva: WHO. Retrieved from: http://www.who.int/mediacentre/factsheets/fs311/en/index.html.

11 Intellectual Property Rights and Inequalities in Health Outcomes

Carlos M. Correa[1]

INTRODUCTION

The intensification of economic globalization that has taken place in recent decades has been facilitated by the internationalization of intellectual property institutions. Although this process started at the end of the nineteenth century, it was accelerated in the twentieth century by the adoption of the Agreement on Trade-Related Aspects of Intellectual Property Rights (TRIPS Agreement) developed and negotiated in the context of the General Agreement on Tariffs and Trade (GATT) Uruguay Round (1986–1994) (World Trade Organization, 1994). The internationalization of intellectual property rights (IPRs) regimes has increasingly limited the room left to countries to exercise their sovereign rights and discharge their obligations in public health, including those subsumed under the right to health (Cullet, 2003; Yamin, 2003; Reinharz & Chastonay, 2004). On the one hand, IPRs promote innovation in pharmaceuticals but, on the other hand, they limit access to the resulting products. In addition, such rights only promote certain types of research and development (R&D)—those addressed to the most profitable markets.

This chapter explores inequalities in health outcomes emerging from the existing IPRs regime. First, it considers the internationalization of the IPRs system and in particular the issues arising from the adoption of minimum standards of IPRs protection contained in the TRIPS Agreement. Second, it briefly examines some features of innovation in the pharmaceutical field and the changes underway in the predominant business model for R&D. Third, it discusses the role of patents in pharmaceutical R&D, particularly with regard to diseases prevailing in developing countries. Fourth, the chapter explores issues relating to IPRs and access to medicines. These include how policy interventions can improve such access through compulsory licenses, as well as the limitations of the existing international framework on the matter. Finally, the implications of recently negotiated free-trade agreements are briefly discussed.

INTERNATIONALIZATION OF INTELLECTUAL PROPERTY

Historically, countries developed their IPRs regimes in accordance with their own interests and levels of development. However, the system gradually began to be internationalized in the late nineteenth century, when two ground-breaking international conventions were adopted: the Paris Convention on the Protection of Industrial Property (1883) and the Berne Convention for the Protection of Literary and Artistic Works (1886). The Madrid Agreement for the Repression of False or Deceptive Indications of Source on Goods was adopted in 1891. With the exception of revisions of the Paris Convention, several decades passed with little change.

During the 1970s, in the context of new perspectives on development, developing countries sought to reverse the trend towards the expansion of IPRs and proposed a revision of the Paris Convention. A major goal of the revision was to amend Article 5A to promote use of the patented inventions in the countries of registration (Roffe & Tesfachew, 2001, p. 388). Not only did this initiative fail; it also caused developed countries to take the offensive once again and propose a new and ambitious instrument in the framework of GATT which eventually led to the adoption of the TRIPS Agreement in 1994. This was followed by the adoption of the Trademark Law Treaty (1994), WIPO Copyright Treaty (1996), WIPO Performers and Phonograms Treaty (1996), and Patent Law Treaty (2000). This new wave of agreements confirmed that the move towards trade liberalization and an increasingly intensive use of knowledge in all spheres of human activity was "accompanied by a heretofore unrecognized rise in 'entry barriers' that impede access to knowledge" (Coriat, 2002, p. 1).

Although after the year 2000 no new international agreements on IPRs were adopted, efforts to create international standards have continued in the area of patents through a World Intellectual Property Organization (WIPO) initiative to develop a Substantive Patent Law Treaty (Correa & Musungu, 2002) and rights related to copyright in the area of signal-based broadcasting through the adoption of a new treaty on the matter under the auspices of WIPO.[2] In addition, a number of free-trade agreements (FTAs) that contain high levels of IPRs protection have been adopted since then. Negotiating such agreements has allowed the United States to gain concessions on a bilateral basis that were unlikely to be reached in a multilateral framework where developing countries have become increasingly reluctant to support a further elevation of IPRs standards (World Intellectual Property Organization Secretariat, 2004).

FROM DOMESTIC FLEXIBILITY TO INTERNATIONAL AGREEMENT—THE NEW SCENARIO

The adoption of the TRIPS Agreement represented a significant step in the internationalization of the IPRs system, because all World Trade Organization (WTO) members are bound to comply with the minimum standards the agreement set forth in the main areas of IPRs protection (Howse, 2007). The TRIPS Agreement introduces for the first time in an international treaty an obligation to protect efficacy and safety data against unfair commercial use (Article 39.3) (Howse, 2007). With regard to patents, the agreement obligates members inter alia to grant product patents in all fields of technology (including pharmaceutical), specifies the exclusive rights to be granted, sets outs conditions for exceptions to exclusive rights and compulsory licenses, and strengthens process patents through the reversal of burden of proof. It also contains some flexibilities, such as the possibility of determining what qualifies as an invention, how compulsory licenses are granted, and the allowance for parallel imports.

The agreement put an end to the significant leeway countries had to design their national systems under those international conventions established between the end of the nineteenth century and the 1980s. When today's industrialized countries were in the process of development, they enjoyed great flexibility in designing their own IPR systems. Mark Twain's personal fight to have his copyright recognized internationally provides a telling example. Twain tried to register his name as a trademark in order to prevent his novels being freely copied; the books of British authors, in particular, were legally copied during most of the nineteenth century. In 1842, Charles Dickens toured the United States pleading for international copyright, and in 1843 he published *American Notes* in which he expressed his frustration with U.S. law. Fifty thousand pirated copies were sold within three days in the United States. His *A Christmas Carol* sold at that time for the equivalent of $2.50 in London and for six cents a copy in the United States (Vaidhyanathan, 2001).[3] Foreign authors did not receive copyright protection in the United States until 1891.

In the case of patents, as a net importer of technology between 1790 and 1836, the United States restricted the issue of patents to its own citizens and residents. Even in 1836, patent fees for foreigners were fixed at ten times the rate for U.S. citizens. In many European countries (such as France, Germany, and Switzerland) that are proponents of strong patent protection today, pharmaceutical product patents were only recognized after the 1960s. Portugal, Spain, and the Nordic countries waited until the 1990s.

Under the Paris Convention for the Protection of Industrial Property, contracting parties were permitted to exclude patent protection in certain sectors (such as pharmaceuticals), determine the duration of patent rights, limit the exclusive rights conferred, and grant compulsory licenses for a variety of reasons, including lack of local working of a patent, that is, the patent holder not industrially executing the invention in the country of grant. In fact, the most successful cases of industrial and technological development in recent history took place in a flexible framework of IPRs protection, such as witnessed in Japan and Korea. The more recent robust development of the Indian pharmaceutical industry, which has become a major world supplier of cheap generic medicines and active ingredients, was also possible in the absence of pharmaceutical product patents (Chaudhuri, 2005).

This flexibility was reduced dramatically with the adoption of the TRIPS Agreement, which is essentially the outcome of well-organized campaigns by a few industries, notably pharmaceutical, entertainment, software, and semiconductors (Sell, 2003). In particular, the TRIPS Agreement represented a major victory for the pharmaceutical industry, which had worked hard to expand the patent protection of products that were excluded from patentability in most developing countries at the time the TRIPS Agreement negotiations were launched in GATT in 1986—a time at which over fifty countries did not recognize patent protection for pharmaceuticals.

Under the TRIPS rules much of the flexibility that developed countries enjoyed to design their own systems of IPRs is no longer permitted for developing countries. Although arguments about increased technology transfer, foreign direct investment to, and innovation in such countries were made during the negotiations by the proponents of the agreement, it was obviously intended to benefit those countries and industries with greater capacity to generate new knowledge and information. An early study concluded that

> patent harmonization has the capacity to generate large transfers of income between countries, with the USA being the major beneficiary ... These transfers significantly alter the perceived distribution of benefits from the Uruguay Round, with the USA benefits substantially enhanced, while those of developing countries and Canada considerably diminished. (McCalman, 1999, p. 30)

McCalman's findings have been widely confirmed by recent statistics. Although there is no conclusive evidence of an increase in the flows of production technologies to developing countries, there has been an impressive rise in world royalty payments. North America and Europe account for more than two-thirds of all payments, followed by Asia and Latin America; royalty payments grew from $61 billion in 1998 to $120 billion in 2004, of which the United States was the main beneficiary (World Bank, 2000, 2007).

INNOVATION IN PHARMACEUTICALS

While public R&D institutions have been the main source for discoveries of potential pharmaceutical use, the pharmaceutical industry has mainly funded and carried out the development phase of pharmaceutical products, including costly and lengthy clinical trials. The public sector accounts for around 44 percent of the total funding for health research, while the private for-profit sector funds around 48 percent (Burke & de Francisco, 2004).[4]

Much incremental innovation takes place in the industry by way of (often marginal) modifications of existing processes or products or the ways products are administered. Patents on these minor modifications are generally applied for as part of a strategy to delay generic competition that is often referred to as "evergreening." The industry's innovation performance is measured, however, by the new chemical entities it is able to develop and have approved by health authorities.

The development of new chemical entities for pharmaceutical use as indicated in Figure 11.1 presents a worrisome picture. The number of such entities delivered per year has fallen substantially since the 1990s,[5] thereby increasing the average cost of developing new drugs. That decline seems paradoxical for three main reasons. First, since the 1980s and particularly as the implementation of the TRIPS Agreement was completed in developed and developing countries,[6] patent protection allowed companies to increase income generation worldwide through the exercise of stronger and, in some cases, longer patent rights and data exclusivity.[7] Second, a new set of scientific and technological tools—such as genomics, proteomics, and combinatorial chemistry—has the potential to speed up drug discovery. Mass screening of potential drug candidates has been substituted by more efficient methods enabling the rational design of drugs. Third, the pharmaceutical industry continues to be one of the most profitable sectors of the global economy, fourth only after mining, crude-oil production, and commercial banking (Angell, 2004; Commission on Intellectual Property Rights, 2006). Moreover, funds allocated to R&D have increased since the last decade. The fall in innovative productivity may indicate a crisis in the model of drug development carried out by large pharmaceutical companies: while the overall level of investment has risen dramatically, the number of new products has not increased (Charles River Associates, 2004; Commission on Intellectual Property Rights, 2006). Large firms find it more difficult to maintain a continuous pipeline of new and commercially viable products. Instead, they depend for new drugs on advances made by small biotechnology companies, while certain segments of biomedical research are undertaken in cooperative ways following an "open-access" model, and many of the clinical studies are done by specialized contractors. Open-access models of innovation may be increasingly applicable to biomedical research as computational models utilizing genetic information become more important as part of the product development process (Maurer, Rai, & Sali, 2004).

In response to the decline in innovative performance, some pharmaceutical companies are moving towards a disaggregated business model focusing on a few areas of core competence (discovery, development or marketing). At the same time, they are outsourcing other activities with biotech companies, contract research organizations, independent drug-development firms, and freelance sales organizations (*Economist*, 2007). Companies are streamlining their pipelines, focusing on fewer

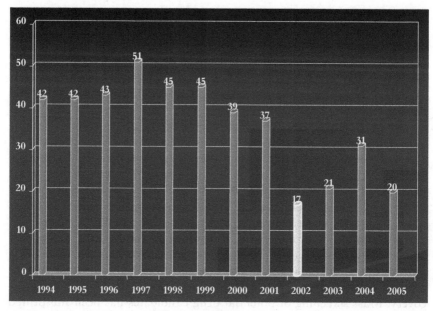

Figure 11.1 Development of new chemical entities for pharmaceutical use, 1992–2004.

Source: US FDA

diseases, and licensing in (i.e., obtaining from other companies under license agreements) more drug candidates. Thus, many large pharmaceutical companies have introduced drastic reorganization of their R&D activities. Years ago, GlaxoSmithKline took the lead by dividing R&D into therapeutic areas and setting up seven Centres of Excellence for Drug Discovery (CEDDs). Roche will also create five Disease Biology Areas (DBAs) for oncology, virology, inflammation, metabolic diseases, and central-nervous-system disorders, which will cover everything from drug discovery to medical proof of concept to marketing (Nagle, 2007). The biggest pharmaceutical company, Pfizer, recently announced up to five R&D site closures and an increasing reliance on outsourcing and in-licensing (Nagle, 2007). Once believed to hold unique competence to develop new drugs, large firms may still retain an unparalleled financial capacity to bear the cost and risks of drug development. However, new actors have emerged that can make better use of new scientific and technological tools, and more efficiently carry out preclinical and clinical trials as well as the complex procedures of marketing approval.

There are other challenges to the existing model of drug development. One is the growing concern about the conflict of interest underlying the development of data regarding drug efficacy and safety. Lewis, Reichman, and So (2006, p. 1) have observed that

[S]o long as drug companies retain primary responsibility for conduct-
ing or funding clinical trials, they will be tempted to selectively disclose
information and to avoid research programs that could reveal unfavorable outcomes. Nor would a disclosure requirement alone ensure
that the stakeholding company will conduct all the tests deemed most
beneficial to public safety. . . . There are few incentives to undertake
costly testing (phase IV clinical trials) if the results might only serve
to narrow use of the drug to a smaller subgroup of patients or prove
unfavorable to its continued use.

For this reason, these authors suggest the "establish[ment of] an independent testing agency to conduct clinical trials under specified conditions of
transparency. . . . This separation of clinical trials from sponsorship could
attenuate the conflict of interest problem" (Lewis et al., 2006, p. 1).

Another effect attributable to the decline in innovative capacity is the
proliferation of secondary patents (such as on polymorphs, isomers, formulations, new uses, etc.) relating to existing drugs which are strategi-
cally used to keep competitors out of the market through administrative
measures or costly litigation (Federal Trade Commission [FTC], 2002).[8]
Through the acquisition of such patents—in some cases fraudulently[9]—
companies are often able to significantly delay the entry of generic competition and maintain high profits on old drugs, to the detriment of consumers
and governments.

In sum, there are important changes in the innovation path and in the
R&D model for pharmaceutical products. Such changes do not affect
the industry's significant reliance on patents for funding R&D and setting limits to generic competitors. On the contrary, they have increased
the value of patents, including those on minor developments, as income-
generating tools.

PATENTS IN THE PHARMACEUTICAL INDUSTRY

The pharmaceutical industry, with sales exceeding US$400 billion annu-
ally, is highly globalized. The major companies operate through subsidiaries
and trade in active ingredients or formulated products in many countries,
while some also hold R&D facilities in several countries. Large pharmaceutical companies acquire patent rights globally, including in poor countries, with few exceptions made in the case of the least developed countries
(LDCs).[10] The advantages of a global patent regime for the industry are
obvious; under patents and other forms of IPRs, such as trademarks, they
can charge prices substantially higher than marginal costs.

There seems to be little doubt that patents play a key role in funding the
activities of the industry and particularly that they provide a stimulus for
R&D. However, this statement needs to be qualified in two respects.

On the one hand, innovation essentially depends on the outcomes of commercial activities in developed countries. Although industry has relentlessly sought to ensure patent protection for its products in developing countries, these countries account for only about 10 percent of global sales (in value) and for 5 to 7 percent of the global industry's profits (Pharmaceutical Research and Manufacturers of America, 2005). The extension of pharmaceutical patents to developing countries under the TRIPS Agreement is likely to have no significant impact on the development of new medicines (Scherer, 2004). Scherer examined whether global welfare is better served by a uniform worldwide system of pharmaceutical product patents or by international rules allowing low-income nations a "free ride" on the discoveries of firms in rich nations. Key variables included the extent to which free riding reduces the discovery of new drugs, the rent potential of rich as compared to poor nations, the ratio of the marginal utility of income in poor as compared to rich nations, and the competitive environment within which R&D decisions are made. Scherer found that, under plausible conditions, global welfare would be better served by allowing free riding by poor countries (Scherer, 2004).

On the other hand, patents foster R&D relating to diseases that predominantly affect rich countries. Patents only work as incentives where profitable markets exist. As noted in the report of the Commission on Intellectual Property Rights, Innovation and Public Health (CIPIH):

> Where the market has very limited purchasing power, as is the case for diseases affecting millions of poor people in developing countries, patents are not a relevant factor or effective in stimulating R&D and bringing new products to market. . . . For developing countries, where the demand is weak—but not the need—there is little incentive to develop new or modified interventions appropriate to the disease burden and conditions of the country. (Commission on Intellectual Property Rights, 2006, pp. 34–6)

This is the logical consequence of the nature of patents. They confer an incentive that may only be realized when the appropriate conditions exist in terms of human resources, capital, and expected returns.

There have been expectations about the new impetus to R&D, especially in the area of Type II and III diseases,[11] which may emerge in innovative developing countries such as India. However, available evidence indicates that, despite an increase in R&D expenditure by large local pharmaceutical companies, their effort is small compared to large multinational companies and is concentrated on drugs of interest in rich markets. Moreover, the model that Indian companies have adopted is to develop new molecules and license them out to large pharmaceutical companies at an early stage of development in order to avoid the heavy costs of clinical trials and regulatory approvals (Chaudhuri, 2005).

In brief, patents do contribute to the development of new treatments where large profitable markets exist. Lack of demand to treat the diseases of the poor makes patent protection irrelevant for Type III diseases and only relatively important for Type II diseases. Hence, patents may deepen the existing inequalities between rich and poor, as they generate an incentive to develop and market profitable drugs and not those badly needed to address the health problems of the greatest portion of the world population. Alternative mechanisms to promote pharmaceutical innovation are needed, especially for diseases of the poor.

Several public-private partnerships (PPPs) have been established to develop products needed in developing countries. For example, a partnership between Drugs for Neglected Diseases Initiative and Sanofi-Aventis, which has developed a fixed-dose combination of artesunate-amodiaquine, has submitted the drug for registration in twenty-three sub-Saharan African countries with current registration in twelve of these countries (Drugs for Neglected Diseases Initiative [DNDi] & Sanofi-Aventis, 2008). There are, however, serious concerns about the sustainability of such initiatives (Commission on Intellectual Property Rights, 2006), and a discussion of alternative mechanisms to promote innovation has been started by the World Health Organization (WHO). In 2008, the World Health Assembly adopted a draft global strategy and plan of action on public health, innovation, and intellectual property that, inter alia, encourages governments to consider new ways to stimulate research and development into health treatment for diseases that disproportionately affect developing countries (ICTSD reporting, 2008). The alternative mechanisms proposed include:

1. Market exclusivity for a limited period modeled on the "orphan drug" scheme applied in the United States under the Orphan Drug Act of 1983. Although this approach apparently has been successful in the United States, it seems to work when purchasing power is high (Commission on Intellectual Property Rights, 2006). In addition, the conferred exclusivity may, unless other measures are implemented, deny low-income patients access to new drugs.

2. Rewards in the form of prizes for the development of medicines to address diseases prevailing in developing countries. Such a scheme might be used more generally to encourage the development of new drugs without subjecting them to exclusive rights under patents. Stiglitz has proposed the establishment of a medical prize fund "for those who come up with a vaccine or cure for the kinds of diseases that afflict those in developing countries" (2007).

3. Advance purchase commitments that guarantee the future purchase of certain quantities of a product to be developed at an agreed price, with further reduction after a period of time. This mechanism is likely to work best when a molecule has already been identified and the risk involved in R&D is relatively low (Barder, Kremer, & Levine, 2005).

4. Open source schemes, particularly for the identification of new candidate molecules (Kepler et al., 2006). This approach may foster advances in early phases of the R&D cycle of pharmaceuticals.
5. A new international treaty on medical research, proposed by a number of nongovernmental organizations (NGOs) and governments to ensure sustainable funding for R&D in pharmaceuticals (Kepler et al., 2006).[12]

Some of these proposals, particularly the scope for open-access initiatives, may be further explored in the context of the World Intellectual Property Organization (WIPO) Development Agenda originally proposed by Argentina and Brazil in 2004. In September 2007, for example, the WIPO Assembly adopted forty-five of the recommendations under discussion (World Intellectual Property Organization, 2008).

ACCESS TO MEDICINES

Like any other incentive mechanism, the way patents work depends on the context in which they are applied. In countries lacking capital and required scientific and technological infrastructure, patents operate as a levy collection mechanism and not as a stimulus of local R&D. Patents restrict the extent of the diffusion of innovations by imposing monopolistic prices on consumers and royalties on technology users. The more isolated the product is from competition with possible substitutes, the higher the prices and the charges that can be levied. This obviously reduces the benefits that would have accrued to society at large and to patients in particular had the innovation been made available to competitors to manufacture generic products. The price increases introduced by patent protection may be extraordinarily high. In India, where pharmaceutical product patents came into force only in January 2005, the cost of treatment against leukemia, for instance, might be several times higher if a patent were to be granted on a crystalline form of the main available treatment (imatinib).

Another illustration is found in the evolution of the prices of patented antiretrovirals (ARVs). In 2000, the cost of treatment per patient per year was more than US$10,000. Competition by Indian generic firms made available the same ARV treatment in 2001 for less than US$400 and the prices of both the originator's and generic drugs continued to fall thereafter. At the time, this lower cost treatment was possible because India did not recognize pharmaceutical product patents and was able to produce generic versions of products which were under patents elsewhere. However, as of January 1, 2005, India was bound to grant such patents (including for patents validly filed after January 1, 1995). Hence, in the future no alternative supply will exist for new drugs, and patent owners may charge prices that high- and middle-income consumers are able to pay. Unless national legislation provides for effective TRIPS-consistent mechanisms to control prices of patented medicines, such as compulsory licenses, a large portion of the poor population in developing countries may be deprived of access to drugs.

High pricing of medicines has human rights implications, particularly through the restriction of domestic autonomy to provide access to needed treatments. These implications are increasingly recognized as a core duty under the international human right to health (Hunt, 2006). Indeed, the CIPIH report recognizes this right and the duties it imposes on states with respect to medicines. Similarly the UN Special Rapporteur on the Right to Health issued, in September 2007, draft *Human Rights Guidelines for Pharmaceutical Companies in Relation to Access to Medicines*, which, inter alia, demand that the company's corporate mission statement "expressly recognize the importance of human rights generally, and the right to the highest attainable standard of health in particular, in relation to the strategies, policies, programs, projects and activities of the company" and that the company "should integrate human rights, including the right to the highest attainable standard of health, into the strategies, policies, programs, projects and activities of the company" (p. 4).[13]

Conventional economic theory suggests that, to encourage innovation, competition based on price and quantity may have to be temporarily restrained. This would reduce *static efficiency* but bolster *dynamic efficiency* by increasing the likelihood of innovators recovering their R&D investment (United Nations Conference on Trade and Development Secretariat, 1998).[14] The static-dynamic efficiency rationale applicable in a developed society, however, does not necessarily hold when strong inequalities exist. High levels of IPRs protection may have significant negative *allocative* consequences in developing countries without contributing to, or even impeding, their technological development (Stiglitz, 1999). In the case of pharmaceuticals, while consumers in developing countries contribute to the R&D budgets of pharmaceutical companies, these companies concentrate their research on profitable drugs for developed countries and neglect those needed by the poor in developing countries (Commission on Intellectual Property Rights, 2006). As a result, while patents play an important role in funding R&D for certain types of pharmaceuticals, they significantly affect access to the innovations they promote (Chaudhuri, 2005). The concerns about the implications of patents on access to drugs have been voiced by developing countries and NGOs in many forums.

Such concerns were reflected in the Doha Ministerial Declaration on TRIPS and Public Health (World Trade Organization, 2001). The declaration recognized the "gravity" of the public health problems afflicting many developing countries and LDCs, especially, but not limited to, those resulting from HIV/AIDS, tuberculosis, malaria, and other epidemics. As well, it recognized concerns about the effects of intellectual property protection on prices (World Trade Organization, 2001). The Doha Declaration confirmed some of the flexibilities allowed by the TRIPS Agreement, such as the possibility of granting compulsory licenses and of permitting the parallel importation of patented products. A key paragraph (Paragraph 4) in the Doha Declaration states:

> We agree that the TRIPS Agreement does not and should not prevent Members from taking measures to protect public health. Accordingly, while reiterating our commitment to the TRIPS Agreement, we affirm that the Agreement can and should be interpreted and implemented in a manner supportive of WTO Members' right to protect public health and, in particular, to promote access to medicines for all.

Compulsory licenses, as next discussed, may be an important instrument to increase access to medicines under patent protection. Indeed, UN bodies such as the Commission on Human Rights have recognized compulsory licensing as a mechanism for developing countries to fulfill their obligations under the right to health (see, for example, United Nations High Commissioner for Human Rights, 2001).

COMPULSORY LICENSES

A compulsory license is an authorization given by a government (through the administration or a court) for the use, by a third party, of a patent (or other intellectual property rights) without the consent of the titleholder. The concept of compulsory licenses also encompasses governmental noncommercial use, that is, the use by or under the authority of the government of a patent. In conformity with Article 31 of the TRIPS Agreement, national laws can provide for the compulsory use of a patent by the government or by a third party. Government use and compulsory licenses mitigate the legal power conferred by a patent and can be an important instrument to ensure access to drugs at affordable prices.

Although the granting of compulsory licenses was contemplated in the Paris Convention for the Protection of Industrial Property as early as 1925, few such licenses have been granted, except in the United States, where, despite the US government's active defense of patents held by US companies abroad, thousands of patents have been subject to compulsory use by the government or to remedy anticompetitive practices (Correa, 1999; Reichman & Hasenzahl, 2003).[15] Many developing countries, especially those that followed British patent law, have provided for the granting of such licenses. However, until recently, the compulsory license system remained unused. Many developing countries have been sensitive to pressures from developed countries not to grant such licenses (Outterson, 2005).

While compulsory licensing is compatible with the TRIPS Agreement, provided that the conditions set out in Article 31 are met, developing countries sought to confirm their right to issue them and determine the grounds for their use through the Declaration on the TRIPS Agreement and Public Health (Paragraph 5(b)). This confirmation was likely instrumental in encouraging a number of developing countries to grant compulsory licenses (see Table 11.1). Brazil also threatened the granting of such licenses, which eventually led to a substantial reduction in the prices charged by patent owners for some antiretrovirals (ARVs) (Commission on Intellectual Property Rights [CIPR], 2002).

As indicated in Table 11.1, in some cases compulsory licenses have been granted to allow the local manufacture of patented drugs, while in others the objective is to import cheaper versions of them. Both means are fully compatible with the TRIPS Agreement. Malaysia, for example, was the first country to issue a license and to exercise the "government use" or "Rights of Government" provisions,[16] a special type of compulsory license issued following the adoption of the Doha Declaration on the TRIPS Agreement and Public Health in 2001 (Ling, 2006). In most cases, compulsory licenses or government use have been granted for ARVs. But there is no reason to limit the use of such mechanisms to ARVs. Thailand is the first developing country to target other types of products—those for the treatment of heart diseases (Ministry of Public Health & National Health Security Office, 2007).[17] Remuneration paid to patent owners ranges from 0.5 to 4 percent of the value of the products produced under license. In most cases, the resulting price reductions are significant, thereby allowing governments to increase the number of patients treated.

However, countries in need of cheaper versions of patented pharmaceuticals may increasingly face a situation in which they lack manufacturing capacity to produce them while foreign supplies are unavailable. Due to lack of technical capacity, adequate equipment, human resources, high costs of production, or other obstacles, many developing countries and LDCs cannot produce the active ingredients needed to manufacture pharmaceutical products. While these countries may issue compulsory licenses to import generic versions of patent-protected medicines, TRIPS rules impose constraints on the production and export of products patented in the supplier country. Paragraph 6 of the Doha Declaration recognizes that WTO members with insufficient or no manufacturing capacities in the pharmaceutical sector could face difficulties in making effective use of compulsory licensing under the TRIPS Agreement. It instructed the Council for TRIPS to find "an expeditious solution to this problem." After long and difficult negotiations, the council reached a consensus agreement that was adopted as the Decision of the General Council of the World Trade Organization on 30 August 2003 (the WTO Decision). It stipulates several conditions to be met in order to make use of the waivers it provides for exporting and importing countries.

Table 11.1   Compulsory Licenses and Government Use of These in Developing Countries

Country and Date Compulsory License Adopted	Type of Authorization	Products	Cost Reduction	Remuneration to the Patent Owner
Zimbabwe May 2002	Based on a declaration of emergency, it empowers the minister to authorize the use of patented inventions by any government department or third party, for the service of the state	ARVs	From US$197–237 per year to US$180	n.a.
Malaysia November 2003	It authorizes the local distributing agent for an Indian manufacturer to import from India, for the purpose of supplying public hospitals for two years	ARVs	From US$315 to US$58 per month	4% value of stocks actually delivered
Mozambique April 2004	Compulsory license to enable local manufacturing	ARV fixed dose combination	2% total turnover	
Zambia September 2004	Compulsory license for local manufacturing	ARV	2.5% total turnover	
Indonesia 2004	It authorizes the minister to appoint a pharmaceutical factory as the patent exploiter for and on behalf of the government	Nevirapine and lamivudine	Fixed dose combination produced for US$38 per month	0.5% net sales
Ghana October 2005	Government use	ARVs	From US$495 to US$235 per year	n.a.
Thailand November 2006 January 2007	Government use	Efavirenz Plavix Kaletra	From US$41 to US$22 per month	0.5% sales value
Brazil May 2007	Public interest	Efavirenz (600 mg)	From US$1.59 to US$0.45 per dose (saving of US$30 million in 2007)	n.a.

Source: Elaborated on the basis of Oh, 2006, and Khor, 2007 (n.a.= information not available).

A few countries have enacted legislation to implement the WTO Decision as potential exporters, namely, Canada, Norway, India, the Netherlands, and Iceland. On 17 May 2006, the European Parliament and Council adopted Regulation (EC) No. 816/2006 on compulsory licensing of patents relating to the manufacture of pharmaceutical products for export to countries with public health problems. Based on a proposal by the European Commission on compulsory licensing of patents relating to the manufacture of pharmaceutical products for export to countries with public health problems (Commission of the European Communities, 2004), the regulation incorporated a number of additional conditions to those already imposed by the WTO Decision, but ultimately took a largely positive approach (Abbott & Reichman, 2007).

A major hurdle in the mechanism set up by the WTO Decision is the need for potential suppliers to undertake prior negotiations with the patent owners (the Canadian and EU implementation regulations, for instance, provide for a thirty-day period for negotiations). This may significantly delay the granting of a compulsory license. In addition, since the simple offer for sale may infringe patent rights (specifically Article 28.1 of the TRIPS Agreement), firms willing to tender for the supply of drugs to beneficiary countries may not do so before obtaining a compulsory license in the exporting and, if needed, the importing countries. Obviously, few firms would be prepared to bear the cost of obtaining such licenses before a firm commitment to purchase their products has been made.

As a condition for use of the WTO Decision, potential importing countries must give notice of their intention to do so (Correa, 2004). So far, no country has done so and the WTO Decision has never been applied. This is a worrisome signal as to the effectiveness and feasibility of the mechanism. Despite this, in December 2005 the WTO Decision was incorporated as a new article (31*bis*) of the TRIPS Agreement, with the intention of it becoming a permanent mechanism. Such incorporation is, however, subject to ratification (in accordance with WTO rules) by member states, which so far have not rushed to do so.[18]

In sum, the Doha Declaration was a politically and socially important initiative that seemed to reaffirm the need to give priority to public health over commercial interests inherent to the acquisition and exercise of intellectual property rights. However, its practical implementation with regard to compulsory licenses has been strongly influenced by the commercial interests it was intended to counterbalance.[19]

FREE-TRADE AGREEMENTS

At the same time the Doha Declaration was negotiated and adopted, the United States initiated negotiations of bilateral and regional FTAs with more than twenty countries. The FTAs incorporate TRIPS-plus requirements. Agreements were entered into with Jordan, Chile, Singapore, Morocco, the

Central American countries and the Dominican Republic, Bahrain, Oman, Peru, and Colombia. Some of these agreements have already been ratified by the US Congress.[20] Other FTAs have been signed by or are under negotiation between developing countries and the European Union (EU) or the European Free Trade Association (EFTA).

The common pattern in these FTAs is that they further elevate the level of protection virtually in all areas of IPRs, notably copyright and patents. In the case of the US FTAs, partner countries are obliged inter alia to grant patents on plants, extend the patent term in certain circumstances, and adopt the "utility" standard for patentability (in place of the narrower requirement of industrial applicability[21]). They are also obliged to grant exclusive rights in respect of test data on pharmaceuticals and agrochemicals. In some cases, the protection enforceable under these FTAs is greater than that applicable in the United States itself (Abbott, 2006). Paradoxically FTAs do not seem to generate any obligation within the United States, leading to a situation in which US companies will receive more extensive IPR protection in FTA signatory countries, including many poor countries, than in the United States (Abbott, 2006). These FTAs may have significant implications on access to medicines while, for reasons explained earlier, they are unlikely to have any impact on R&D investment. Governments seek, however, to sign FTAs in order to get permanent free access to the big US market, or retain current preferential conditions of access, with the expectation of gains in other trade areas.

The US FTAs further obligate partner countries to extend patent terms to compensate for delays in marketing caused by approval procedures for medicines and "unreasonable" delays in the examination of patent applications. Most agreements do not mention whether extensions to compensate for delays apply only to the country where the medicine is sought (a seemingly legitimate interpretation) or whether delays in the country where first approval was obtained should also be calculated. No maximum period is provided for the extension, unlike the current law in the United States, where some time limits are provided.[22] As a result of these extensions, which may be cumulative, patents for medicines may last much longer than the twenty years required under Article 33 of the TRIPS Agreement.

In a significant departure from the TRIPS standard,[23] the US FTAs also obligate the parties to grant "data exclusivity" for at least five years starting from the date of approval of a pharmaceutical product. This is granted irrespective of whether or not the product is patented and whether or not the relevant test data are undisclosed. Such exclusivity will also apply irrespective of whether the national health authority requires the submission of the data; that is, even in cases where it relies on an approval made in a foreign country. In addition, the Central America–Dominican Republic–United States Free Trade Agreement (CAFTA-DR) and those signed with Peru and Colombia provide for a five-year waiting period. According to Article 15.10.1(b) of CAFTA, a signatory country may require the person providing information in another territory to seek approval in that country within five years of obtaining marketing approval in the other territory. If narrowly interpreted, this provision may allow the originator of test data who obtained approval for a medicine in a foreign country to delay up to five years an application for the approval of the same medicine in a country signatory of the FTA.

The implications of data exclusivity will be significant, particularly in countries that only recently introduced patent protection for pharmaceutical products, since medicines that are now off-patent will become subject to exclusive rights. These provisions create an effective barrier to generics competition, since even where a product is off-patent, no marketing approval can be granted to a generic manufacturer unless it replicates the full set of test data necessary to obtain approval. This is costly, time-consuming, and questionable under ethical rules, such as those of the Helsinki Declaration and its amendments (World Medical Association, 2004). A study for Peru relating to forty-three pharmaceutical products estimated that their average price would have been between 94.3 percent and 114.4 percent higher if they were subject to data exclusivity (Apoyo Consultoría, 2005).

The US FTAs also require a *linkage* between drug registration and patent protection that is absent in the TRIPS Agreement. As a result, if broadly interpreted, the national health authority may be required to refuse marketing approval to a generic version of a product if a patent on it is in force, except by consent or acquiescence of the patent owner. In addition, such authority must inform the patent owner about applications for the approval of generic products. Parties may, however, narrowly interpret the "linkage" obligation, for instance, by limiting it to patents over active ingredients (excluding formulations, polymorphs, isomers, doses, etc.), and put on the patent owner the burden to judicially request the suspension of third parties' approval procedures, as is the case in the United States.

Some US FTAs restrain WTO member states' freedom, confirmed by the Doha Declaration, to determine the grounds for compulsory licenses. Thus, in the case of the FTAs with Jordan, Australia, and Singapore, such grounds are limited to cases such as anticompetitive practices, public noncommercial use, national emergency, or other circumstances of extreme urgency. This limitation, which openly contradicts the Doha Declaration, did not appear in other US FTAs with developing countries after the adoption of the declaration. US FTAs with Australia, Singapore, and Morocco limit parallel importing of medicines and other products, that is, importing without the consent of the patent owner a patented product that has been legitimately put on the market abroad. Finally, some US FTAs, such as the one with Morocco, require the recognition of patents over the "second indication," that is, a new therapeutic use of a known medicinal product. This unnecessarily expands the scope of patentability and ignores the right, recognized by the TRIPS Agreement, to exclude the patentability of therapeutic methods.

So far the European Union has included a few provisions in trade agreements with other partners, mainly the obligation to adhere to intellectual property conventions, such as the Budapest Treaty and the international convention establishing the International Union for the Protection of New Varieties of Plants (UPOV). Some bilateral agreements, such as those entered into with South Africa (1999), Tunisia (1998), and the Palestinian Authority (1997), require them to ensure adequate and effective protection of intellectual property rights "in conformity with the highest international standards" (Drahos, 2002, pp. 14–18). Currently the EU is engaged in negotiations with six regions in Africa, the Caribbean, and the Pacific. These include more elaborated chapters on intellectual property, including TRIPS-plus substantive and enforcement provisions. However, unlike the US FTAs, the drafts under consideration do not seem to include higher substantive standards of protection on medicines.

In sum, US FTAs significantly increase the level of IPRs protection for medicines and, hence, the power of large pharmaceutical companies to charge higher prices in signatory countries. There is no justification for this in terms of additional R&D, since the markets of partner countries are relatively small and the additional income will make no difference to the global R&D budgets of these companies.[24] However, the increase in the cost of medicines may have a disproportionately high impact on the population of poorer countries. In some countries, such as Colombia and Peru, the ministries of health, which actively participated in the FTA negotiations without having sufficient power to influence their outcome, requested that their governments provide compensatory funds in order to face the increased costs of medicines. At least in the case of Peru, such measures were never actually implemented.

CONCLUSIONS

The intellectual property system has undergone a gradual but steady process of internationalization. A web of international treaties today supports global R&D, production, and trade. In the case of pharmaceuticals, such treaties, in particular the Patent Cooperation Treaty (PCT) and the TRIPS Agreement, provide large companies procedural means and substantive rights to exploit their innovations practically worldwide.

The international treaties entered into at the end of the nineteenth century and for most of the last century gave countries leeway to exercise their sovereignty in health-related matters. The TRIPS Agreement has dramatically changed that scenario by imposing a number of minimum standards, particularly in the area of patents.

Patents have played an important role in encouraging investment in pharmaceutical R&D. However, the innovative productivity of the industry is drastically declining, despite new scientific and technological tools available for drug development. In addition, patents only work as incentives where profitable markets exist. Other mechanisms need to be established and initiatives supported (such as "open-access" models) to encourage more R&D in diseases disproportionately affecting developing countries.

Likewise, policy interventions are needed to mitigate the negative impact of IPRs on access to medicines by the poor. Compulsory licenses provide one such measure. A growing number of developing countries have made use of these licenses, particularly to increase access to HIV/AIDS drugs, but there is nothing in the compulsory licenses system limiting its use to one category of medicines or diseases.

In the future, governments may face difficult challenges to provide access to patented drugs. This is because all WTO member states are now bound to confer product patent protection, and the mechanism set up by the WTO Decision is overburdened by conditions unlikely to encourage the supply of cheap products under patent protection in possible exporting countries.

Finally, despite the moral and political weight of the Doha Declaration, the United States and other developed countries have continued to seek a further expansion of IPRs to the benefit of pharmaceutical companies and other patent holders. The enhanced standards of protection create a disproportionate cost to developing countries that are parties to such agreements.

In sum, the IPRs system does promote research into more effective and efficient treatments. However, its bias is towards diseases of commercial interest. Some developing countries have applied policies to minimize the harm of IPRs, but their capacity to do so is being eroded by the new wave of FTAs. In addition, and most importantly, these countries need to look outside the IPRs system for mechanisms that foster innovation in the treatment of diseases that prevail among their people.

NOTES

1. The author is thankful for the contribution of Lisa Forman.
2. See http://www.cptech.org/ip/wipo/bt/.
3. The arguments articulated during that period in the United States against international copyright may currently suit numerous poor countries. It was argued that expanding literacy demanded cheap yet excellent books; there was no inherent property right in literature; granting copyright to foreigners would give them a monopoly at the expense of US reading public; US publishers and their employees needed the de facto advantage afforded by the absence of protection (Vaidhyanathan, 2001).
4. Given the amount of public funding involved in the creation of new patented drugs, including in some cases foregone tax deductions for R&D, at least part of the income obtained by pharmaceutical companies may be regarded as an inequitable windfall.
5. It is also to be taken into account that most new chemical entities are "me toos," that is, they do not represent a genuine therapeutic innovation. The great majority of new drugs approved annually have therapeutic qualities

similar to those of one or more already marketed drugs. The proportion of drugs considered by the US Food and Drug Administration (FDA) as potentially significant therapeutic advances over existing drugs has declined from 26 percent to 19 percent since the early 1990s (Center for Drug Evaluation and Research, 2005; see also Spector, 2005).

6. Transitional periods were provided for developing countries, economies in transition, and the least developed countries. Developing countries that did not previously recognize pharmaceutical product patent protection could delay its introduction until January 1, 2005, but only a few countries made full use of this possibility.

7. As a result of demands received in the process of accession to the WTO or to satisfy demands of the United States or the European Union, several countries have implemented in the context of FTAs sui generis regimes granting exclusivity over the test data necessary to obtain the marketing approval of pharmaceutical products containing new chemical entities.

8. In order to avoid the proliferation of "low quality" or wrong patents, strict standards of patentability should be applied to assess patent applications. See, e.g., Correa, 2006.

9. See, e.g., Federal Trade Commission (FTC), 2003.

10. Occasionally, pharmaceutical companies fail to patent in other developing countries, such as in the case of oseltamivir, prescribed for avian flu and produced by Hoffman LaRoche under an exclusive license from Gilead Sciences (USA). This drug was not patented, for instance, in Argentina, Indonesia, Philippines, and Thailand by Hoffman LaRoche.

11. Type I diseases are incident in both rich and poor countries, with large numbers of vulnerable populations in each. Type II diseases (often termed *neglected diseases*) are incident in both rich and poor countries, but with a substantial proportion of the cases in the poor countries (e.g., HIV/AIDS and tuberculosis). Type III diseases are those that are overwhelmingly or exclusively incident in the developing countries (Intergovernmental Working Group on Public Health, 2007).

12. See, e.g., http://www.cptech.org/workingdrafts/rndtreaty.html.

13. Available at huachen.org/english/issues/health/right/docs/draftguid150508.doc.

14. *Static efficiency* is achieved when there is an optimum utilization of existing resources at the lowest possible cost. Static efficiency may be subdivided into: *(i) Production efficiency*, which includes technical and nontechnical operating efficiencies, together with transaction cost and X-efficiency savings; *(ii) Allocative efficiency*, which is the allocation of products through the price system in the optimum manner required to satisfy consumer demand. *Dynamic efficiency* is the optimal introduction of new products or products of superior quality, more efficient production processes and organization, and (eventually) lower prices over time (United Nations Conference on Trade and Development Secretariat, 1998).

15. A recent US Supreme Court decision that denied a permanent injunction in a case of patent infringement effectively amounts to the grant of a compulsory license on "equity" grounds. In eBay Inc. *et al.* v. Mercexchange, L. L. C. of May 15, 2006, the Court stated that "the decision whether to grant or deny injunctive relief rests within the equitable discretion of the district courts." This means that an infringement may not necessarily lead to a permanent injunction if the court is convinced, based on equity considerations, that it is not justified.

16. The criteria to determine which patented medicines may be subject to government use are the following: must be listed in the National Essential Drug

List; or necessary to solve important public health problems; or necessary in emergency or extreme urgency; or necessary for the prevention and control of outbreaks/epidemic/pandemics; or life saving; and, if the prices of the medicines are too high to be affordable by the government to supply to the beneficiaries of the national health insurance. The royalties will be between 0.5 percent and 2 percent, depending on the retail value of the products.

17. The Thai decision has been challenged on arguments that the grant of compulsory licenses will jeopardize innovation in pharmaceuticals. The available empirical evidence, however, does not support this contention. Scherer analyzed the extent to which the granting of compulsory licenses in the United States affected R&D expenditures by firms and, particularly, whether such licenses diminished or destroyed the incentives to undertake R&D by patent holders. His statistical findings relating to seventy companies showed no negative effect on R&D in companies subject to compulsory licenses but, on the contrary, a significant rise in such companies' R&D relative to companies of comparable size not subject to such licenses. See Scherer, 2003, p. 107–08; Outterson, 2005, p. 230 (arguing that compulsory licenses need not harm optimal innovation). Indeed, this evidence undermines the argument that no R&D would be carried out if exclusive rights were not granted under patents. Thus, Tandon noted that "firms spend large sums of money on efforts to 'invent around' the patents of their competitors. Under generalized compulsory licensing, these expenditures would be unnecessary, which might increase the welfare benefits" (Tandon, 1982, p. 485).

18. Only sixteen members and the European Union (out of 150 members) have so far accepted the amendment. They are: United States (December 17, 2005); Switzerland (September 13, 2006); El Salvador (September 19, 2006); Rep. of Korea (January 24, 2007); Norway (23 May, 2008).

19. As evidenced, for instance, by the statement read by the chair of the WTO General Council as a condition for the approval of the WTO Decision by the United States. The statement overstated the need for measures to prevent the diversion of cheap drugs from poor to rich countries, and unjustifiably extended differential coloring and shaping conditions to active ingredients. See http://www.wto.org/english/tratop_e/trips_e/gc_stat_30aug03_e.htm.

20. United States–Jordan Free Trade Agreement (2001); United States–Chile Free Trade Agreement, signed at Miami June 6, 2003, and entered into force January 1, 2004 (Chile FTA); United States–Singapore Free Trade Agreement, signed at Washington May 6, 2003, and entered into force January 1, 2004 (Singapore FTA); United States–Morocco Free Trade Agreement, signed at Washington June 15, 2004 (Morocco FTA) and entered into force on July 1, 2005; United States–Dominican Republic–Central America Free Trade Agreement, signed at Washington May 28, 2004, and entered into force August. 5, 2004 (CAFTA-DR FTA). Parties to the CAFTA-DR FTA are Costa Rica, Dominican Republic, El Salvador, Guatemala, Honduras, Nicaragua, and the United States.

21. Under this "utility" standard, any invention which is useful may be patentable, even if not industrially applicable (e.g., business methods, research tools). The "industrial applicability" standard is narrower, as it requires that the invention be usable in an industry (broadly understood).

22. The extension in the United States to compensate for delays in the marketing approval process shall not exceed five years and, in no case, shall exclusivity exceed fourteen years from the date of approval by the Food and Drug Administration (35 U.S.C. § 156). In addition, the extension applies to only one patent per product.

23. The TRIPS Agreement requires members to protect *undisclosed* test data of pharmaceutical (and agrochemical) products against unfair competition (Article 39.3). Under this rule, correctly interpreted, members are not obligated to grant exclusive rights over test data.
24. In May 2007, a bipartisan agreement was reached at the U.S. Congress to amend some of the provisions of the FTAs signed by the United States with Peru and Panama in order to reduce negative impacts on public health.

REFERENCES

Abbott, F. M. (2006). *Intellectual property provisions of bilateral and regional trade agreements in light of U.S. federal law.* UNCTAD-ICTSD Project on IPRs and Sustainable Development Issue Paper No. 12. Geneva: International Centre for Trade and Sustainable Development (ICTSD)/United Nations Conference on Trade and Development (UNCTAD). Retrieved from: http://www.unctad.org/en/docs/iteipc20064_en.pdf.

Abbott, F. M., & Reichman, J. H. (2007). *Access to essential medicines: Lessons learned since the Doha Declaration on the TRIPS Agreement and public health, and policy options for the European Union.* Brussels: European Parliament. Retrieved from: http://www.law.fsu.edu/faculty/profiles/abbott/study_TRIPS.pdf.

Angell, M. (2004). *The truth about the drug companies: How they deceive us and what to do about it.* New York: Random House.

Apoyo Consultoría. (2005). *Impacto de las negociaciones del TLC con EE.UU en materia de propiedad intelectual en los mercados de medicamentos y plaguicidas.* Lima: Apoyo Consultoría. Retrieved from: http://www.cepes.org.pe/apc-aa/archivos-aa/a6febae6efa968397aff3016c880508e/APOYO_TLC_medicamentos_y_agroexportacion.pdf;   http://cies.org.pe/files/tlc/apoyo.pdf.

Barder, O., Kremer, M., & Levine, R. (2005). *Making markets for vaccines: Ideas to action.* Washington, DC: Center for Global Development. Retrieved from: http://www.cgdev.org/doc/books/vaccine/MakingMarkets-complete.pdf.

Burke, M.A., & de Francisco, A., eds. (2004). *Monitoring financial flows for health research 2004* . Geneva: Global Forum for Health Research. Retrieved from: http://www.globalforumhealth.org/Site/002__What%20we%20do/005__Publications/004__Resource%20flows.php.

Center for Drug Evaluation and Research. (2005). *CDER ND as approved in calendar years 1990–2004 by therapeutic potential and chemical type.* U.S. Food and Drug Administration [online]. Retrieved from: http://www.fda.gov/cder/rdmt/pstable.htm.

Charles River Associates. (2004). *Innovation in the pharmaceutical sector: Study undertaken for the European Commission.* ENTR/03/28. Brussels. Retrieved from:http://ec.europa.eu/enterprise/pharmaceuticals/pharmacos/docs/doc2004/nov/eu_pharma_innovation_25–11–04.pdf.

Chaudhuri, S. (2005). *The WTO and India's pharmaceuticals industry: Patent protection, TRIPS, and developing countries.* New Delhi: Oxford University Press.

Commission of the European Communities. (2004). *COM (2004) 737 final. Proposal for a regulation of the European Parliament and of the council on compulsory licensing of patents relating to the manufacture of pharmaceutical products for export to countries with public health problems.* Brussels. Retrieved from: http://www.europarl.europa.eu/oeil/FindByProcnum.do?lang=2&procnum=COD/2004/0258.

Commission on Intellectual Property Rights (CIPR). (2002). *Integrating intellectual property and development policy—report of the Commission on Intellectual Property Rights.* London: Commission on Intellectual Property Rights. Retrieved from: http://www.iprcommission.org/papers/pdfs/final_report/CIPRfullfinal.pdf.

Commission on Intellectual Property Rights, Innovation and Public Health. (2006). *Public health innovation and intellectual property rights.* Geneva: World Health Organization. Retrieved from: http://www.who.int/entity/intellectualproperty/documents/thereport/CIPIHReport23032006.pdf.

Coriat, B. (2002, September). *The new global intellectual property rights regime and its imperial dimension: Implications for "North/South" relations.* Paper prepared for the 50th BNDS Anniversary Seminar, Rio de Janeiro, Brazil.

Correa, C. (1999). *Intellectual property and the use of compulsory licences: Options for developing countries.* Trade-Related Agenda, Development and Equity (T.R.A.D.E.) Working Paper No. 5. Geneva: South Centre. Retrieved from: http://www.southcentre.org/publications/workingpapers/wp05.pdf.

———. (2004). *Implementation of the WHO General Council Decision on paragraph 6 of the Doha Declaration on the TRIPS Agreement and public health.* Geneva: World Health Organization. Retrieved from: http://www.who.int/medicines/areas/policy/WTO_DOHA_DecisionPara6final.pdf.

———. (2006). *Guidelines for the examination of pharmaceutical patents: Developing a public health perspective—a working paper.* Geneva: ICTSD/UNCTAD/WHO. Retrieved from: http://www.iprsonline.org/unctadictsd/docs/Correa_Pharmaceutical-Patents-Guidelines.pdf.

Correa, C., & Musungu, S. (2002). *The WIPO patent agenda: The risks for developing countries.* Working Paper No. 12. Geneva: South Centre. Retrieved from: http://www.southcentre.org/publications/workingpapers/wp12.pdf.

Cullet, P. (2003). Patients and medicines: The relationship between TRIPS and the human right to health. *International Affairs, 79,* 139–60.

Drahos, P. (2002). *Developing countries and international intellectual property standard-setting.* Study Paper 8. London: Commission on Intellectual Property Rights. Retrieved from: http://www.iprcommission.org/papers/pdfs/study_papers/sp8_drahos_study.pdf.

Drugs for Neglected Diseases initiative (DNDi) & Sanofi-Aventis. (2008). *ASAQ: Hope for malaria. DNDi and Sanofi-aventis: An innovative partnership.* http://www.actwithasaq.org/en/asaq3.htm. Retrieved from: http://www.actwithasaq.org/en/asaq3.htm.

Economist. (2007). Billion dollar pills. *Economist,* January 27, 69–71.

Federal Trade Commission (FTC). (2002). *Generic drug entry prior to patent expiration: An FTC study.* Washington, DC: Federal Trade Commission. Retrieved from: http://www.ftc.gov/os/2002/07/genericdrugstudy.pdf.

———. (2003). *FTC charges Bristol-Myers Squibb with pattern of abusing government processes to stifle generic drug competition.* Washington, DC: Federal Trade Commission. Retrieved from: http://www.ftc.gov/opa/2003/03/bms.htm.

Howse, Robert, ed. (2007). *Trade related aspects of intellectual property rights: A commentary on the TRIPS Agreement.* Oxford: Oxford University Press.

Hunt, P. (2006). *The right of everyone to the enjoyment of the highest attainable standard of physical and mental health.* A/61/338. New York: United Nations General Assembly. Retrieved from: http://daccessdds.un.org/doc/UNDOC/GEN/N06/519/97/PDF/N0651997.pdf?OpenElement.

ICTSD reporting. (2008). WHO adopts strategy on public health, innovation and intellectual property. *Bridges Weekly Trade News Digest, 12.* Retrieved from: http://www.ictsd.org/weekly/08–05–28/story6.htm.

Intergovernmental Working Group on Public Health, Innovation and Intellectual Property. (2007). *Draft global strategy and plan of action on public health, innovation and intellectual property. Glossary of terms. Report by the Secretariat.* A/PHI/ IGWG/2/INF.DOC./6. Geneva: World Health Organization. Retrieved from: http:// www.who.int/gb/phi/pdf/igwg2/PHI_IGWG2_ID6-en.pdf.

Kepler, T. B., Marti-Renom, M. A., Maurer, S. M., Rai, A. K., Taylor, G., & Todd, M. H. (2006). Open source research—the power of us. *Australian Journal of Chemistry, 59,* 291–94.

Khor, M. (2007). *Patents, compulsory licences and access to medicines: Some recent experiences.* Penang, Malaysia: Third World Network (TWN). Retrieved from: http://www.twnside.org.sg/title2/IPR/ipr10.pdf.

Lewis, T. R., Reichman, J. H., & So, A. D. (2006). *Treating clinical trials as a public good: The most logical reform.* Law and Economics Workshop (University of California, Berkeley) Paper No. 11. Berkeley: University of California. Retrieved from: http://repositories.cdlib.org/cgi/viewcontent.cgi?article =1147&context=berkeley_law_econ.

Ling, C. Y. (2006). *Malaysia's experience in increasing access to antiretroviral drugs: Exercising the "government use" option.* Penang, Malaysia: Third World Network. Retrieved from: http://www.twnside.org.sg/title2/IPR/ IPRS09.pdf.

Maurer, S., Rai, A., & Sali, A. (2004). Finding cures for tropical diseases: Is open source an answer? *Public Library of Science Medicine, 1,* 183–86.

McCalman, P. (1999). *Reaping what you sow: An empirical analysis of international patent harmonization.* Cambridge, MA: Center for Business and Government, John F. Kennedy School of Government, Harvard University. Retrieved from: http://www.innovations.harvard.edu/showdoc.html?id=5075.

Ministry of Public Health & National Health Security Office. (2007). *Facts and evidences on the 10 burning issues related to the government use of patents on three patented essential drugs in Thailand: Document to support strengthening of social wisdom on the issue of drug patent.* Bangkok: The Ministry of Public Health and The National Health Security Office. Retrieved from: http://www. moph.go.th/hot/White%20Paper%20CL-EN.pdf.

Nagle, M. (2007). Roche revamps R&D for speed. Retrieved from: in-Pharma Technologist.com.

Oh, C. (2006). Compulsory licenses: Recent experiences in developing countries. *International Journal of Intellectual Property Management, 1,* 22–36.

Outterson, K. (2005). Pharmaceutical arbitrage: Balancing access and innovation in international prescription drug markets. *Yale Journal of Health Policy, Law and Ethics, 5,* 193–291.

Pharmaceutical Research and Manufacturers of America. (2005). *Pharmaceutical industry profile 2005. From laboratory to patient: Pathways to biopharmaceutical innovation.* Washington, DC: Pharmaceutical Research and Manufacturers of America. Retrieved from: http://international.phrma.org/publications/ publications/17.03.2005.1142.cfm.

Reichman, J. H., & Hasenzahl, C. (2003). *Non-voluntary licensing of patented inventions: Historical perspective, legal framework under TRIPS and an overview of the practice in Canada and the United States of America.* UNCTAD-ICTSD Project on IPRs and Sustainable Development Issue Paper No. 5. Geneva: International Centre for Trade and Sustainable Development (ICTSD)/United Nations Conference on Trade and Development (UNCTAD). Retrieved from: http://www.ictsd.org/pubs/ictsd_series/iprs/CS_reichman_ hasenzahl.pdf.

Reinharz, H. Y., & Chastonay, P. (2004). *Santé et droits de l'homme* (vol. 1). Geneva: Editions Médecine & Hygiène en collaboration avec la société académique de Genève, Collection Médecine Société (CMS).

Roffe, P., & Tesfachew, T. (2001). *International technology transfer: The origins and aftermaths of the United Nations negotiations on a draft code of conduct.* The Hague: Kluwer Law International.

Scherer, F. M. (2003). Comments. In R. Anderson & N. Gallini (eds.), *Competition policy and intellectual property rights in the knowledge-based economy.* Calgary: University of Calgary Press.

———. (2004). A note on global welfare in pharmaceutical patenting. *The World Economy,* 27, 1127–42.

Sell, S. K. (2003). *Private power, public law: The globalization of intellectual property rights.* Cambridge: Cambridge University Press.

Spector, R. (2005). Me-too drugs. Sometimes they're just the same old, same old. *Stanford Medicine Magazine,* Summer.

Stiglitz, J. (1999). Knowledge as a global public good. In I. Kaul, I. Grunberg, & M. Stern (eds.), *Global public goods: International cooperation in the 21st century* (pp. 308–25). New York: Oxford University Press.

———. (2007). *Times online MBA podcasts in association with IBM: Week 1—making globalisation work.* London: News International Limited. Retrieved from: http://ecours.univ-reunion.fr/ecours/IMG/pdf/mba_stiglitz-4.pdf.

Tandon, P. (1982). Optimal patents with compulsory licensing. *The Journal of Political Economy,* 90, 470–86.

United Nations Conference on Trade and Development Secretariat. (1998). *Empirical evidence of the benefits from applying competition law and policy principles to economic development in order to attain greater efficiency in international trade and development.* TD/B/COM.2/EM/10. Geneva: UNCTAD. Retrieved from: http://www.unctad.org/en/docs/c2emd10r1.en.pdf.

United Nations High Commissioner for Human Rights. (2001). *Economic, social and cultural rights: The impact of the Agreement on Trade-Related Aspects of Intellectual Property Rights on human rights.* No. E/CN.4/Sub.2/2001/13. Geneva: United Nations Commission on Human Rights. Retrieved from: http://www.unhchr.ch/Huridocda/Huridoca.nsf/(Symbol)/E.CN.4.Sub.2.2001.13.En?Opendocument.

Vaidhyanathan, S. (2001). *Copyrights and copywrongs: The rise of intellectual property and how it threatens creativity.* New York: New York University Press.

World Bank. (2000). *World development indicators 2000.* Washington, DC: Author. Retrieved from: http://www-wds.worldbank.org/external/default/WDSContentServer/IW3P/IB/2000/05/25/000094946_00050605490166/Rendered/PDF/multi0page.pdf.

———. (2007). World development indicators [online] 2006. World Bank [online]. Retrieved from: http://devdata.worldbank.org/wdi2006/contents/index2.htm.

World Intellectual Property Organization. (2008). *The 45 agreed recommendations under the WIPO development agenda.* Geneva: World Intellectual Property Organization. Retrieved from: http://www.wipo.int/ip-development/en/agenda/cdip_recommendations.html.

World Intellectual Property Organization Secretariat. (2004). *Proposal by Argentina and Brazil for the establishment of a development agenda for WIPO.* WO/GA/31/11. In WIPO General Assembly, Thirty-First Session, Geneva. Geneva: WIPO. Retrieved from: http://www.wipo.int/documents/en/document/govbody/wo_gb_ga/pdf/wo_ga_31_11.pdf.

World Medical Association. (2004). *World Medical Association Declaration of Helsinki: Ethical principles for medical research involving human subjects.* World Medical Association (WMA). Retrieved from: http://www.wma.net/e/policy/pdf/17c.pdf.

World Trade Organization. (1994). *Agreement on trade related aspects of intellectual property rights 1986–1994 Uruguay round.* Geneva: World Trade Organization. Retrieved from: http://www.wto.org/english/docs_e/legal_e/legal_e.htm#TRIPs; http://www.wto.org/english/docs_e/legal_e/27-trips.pdf.
————. (2001). *Declaration on the TRIPS Agreement and public health.* WT/MIN(01)/DEC/W/2 from the WTO Ministerial Conference, 4th Session, Doha, 9–14 November 2001. New York: World Trade Organization. Retrieved from: http://www.who.int/medicines/areas/policy/tripshealth.pdf.
Yamin, A. E. (2003). Not just a tragedy: Access to medications as a right under international law. *Boston University International Law Journal, 21,* 325–71.

12 Global Governance for Health

Kelley Lee, Meri Koivusalo, Eeva Ollila,
Ronald Labonté, Claudio Schuftan, and
David Woodward

INTRODUCTION

The acceleration of globalization in recent decades has led to widespread efforts to develop appropriate forms of governance to deal effectively with emerging challenges. Intense debates have ensued about the imperfections of existing institutions, as well as the desired features of emerging forms of governance. Global governance for health concerns the institutional settings and relationships in which health goals are collectively agreed upon and pursued by state and nonstate actors. The universal value placed on human health has contributed to considerable institutional innovation, but also to critical reflection on how collective health goals are defined and acted upon.

This chapter reviews the existing evidence concerning the impacts of global governance with particular reference to social determinants of health (SDH). First, it describes institutional actors in terms of their relative roles, power, and authority. This requires an understanding of the changing architecture comprising health-based and non-health-based institutions. Second, it considers how emerging forms of global governance, its various institutions, and the distribution and use of power and authority among them might influence and affect SDH. Third, emerging forms of global governance for health are assessed against "good governance" criteria of coordination and coherence; transparency, and accountability; participation and representation; resource mobilization and allocation; and leadership (United Nations Economic and Social Commission for Asia and the Pacific, 2007). Addressing poor performance within and across global governance institutions is arguably a necessary prerequisite to tackling SDH.

The chapter thus concludes by considering how global governance can play a transformational role in addressing SDH and makes recommendations as to how global governance for health can be more equity-oriented and prohealth.

WHAT IS GLOBAL GOVERNANCE FOR HEALTH?

Governance concerns the agreed actions and means adopted by a society to promote collective action and deliver solutions in pursuit of common goals (Dodgson, Lee, & Drager, 2002). Governance takes place whenever people organize themselves to achieve a shared end through rules and procedures. This can take place at different levels of social organization: community, state/provincial, national, regional, and global. If a local community decides to initiate a campaign to slow traffic speed and improve road safety, this requires some form of governance to organize collective efforts. If a global campaign is initiated to strengthen tuberculosis control, an agreed form of governance is needed to take decisions, for example, on strategy, resource mobilization, and implementation of agreed actions. Unlike government, whose actions are backed by formal authority, "governance refers to activities backed by shared goals that may or may not derive from legal and formally prescribed responsibilities and that do not necessarily rely on police powers to overcome defiance and attain compliance" (Rosenau, 1995, p. 15).

> The concept of governance has gained relevance since 1945 with increased integration of the world economy and proliferation of non-state actors, and raises important questions regarding "how modern societies are governed and, normatively speaking, how they should be governed" as well as questioning the effectiveness of modern governments "when the organization of economic and social life appears systematically to transcend territorial jurisdictions." (McGrew, 2000, p. 130)

Diverse perspectives have been put forth, ranging from the creation of a global government to minimalist laissez-faire forms of governance (McGrew & Held, 2002).

Global governance is "the sum of the many ways individuals and institutions, public and private, manage their common affairs . . . [through] intergovernmental relationships . . . [and] non-governmental organizations (NGOs), citizens' movements, multinational corporations, and the global capitalist market" (Commission on Global Governance, 1995). By extension, global governance for health concerns (a) institutions and practices of global governance specifically created to address health determinants and outcomes, and (b) any institutions and practices of global governance with substantial impact on determinants of health.

Global governance is emergent in certain issue areas (e.g., trade) while remaining weak or nonexistent in others (e.g., health) (Ware, 2006). Importantly the nature, goals, and impacts of emerging forms of global governance remain highly contested (Kickbusch, 2003; Barnett, 2005). While some perceive contemporary developments as progress towards more pluralist and democratic forms of governance, others have grave concerns about the concentration and misuse of power, and the disadvantaging this creates for certain social groups, such as the poor and women (Held, 1995; Falk, 1999).

An integral part of debates about global governance is widespread recognition that its current forms fall short in their capacity to manage globalization effectively. As the World Commission on the Social Dimensions of Globalization reports:

> Global markets have grown rapidly without the parallel development of economic and social institutions necessary for their smooth equitable functioning. At the same time, there is concern about the unfairness of key global rules on trade and finance and their asymmetric effects on rich and poor countries. (International Labour Organization, 2004, p. xi)

Criteria for improved governance (at whatever level) range from a relatively narrow focus on administrative, technical, and economic competence of specific institutions, notably of the state (World Bank, 1994), to broader assessments of how well political systems, encompassing both state and nonstate institutions, function as a whole (Grindle, 2004). For example, the World Bank has emphasized the reform of the state as an enabler of economic growth and development, leading to a focus on reducing state corruption and strengthening public administration (Huther & Shah, 1998; Ng & Yeats, 1999; Wei, 2000; Wolfowitz, 2006). The United Nations Development Program (UNDP), in contrast, has adopted broader criteria for assessing good governance as integral to state, market, and civil society interaction (United Nations Development Program, 1997).

Notions of good governance have not remained static or limited in application. They have developed to incorporate all countries, levels, and a variety of state and nonstate institutions, as well as being applicable to the functioning and processes of a wide variety of organizational forms. Although initially the emphasis on good governance was intended for low- and middle-income countries (LMICs), all nations are now challenged to aspire to broadened criteria of good governance. Moreover, such aspirations are not confined to specific institutions but extend to private companies and civil society organizations (CSOs). There is also widespread acceptance that the appropriate criteria for assessing good governance should go beyond measures of administrative, technical, and economic competence to the functioning of legal systems, democratic institutions and processes, and the development of civil society (Leftwich, 1994; AusAID, 2000; Dobriansky, 2003). These notions of good governance are particularly important in assessing the linkages between global governance, health, and SDH.

THE EMERGING ARCHITECTURE OF
GLOBAL GOVERNANCE FOR HEALTH

Globalization is affecting governance in four fundamental ways. First, it is shifting the distribution of power and authority among different levels of governance. Globalization creates challenges to the capacity of national institutions to govern effectively (see Chapter 5, this volume). While formal authority may largely remain with sovereign states, the power and authority of certain institutions at the national, regional, and global levels have increased.

Second, globalization is increasing the causal connections across different policy spheres and extending connections long recognized at the local/ national levels to the global level. For example, health policy is increasingly affected by policy decisions on trade, environment, migration, security, and agriculture. This requires forms of governance that facilitate multisectoral and multilevel action. In health, efforts have been made to develop approaches that cut across institutional boundaries to address issues of transnational reach (Martin, 2006) or, for example, to attain intersectoral targets, such as those expressed as the Millennium Development Goals (MDGs).

Third, globalization is changing the relative number of institutions belonging to the state, market, or civil society, and the distribution of power and authority among them. Of particular note is the growth in market-based institutions and their relative power within an emerging global political economy. The commercial sector comprises a diverse range of interests and institutions, from small-scale concerns such as local farms and manufacturers to large-scale global concerns such as transnational corporations (TNCs). Economic globalization is characterized by the increased concentration of ownership and global expansion within many sectors, such as food and drink, pharmaceuticals, electronics, automotives, energy, and telecommunications (Braithwaithe & Drahos, 2004). This has given companies sizable resources and capacity to influence not only the functioning of the world economy through transactions but also how it is regulated through institutions of global governance. In some cases, TNCs have become direct participants in global governance through institutional arrangements, notably global public-private partnerships (GPPPs). TNC influence has also been enhanced through lobbying and advocacy, sponsorship of research and policy, and membership of opinion-forming bodies (e.g., commissions).

Similarly, CSOs, which are defined here as the totality of voluntary civic and social organizations that form the basis of a functioning society, have become more important within global governance. In health, CSOs played an instrumental role in the adoption of the International Code on the Marketing of Breastmilk Substitutes (Richter, 2002) and model lists of essential medicines (World Health Organization, 2001). At the United Nations (UN) Conference on Population and Development in 1994, the women's health movement played a prominent role in preparations and deliberations, influencing a shift from population control to reproductive health (Neidell, 1998). Similarly, CSOs were active contributors to the negotiation of the Framework Convention on Tobacco Control and the Doha Declaration on the Trade-Related Aspects of Intellectual Property Rights (TRIPS) agreement and public health (Collin, Lee, & Bissell, 2002).

Notably, "hybrid" institutions have emerged as part of global governance, bringing together state, market, and civil society actors (Figure 12.1). Philanthropic foundations straddle civil society, given their nonprofit activities, and the private sector, where funding may originate. The scale of resources commanded by some foundations today, and the corresponding increase in scale and scope of their activities, suggests unprecedented influence in global health governance. For example, the Bill and Melinda Gates Foundation is among the three biggest donors to global health, including its Grand Challenges in Global Health initiative and contributions to the Global Alliance for Vaccines and Immunization (GAVI).

Since the early 1990s, there have been initiatives, often referred to as global public-private partnerships (GPPPs), that have brought together state, market, and civil society actors. In health, these include the Global Forum for Health Research, GAVI, the Global Fund to Fight AIDS, Tuberculosis and Malaria (GFATM), and the Global Alliance for Improved Nutrition (GAIN), concerned primarily with vitamin and mineral supplementation. One of the key innovations of these organizations has been to involve for-profit organizations directly in decision making, the appropriateness of which has been questioned (Koivusalo & Ollila, 1997; Buse & Walt, 2000; Ollila, 2003; Zammit, 2003; Richter, 2004; Ollila, 2005). There has also been increased attention to new forms of management, with increased emphasis on results-based approaches such as payments for progress (Barder & Birdsall, 2006), pilot funding, rapid measurable results, monitoring and evaluation, exit strategies, and implementation of and/or research on new technologies. Given the emphasis of GPPPs on short-term and quantifiable measures, there remain considerable concerns about the extent to which they are appropriate governance vehicles to address SDH.

Fourth, global governance in its emergent form has been characterized by shifts in power and authority within and across countries and institutions. Among those institutions directly concerned with SDH, the relative decline of the World Health Organization's (WHO) authority and power has been observed alongside the rise of the World Bank through its health sector lending since the 1980s (see Chapter 8, this volume), and the proliferation of GPPPs. Beyond the health sector, the increasing power of multilateral and regional trading systems, the Organization for Economic Cooperation and Development (OECD), and the Group of Eight (G8) can also be compared with the corresponding decline of the United Nations Conference on Trade and Development (UNCTAD), the Group of 77, and the Non-aligned Movement since the New International Economic Order debates of the 1970s.

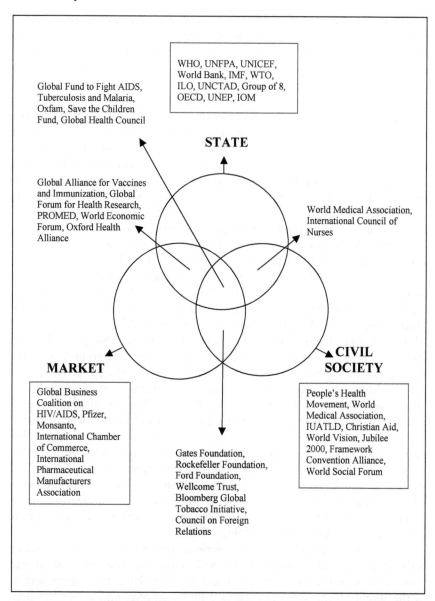

Figure 12.1   Selected global institutions with an impact on the social determinants of health.

IDENTIFYING KEY GLOBAL HEALTH GOVERNANCE ACTORS

There is a broad range of global institutions concerned with SDH. Historically, WHO has played a lead role as the UN specialist agency for health since its creation in 1948. Other UN organizations have included health issues as part of broader mandates concerning children (United Nations

Children's Fund–UNICEF), agriculture/food (World Food Program–WFP, Food and Agriculture Organization–FAO, and International Fund for Agricultural Development–IFAD), population (United Nations Population Fund–UNFPA), and development (United Nations Development Program–UNDP). The mandates of these institutions remain a subject of debate over how narrowly or broadly they should be defined, and thus whether specific initiatives should tackle SDH. Broadly defined examples include UNICEF's campaign on child poverty (UNICEF, 2005), UNDP's work on global trade (Malhotra, 2002), and UNFPA's promotion of gender equality (Microcredit Summit Campaign/United Nations Population Fund, 2005). In addition, UNICEF examined the health effects of structural adjustment programs and globalization during the 1980s (Cornia, Jolly, & Stewart, 1987). The International Labour Organization (ILO) Program on Safety and Health at Work and the Environment (Safe Work), and its activities concerning social security and health insurance, are relevant here, as is its facilitation of the 2004 World Commission on the Social Dimension of Globalization.

Non-health-focused institutions are concerned with a wide range of issue areas that indirectly affect SDH. These institutions may address specific health issues, as part of their mandates concerning, for example, trade and investment, education, housing, or employment. They also influence SDH through the pursuit of these core mandates. The most important non-health-related institutions in global governance, in terms of impacts on SDH, are those concerned with governance of the world economy. These are led by the international financial institutions (IFIs) and the World Trade Organization (WTO), and their regional counterparts, along with the OECD and G8. The International Monetary Fund (IMF) and World Bank play a critical role in providing and catalyzing external financing for developing countries, with the mandate to prevent and resolve debt and financial crises which have had major effects on SDH in recent decades (see Chapters 7, 8, and 9, this volume). The nature of their response to debt and financial crises and the conditions attached to their loans give them considerable, if not controversial, influence over policymaking processes in many developing countries for extended periods of time. The IMF and World Bank are also major sources and commissioners of research, the latter having consciously established a role as a self-styled "Knowledge Bank" since 1996 (Cohen & Laporte, 2004), although independent evaluation studies have raised concerns about the validity and credibility of its knowledge (Banerjee, Deaton, Lustig, Rogoff, & Hsu, 2006). While SDH may be explicitly or implicitly recognized as important by existing institutions of global governance, the solutions they put forth generally have focused on selective health care interventions to alleviate disease consequences, rather than measures to address the multiple pathways by which social conditions influence health outcomes (Solar & Irwin, 2006). This tendency may be understandable from an institutional perspective, in terms of focusing activities and avoiding "mandate creep," but hinders the production of an evidentiary base and policy recommendations for addressing SDH.

Beyond the UN system, a variety of health-focused GPPPs have joined the global governance scene. As new initiatives, they have attracted public attention to specific causes, such as the need for certain technologies (e.g., vaccines, supplements), the neglect of specific diseases, gaps in global health research, or the plight of certain populations. Analyses of GPPPs to date have raised concerns about their vertical (disease-focused) approach, longer-term sustainability, undermining of local health systems, capacity to achieve measurable results, and contribution to fragmenting global health governance (Ollila, 2003, 2005). Critical assessment of the governance of GPPPs continues to be outpaced by their creation and operation.

Overall, there are clear tensions within and across health-focused organizations on what should be the priorities in health development and how they should best be achieved. In general, attention to SDH has increased within some organizations but remains challenged by a continued emphasis on biomedical and vertical approaches to health. Non-health-focused institutions play an important if indirect role in shaping SDH as part of their core mandates concerning, for example, trade and investment, education, housing, or employment. Whether or not health-focused institutions influence SDH depends on a number of factors.

First, there appear to be no minimal legal obligations for these institutions to consider health and/or its broad determinants. The development of international human rights law could inform a strengthening of global governance for SDH, although human rights treaties are binding on state parties and not on multilateral institutions per se. It may be argued that human rights instruments do apply to institutions indirectly through obligations binding the member states of these institutions to citizens' rights in their own and other countries (Hunt, 2005a, 2005b). This argument has been advanced with respect to the WTO and its member states, but could also be applied, for example, to the IMF and the World Bank. However, Fidler (2005b) notes that international trade law, including aspects directly related to health, is more developed than international health law. Unlike most international obligations, including human rights treaties, WTO agreements are also backed by sanctions, so national governments have an incentive to give greater weight to these obligations. Furthermore, trade relations are often asymmetrical, taking place between more and less economically powerful countries. Sanctions that may arise from these relations are highly inconsistent in their effectiveness, and often have inequitable consequences across countries (Stiglitz & Charlton, 2004; Birdsall, 2006).

Second, to what extent are health objectives compatible with the mandates and declared goals of non-health-focused institutions? There are measures within certain multilateral trade agreements to limit potentially adverse health effects, as well as proactive measures taken to protect health, such as the clarifications provided by the Doha Declaration and Paragraph 6 decision for the TRIPS Agreement (Bloche 2002) (see

Chapter 11, this volume). The asbestos dispute between the European Union (EU) and Canada also suggests that health protection measures can pass the dispute settlement process (Ranson et al., 2002; Koivusalo, 2003) (see Chapter 5, this volume). However, the scope for applying public policy interventions may depend on how such key concepts as "public health emergency," "least trade restrictive," "sufficient scientific evidence," and "services supplied in the exercise of government authority" are interpreted (Woodward, 2005). The WTO decision regarding the beef hormone dispute among the EU, the United States (U.S.), and Canada suggested that the WTO's interpretation of the standard of scientific evidence to uphold the EU's ban was particularly stringent. Similar concerns were raised by the WTO decision on the case brought by the United States, Canada, and Argentina ruling against stringent EU regulation of genetically modified organisms. Even the flexibilities under TRIPS remain problematic given the lack of consensus over their scope, and the capacity for LMICs to exercise them (see Chapter 11, this volume). Moreover, there remains limited analysis of the health protections available under the growing number of regional and bilateral trade agreements that create so-called WTO-plus measures, for example, because they provide stronger intellectual property protection than TRIPS.

The impact of standards-setting bodies on SDH is also important to consider. One example is the Codex Alimentarius Commission (or Codex), a joint body created by WHO and FAO in 1963 "to develop food standards, guidelines and related texts such as codes of practice."[1] In 1995, as part of the Uruguay Round under the General Agreement on Tariffs and Trade (GATT), the status of the Codex was elevated to that of a binding regulatory body. Critics argue that the dominant role of large-scale commercial producers has led to standards being set too low to adequately protect consumers' health. Conversely, setting higher standards has the potential to bolster the competitive position of larger producers who are better placed to meet these standards and consequently may negatively affect small producers, with potentially adverse effects on poverty. Enhancing the health equity effects of international standards requires taking into account both direct (biomedical) and indirect (SDH) health effects. Too much emphasis on economic benefits will result in standards too low to protect health, while a purely biomedical perspective may set them too high for economic-related health benefits to be realized. This represents a strong case for raising the profile of SDH relative to both, and of institutionalizing this in the global governance system negotiating and resolving disputes related to trade rules.

A more promising link with SDH is the inclusion of health issues within broader development initiatives. At the World Summit for Social Development in 1995, governments reached consensus on "the need to put people at the center of development." The subsequent Copenhagen Declaration adopted 10 commitments central to SDH, including poverty reduction, full employment, and social integration, which were also reconfirmed in the General Assembly resolution in 2000 (United Nations, 1995, 2000). These commitments have been largely subsumed by the health goals included within the MDGs, intended as a framework for targeting development assistance in key priorities. The Millennium Declaration, however, provides some basis for the importance of global governance for SDH in emphasizing that "We recognize that, in addition to our separate responsibilities to our individual societies, we have a collective responsibility to uphold the principles of human dignity, equality and equity at the global level" (United Nations, 2004). Depending on the context and how MDGs are used, they could provide a potential, albeit still unproven, tool for addressing SDH, with three of its goals explicitly addressing health, and four additional goals closely related to broader SDH (UN Millennium Project, 2005).

Third, it is not yet clear that there is sufficient evidence and potential for actions linking a nonhealth policy domain with SDH. Over the past decade, there have been many, mostly unheeded, efforts to give attention to the social impacts of globalization, including health, notably the ILO's World Commission on the Social Dimension of Globalization (International Labour Organization, 2004). The vision put forth by the commission is

> a process of globalization with a strong social dimension based on universally shared values, and respect for human rights and individual dignity; one that is fair, inclusive, democratically governed and provides opportunities and tangible benefits for all countries and people. (International Labour Organization, 2004, p. ix)

The World Social Forum (WSF) similarly has sought to challenge current forms of globalization. It is described as

> an open meeting place for reflective thinking, democratic debate of ideas, formulation of proposals, free exchange of experiences and inter-linking for effective action, by groups and movements of civil society that are opposed to neo-liberalism and to domination of the world by capital and any form of imperialism, and are committed to building a society centered on the human person. (World Social Forum, 2006)

In addition, there is now substantive empirical evidence analyzing the impact of globalization on poverty, labor-market restructuring, income inequalities, physical environments, health systems, and financial flows (Pangestu, 2001; Lee & Vivarelli, 2006; Labonté & Schrecker, 2007a, 2007b, 2007c). Health has also been included in research and policy on global public goods (Smith, Beaglehole, Woodward, & Drager, 2003).

"GOOD" GLOBAL GOVERNANCE TO ADDRESS
SOCIAL DETERMINANTS OF HEALTH

The links between specific principles of good governance and SDH can be considered in two ways: first, the quality of governance within individual institutions which shape their decisions and activities; and second, how these institutions collectively contribute to the governance of an increasingly globalized world.

Policy Coherence and Coordination

Weak policy coherence and coordination in health cooperation have long been recognized. Efforts to improve coherence and coordination have been hindered foremost by the absence of any overarching authority in global governance above sovereign states. Key institutional actors concerned with global governance operate largely independently of one another, formally accountable to certain constituencies such as powerful donor governments, but not to a higher level of authority. There are fundamental differences in goals, expertise, value bases, constituencies and resources, and variations in power and influence among a diversity of institutions. Deacon et al. (2003) observe fragmentation and competition among the World Bank, WTO, the UN system, the G8, and other groupings of countries, and national social development initiatives. The current global architecture is, in short, a complex array of independent, unequal, and even competing institutions.

Within the health sector, the need for better coordination is recognized as a long-standing challenge. There is substantial evidence of the imperfections of the global governance architecture in the form of duplication of effort, overlapping mandates, gaps in effort, and undue transaction costs imposed on recipient countries (Lee, Collinson, Walt, & Gilson, 1996; Buse & Walt, 1997; van Diesen & Walker, 1999; Walt, Pavignani, Gilson, & Buse, 1999; Martinez, 2006). The WHO Constitution states that one of its functions is "to act as the directing and coordinating authority on international health work" (Paragraph 2(a)). However, dissatisfaction by some donor governments with certain WHO activities from the late 1970s deemed "political," notably Health for All by the Year 2000, essential drugs, and regulation of breast-milk substitutes, led some major donors to support the freezing of WHO resources, as well as the creation of alternative institutions. The World Bank, governed by an economically weighted voting system, in contrast with WHO's one-country, one-vote system, subsequently asserted its leadership role for new health-related activities, notably the promotion of market-oriented health sector reforms from the 1980s (see Chapter 8, this volume).

The perceived need for improved policy coherence has arisen more recently from efforts to address key health issues through intersectoral cooperation. Globalization has blurred policy domains by creating greater linkages across issue areas, as well as levels of governance. According to the United Kingdom (UK) Department for International Development (UK DFID) (United Kingdom Department for International Development, 2006), policy coherence "is achieved when policies across a range of issues (for example, trade, migration, security) support, or at least do not undermine, the attainment of development objectives." Similarly, the OECD (Organisation for Economic Cooperation and Development, 2003, p. 2) defines policy coherence as "systematic promotion of mutually reinforcing policy actions among government departments and agencies creating synergies towards achieving the agreed objectives." The lack of policy coherence, according to UK DFID (United Kingdom Department For International Development, 2006), weakens the efficiency and impact of aid. This occurs through:

1. Lost opportunities for complementarities when policies contradict each other.
2. Too few mechanisms to systematically detect and resolve policy conflicts, and the difficulty of balancing legitimate domestic and global interests when such conflicts become apparent.
3. Insufficient political pressure for change, both at the domestic level (with limited public awareness of the impact of different policies and trade-offs made by government) and internationally (with limited fora for low-income countries to hold rich ones to account).
4. Complex decision-making systems where multiple domestic interests compete alongside multilateral agendas, special interest groups, and developing partners.

There have been ongoing efforts since the early 1990s to improve coherence and coordination in health development as part of a "new architecture of aid." For example, within individual countries, the sector-wide approach (SWAp) has been adopted to bring together institutions concerned with health development. A SWAp is defined as

> a process in which funding for the sector—whether internal or from donors—supports a single policy and expenditure program, under government leadership, and adopting common approaches across the sector. It is generally accompanied by efforts to strengthen government procedures for disbursement and accountability. A SWAp should ideally involve broad stakeholder consultation in the design of a coherent sector program at micro, meso and macro levels, and strong co-ordination among donors and between donors and government. (United Kingdom Department for International Development, 2001, p. 1)

While focused on the health sector per se and thus not an instrument for addressing SDH, SWAp offers ideas for strengthening institutional links across multiple sectors (see Chapter 7, this volume). Other UN initiatives include the Common Country Assessment, UN Development Assistance Framework, and UN Resident Coordinators. Joint efforts by the WHO and the ILO on ensuring decent working conditions in the Americas illustrate further the potential for strategic and operational collaboration (International Labour Organization, 2006).

Another approach is to strengthen coordination of institutions across targeted populations or health issues. The Integrated Management of Childhood Illness is an integrated strategy by the WHO and UNICEF that focuses on promoting and protecting the well-being of the whole child, taking into account the variety of factors that put children in the developing world at serious risk, emphasizing prevention of disease through immunization and improved nutrition (World Health Organization, 1999).

It is widely acknowledged that impacts on health and health determinants arise from policies dealing primarily with matters other than health (Ståhl, Wismar, Ollila, Lahtinen, & Leppo, 2006). This is especially important and notable in areas where health impacts have not traditionally been considered, such as economic, trade, and industrial policies. By definition, efforts to address SDH require engagement with nonhealth sectors, implying a need to redress the shortfalls in global institutional coordination and coherence. The most prominent of these initiatives is the MDGs. Similarly, to reduce poverty more effectively, the Poverty Reduction Strategy (PRS) approach emphasizes cross-sectoral collaboration (a) to identify effective strategies to reduce poverty; and (b) to modify external partnerships and assistance (World Bank, 2006). Who identifies effective strategies remains a contentious issue; however, a number of observations can be made about efforts to date:

1. Although strong consensus exists for such improvements, the effectiveness of such efforts remains dependent on the degree to which powerful interests are willing to submit to coordination efforts. There has been a tendency for such interests to create new institutional mechanisms where they retain dominance, rather than to redistribute power among a wider range of stakeholders within existing mechanisms. For example, donor support for the creation of the Joint United Nations Programme on HIV/AIDS (UNAIDS) stemmed from dissatisfactions with the WHO. The US government decision, in turn, to establish the US President's Emergency Fund for AIDS Relief (PEPFAR), rather than contribute to UNAIDS or to meet its full one-third permitted share to the Global Fund or UNAIDS, has resulted in additional, even competing, institutional structures.

2. Health appears to be well recognized in broader development initiatives of some institutions. However, health is normally framed within the context of health services and technologies, while SDH remain largely unrecognized. Moreover, policy coherence is hindered by the

uneven level of development of global governance across different sectors. Economic globalization has led to a strengthening of the influence of global institutions with mandates relating to trade and finance, reflecting their importance to high-income countries and corporate interests. At the same time, health-based normative and standard-setting work has not developed to the same degree and speed (Fidler, 2005a).

3. There is a clear tension among competing ideological perspectives, interests, and goals in health development and the optimal use of limited resources through coordinated action. How can SDH be addressed best?

4. There remains a need at the global level for a central body to act as a key reference point, for example, to consolidate technical knowledge, monitor global trends in health, and serve as a venue for policy debate, putting SDH at center stage. This presents an important and challenging opportunity for the WHO.

5. Comparative assessment of the effectiveness of various initiatives to improve coordination and coherence is needed. The proliferation of new coordinating mechanisms, particularly those for disease-focused initiatives, has outpaced any critical evaluation.

6. The nature of contemporary global governance relevant to SDH cannot be described as a "system" per se. Rather, it is a set of institutions evolving from a base established in the 1940s, through ad hoc changes determined by changing circumstances, historical precedent, an ideological orientation, and the current and historical unequal distribution of power and resources. As a result, existing institutions are neither an expression of the collective will of the global community nor a beneficiary-centered strategic approach to addressing common needs.

TRANSPARENCY AND ACCOUNTABILITY

Mechanisms of transparency and accountability in public policy are fundamental to the effective functioning of democratic political systems.

One clear divide among the various institutions concerned with SDH is whether their accountability relates primarily to people or to the funds that they receive from donors. Accountability within the UN system is primarily based on the principle of one nation, one vote. In practice, this is undermined to some extent by the degree to which institutions receive voluntary contributions from donors. In the case of the WHO, for example, such contributions are substantial, leading to concerns about the disproportionate influence of donor states on policymaking. In the case of IFIs in which voting power is weighted by member states based on level of financial contribution, formal accountability has been skewed heavily in favor of high-income countries at the expense of low- and middle-income countries, which are most affected by their policy decisions. Additionally, the IFIs have long been challenged for their lack of transparency, a criticism also leveled at the WTO, although there has been increased attention to improving the transparency and accountability of global institutions in recent years. For example, the IFIs Transparency Resource has developed 250 indicators for assessing transparency from their perspective within the international financial institutions.[2] Similarly the One World Trust (Blagescu & Lloyd, 2006) has developed a Global Accountability Index to individually assess "thirty of the world's most powerful organizations from the corporate, inter-governmental, and non-governmental sectors" including the WHO, the World Bank, Nestlé, Pfizer, and the International Federation of the Red Cross and Red Crescent Societies (IFRC). Four core accountability dimensions are identified as critical to managing accountability claims from both internal and external stakeholders: transparency, participation, evaluation, and complaint and response mechanisms. The report concludes that global governance today is defined not by unaccountable organizations but by "organizations that are either accountable to the wrong set of stakeholders, or focus their accountability on one set of stakeholders at the expense of others" (Blagescu, de Las Casas, & Lloyd, 2005).

Implicit or explicit assumptions of stakeholder accountability underpin recent efforts to engage with institutional actors within the state, the market, and civil society in policymaking. The result has been a proliferation of "partnerships" and global public policy networks (GPPNs) seen as a less formal participatory, yet more integrated, approach to global governance (Reinicke, Deng, Benner, & Witte, 2000). In this context international organizations are cast in the role of convenors, platforms, networkers, and, at times, part financiers of GPPNs. A good example is the work of the Global Public Policy Institute, a nonprofit think tank based in Berlin, which seeks to strengthen "strategic communities around pressing policy challenges by bringing together the public sector, civil society and business."[3] In global health, examples include the Healthy Cities Networks, Global Network of People Living with HIV/AIDS, and the (Tobacco) Framework Convention Alliance.

Despite this apparent broadening of stakeholder involvement, a more systematic and critical assessment of the representativeness, quality of transparency, and accountability remains needed for most global institutions concerned with SDH. The focus to date has largely been on improving financial and program accountability, notably to major funders of global initiatives, rather than to a broad range of stakeholders, especially beneficiaries. The current global governance architecture related to SDH lacks agreed definitions and measures of transparency and accountability. Which processes should be transparent? For what should an organization be accountable and to whom? Should a regulatory global agency be accountable to global stakeholders that it aims to regulate? To whom and for what are global CSOs, networks, and corporations accountable, apart from the national laws that might regulate them, or the interests of their own members?

Among health-focused organizations, the Global Fund, corporate associations (e.g., International Federation of Pharmaceutical Manufacturers and Associations–IFPMA), and various global public-private partnerships remain largely outside wider public scrutiny. Large foundations such as the Gates Foundation operate independently given their substantial resources. Large transnational nongovernmental organizations (NGOs) are answerable to boards of directors and funders, rather than to the communities they serve. Even intergovernmental organizations, led by WHO, must reflect on who their stakeholders are (beyond member states) and how they should engage with them. The fate of the much anticipated but problematic Civil Society Initiative of the WHO, criticized for failing to distinguish between CSOs and corporate interest groups, remains unclear. Perhaps most importantly there are questions to be raised about the narrow range of stakeholders served by key institutions such as the OECD and G8. Finally, in keeping with generally accepted principles of democracy and/or of good governance, an overall system of "checks and balances" must evolve. Its purpose would be to ensure collective transparency and accountability across the diverse institutions as a key feature of any system of global governance.

PARTICIPATION AND REPRESENTATION

There have been more institutional actors involved in global health since the 1990s, but the degree to which this reflects greater political pluralism or elitism must be critically assessed. The quality of participation and representation within key global health institutions remains disappointing. Of ongoing concern are the imbalances in power between donors and beneficiaries. While these imbalances may seem to be an intractable reflection of broader power politics, institutional structures that maintain the imbalances remain unaddressed. Continued failure to reform the decision-making processes of the IFIs is the most prominent example. Beyond formal mechanisms that grant de jure (e.g., voting power) representation are structurally embedded de facto means of representation (e.g., financial dependence, commercial pressure within WTO) which maintain inequities in participation and representation.

The greater participation of nonstate actors in global governance is seen by many as enhancing representation. However, nonstate actors have included commercial entities seeking to further their economic interests. For example, industry participation in the Codex has raised concerns about the protection of consumer interests. So-called astro-turf (false grassroots) organizations (e.g., patient groups funded by industry) have proliferated, raising concerns about conflicts of interest. The funding of front groups by the tobacco industry, such as the International Tobacco Growers' Association (ITGA), is well documented. The ITGA describes itself as "a non-profit organization founded in 1984 with the objective of presenting the cause of millions of tobacco farmers to the world."[4] In practice, it is "a public relations vehicle created in the 1980s by the tobacco industry to front its lobbying against international tobacco control initiatives by giving the industry a human face and a Third World grassroots voice" (Must, 2001, p. 2).

RESOURCE MOBILIZATION AND ALLOCATION

How can the quality of governance concerning the mobilization and allocation of global resources be assessed in terms of their impact on SDH? How can the global governance of financing be improved?

One key matter concerns how decisions are taken regarding the use of funds. This is directly related to the source of funding and how they are managed. Among health-related organizations, WHO's regular budget funds, over which the organization has discretionary control, have remained static and are even shrinking in real terms, totaling US$915 million in 2006. In contrast, extrabudgetary funds, over which donors choose to exert varying degrees of control, have grown in relative terms since the early 1990s, reaching US$2,398 million in 2006 (Lee & Buse, 2006). Along with concerns about the sustainability of extrabudgetary funds, there are questions about the WHO's capacity to establish a coherent work program given this skewed funding structure. For donors seeking to demonstrate accountability to domestic constituencies, and able to disproportionately influence decision-making processes through their financial clout, funds tend to be earmarked for vertical disease-focused activities (Vaughan et al., 1995; Lucas et al., 1997). As a result, longer-term and large-scale funding to tackle structural factors that contribute to ill health receives limited support (Shiffman, 2006). For example, substantial extrabudgetary funds have been given to the Expanded Program on Immunization and GAVI to immunize against major childhood diseases. However, limited efforts have been made to address the social conditions, such as poverty, poor housing, and poor sanitation, by which children become more prone to such diseases.

The UN system as a whole has long faced concerns about major financial contributors using funding as a political tool. There are three main categories of UN expenditure: the *regular budget*, which is financed by mandatory assessment of member states; the *peacekeeping budget*, which is separate from the regular budget but also financed by assessment; and *voluntary contributions*, which finance most of the humanitarian relief and development agencies such as UNDP, UNICEF, and UNFPA, which are not considered core UN activities. Under this system, member states share in the financial support of core activities, but each country pursues its own priorities in the other budgets. The refusal of some member states to pay their assessed contributions in full or on time has affected growth of the UN budget, thus limiting expenditures in health or SDH programs. This is illustrated by the terms of the Helms-Biden Act, whereby the U.S. government has offered to pay a proportion of its UN arrears (US$1.3 billion) in return inter alia for reducing US assessed (from 25 percent to 22 percent) and peacekeeping contributions, and no growth of the UN budget in real terms. Substantial arrears of US$244 million, not covered by the Act, remain outstanding, including US$214 million to various UN organizations (Biden, 2001). UN funding to address SDH falls largely under voluntary contributions, leaving initiatives subject to the decisions of donors.

Given financial uncertainty and shortfalls, there have been efforts to secure alternative sources of funding for development purposes. One source has been the initiation of innovative funding mechanisms, such as the International Finance Facility and United Nations International Drug Purchase Facility (UNITAID), to generate additional resources, support acquisition of vital supplies, or provide increased bargaining power for countries in need. Another example is the Pan American Health Organization (PAHO) Revolving Fund for Vaccine Procurement, created in 1979, to: provide countries with affordable vaccines; enable uninterrupted procurement of supplies; facilitate use of local currency; allow cost-effective bulk purchasing; assure product quality; and permit urgent orders to be met (Pan American Health Organization, 2000).

An increasingly important funding source for global health has been the private sector and civil society. Philanthropic organizations, which encompass the two spheres, have become especially prominent in global health since the 1990s (Cohen, 1999) with the scale of their resources raising familiar questions about the governance of such funds. As well as concerns about donor-driven decision making, existing problems of coordination, short-term emphasis on disease-focused interventions, and the creation of undue burdens on recipient countries may be worsening (Barder & Birdsall, 2006).

Finally, there has been substantial funding of GPPPs since the mid-1990s, largely targeted at specific diseases or health issues (Buse & Walt, 2000). Given their disease-focused nature, existing GPPPs are unlikely to be appropriate mechanisms to tackle SDH. There is also potential conflict of interest between the need to tackle issues such as poverty and inequality through fundamental structural change, and the vested interests of private sector "partners" in the existing economic order.

Overall there remain stark irrationalities in funding, both within and across SDH-related institutions. As long as funding for development purposes remains voluntary, and major donors earmark such funds, limited global resources will be available to address SDH. Moreover, the funding decisions of health-related institutions are likely to have only marginal effect unless there are fundamental changes by major shareholders in underlying global economic, and political structures that impact on SDH, notably the IFIs.

LEADERSHIP IN GLOBAL GOVERNANCE AND
SOCIAL DETERMINANTS OF HEALTH

Leadership can be defined as "the ability of an individual [or institution] to influence, motivate, and enable others to contribute toward the effectiveness and success of the organizations of which they are members" (House, 2004, p. 15). As the recognized exercise of authority, leadership is clearly lacking among health- and non-health-focused institutions relevant to SDH. With formal authority residing with sovereign states, intergovernmental organizations remain subject to their will. State compliance with international treaties, such as the Framework Convention on Tobacco Control (FCTC), depends on acquiescence by states, with sanctions for noncompliance often nonenforceable. There are few examples of states conceding their sovereignty to "supranational" organizations with higher powers. Certain functions of the EU are examples, along with multilateral trade agreements.

In the absence of overarching legal or political authority at the global level, other forms of leadership become important. Technical leadership in health can be identified as broadly residing in the WHO, which is widely recognized as having access to unrivaled technical knowledge and expertise. Member states, notably low- and middle-income countries, look to the WHO to undertake a wide range of activities, such as assigning nomenclature, issuing guidelines and standards, and reviewing and coordinating research. While other institutions hold specialist expertise on selected areas, the WHO and its extensive global networks can provide broadly based health expertise. The key question is whether technical leadership alone is sufficient to achieve real progress on SDH.

Moral or ethical leadership can also be considered an important factor in global governance. Such power arises from shared support of certain values and principles seen as underlying decision making and action. It is clear that fundamental decisions that affect SDH all have normative dimensions involving (for instance) allocation of scarce resources, access to health care, and priority setting across populations and their needs. During its first two decades, the WHO's strong biomedical focus brought limited engagement with such value-laden choices. By the 1970s, an attempt to address broader determinants of health was driven by principles of social justice, fairness, and equity. These included such groundbreaking initiatives as primary health care (PHC), the essential medicines list, and the International Code on the Marketing of Breastmilk Substitutes. Some high-income countries argued that the WHO was engaging inappropriately in "political" issues. Others applauded its moral courage and leadership, and encouraged its role as "the world's health conscience" (Kickbusch, 1997). CSOs representing vulnerable and marginalized populations are seen as playing a similar role. Advocates of the human rights–based approach see this framework as a much needed return to an ethical and political focus indispensable for revitalizing the WHO's leadership role in global health. Thus, the moral and ethical perspectives of different global institutions compete today for leadership amid a more crowded policy space in global health (Lee & Buse, 2006; Horton, 2006).

Finally, leadership unequivocally arises from control of financial and other resources. While the WHO may exert technical and moral leadership, its relatively limited resources and human rights orientation prevent it from exercising this leadership effectively. Moreover, the growth of health sector lending by the World Bank, together with the creation and funding of GPPPs, has undermined the WHO's capacity to carry out its mandate with commensurate policy decisions and actions.

Overall no single institution is recognized as providing decisive leadership in global governance related to SDH. Instead, there are different forms of leadership that reside in specific institutions. While this may be seen as a rational division of labor based on comparative advantage, in practice it is more a misalignment of different types of authority. The World Bank has relatively substantial resources to address SDH, but it is mistrusted in many countries and large portions of the NGO community, not least because of the shortcomings in its governance structure. The WHO has recognized technical expertise, but limited financial means and has to rely on other institutions to apply this expertise. More problematic is the perceived erosion of the WHO's ethical authority. While Bale (Bale, 2003) calls for the WHO to "build partnerships with the pharmaceutical industry," Hardon (2003) argues that the WHO has come under undue commercial influence at the expense of equity-focused policies. Horton (2003) warns of "a damaging reinterpretation" of the WHO's historically important role in setting norms and standards for the global health community by development agencies and donors, which define WHO's work within the context of human development and its chief purpose as being an instrument to achieve the MDGs. The diversity of institutional actors concerned with SDH, in short, is accompanied by a split of ideologies and value systems underlying their actions. Consensus around certain normative principles, such as social justice and equity, has strengthened in many institutions, though actions have not necessarily always followed. At the same time, other value systems, such as economic and managerial efficiency, remain dominant.

CONCLUSIONS

The emergent global governance architecture relevant to SDH can thus be characterized as follows:

1. "Thick" governance in certain issue areas, notably economic relations such as trade, investment, and finance, but "thinner" governance in other issue areas, notably the social sectors. Despite increased recent attention to selected global health issues, resulting in the creation of various individual initiatives, addressing SDH has not yet been given sufficient priority in the building and running of effective global governance institutions.

2. The relative balance of power among state, market, and civil society institutions has shifted radically in recent decades. The private sector (market), civil society, and philanthropy have gained more prominent roles at the global level, including institutions concerned with global health, while state institutions have seen a relative decline.

3. Within each type of institution, there is a greater concentration of power in fewer hands at the global level. Large transnational corporations, major industrialized countries, and mostly Northern-based "international" non-governmental organizations have come to dominate global governance, while many developing country governments, small businesses, and southern NGOs and CSOs remain marginalized by the current architecture. Economic globalization defined by economic growth has been prioritized over social and environmental protection.

4. A certain degree of innovation has characterized some mechanisms in global institutions concerned with SDH. However, these innovations to broaden representation in global governance of nonstate actors, most notably the corporate sector, have been accompanied by the simultaneous reduction of the power of competent UN bodies. And in that way they have been conducive to further fragmentation and confusion of global governance on these essential health issues.

Through poverty-reduction strategies and the MDGs, there has been increased attention to SDH within a number of institutions. However, there remain concerns that these initiatives have lacked genuine commitment and been narrowly interpreted in their implementation, focusing on technical interventions and measurable outcomes rather than on underlying structural factors. Where powerful nonhealth interests prevail, there are profound difficulties in gaining sufficient attention and political priority for health issues in general and for SDH in particular.

In summary, when assessed against key criteria of good governance, global institutions show a number of weaknesses that are detrimental to tackling SDH:

1. The long-standing *problems of coordination and coherence,* characterizing global institutions in general, extend to institutions concerned with SDH. The resulting patchwork of mandates, activities, authority, and resources reflects the absence of an agreed plan or strategic vision to tackle SDH.

2. The key global *institutions affecting SDH have inadequate systems of transparency and accountability.* A more critical evaluation of transparency and accountability mechanisms is still needed. Foremost, there is need for an overall system of "checks and balances" within and across global institutions to ensure collective transparency and accountability.

3. There have been some efforts to *diversify representation* within global institutions concerned with SDH, but limited efforts to *redistribute power* within them.

4. Resources for global health have increased in recent years (e.g., to GPPPs and to initiatives to strengthen cooperation on global health issues such as pandemic influenza). However, *the governance of resource mobilization and allocation has remained firmly under the control of major donors.* Decisions continue to reflect accountability to foreign and economic policy goals, and to favor short-term projects and measurable outcomes.

5. There is a *distinct lack of overall leadership* among global institutions affecting SDH in terms of formally recognized authority.

At the national level there is strong evidence that good governance is an important factor in addressing SDH. Evidence on the strengths and weaknesses in national governance for SDH might be applied to global governance, where there is a need for fuller assessment of how good governance could contribute to tackling SDH.

Our findings suggest the need for a fundamental review of the structure of global governance in the context of the needs, priorities, and political culture of the early twenty-first century. Such a process would clearly have to go beyond SDH to other concerns not recognized as priorities in the 1940s, such as environmental sustainability. However, SDH must clearly play a central role in the process. Building global institutional and intergovernmental support for such a large but important initiative requires the WHO to promote this goal among its member nations and its global institutional partners.

Such a reform process first requires a more critical, detailed, and systematic assessment of health and non-health-focused institutions, individually and collectively, in terms of their de facto concern and impact on the various SDH, and the effects of their governance structures in this context. The WHO could similarly assume institutional leadership in undertaking this assessment, working with partner institutions, CSOs, and independent researchers/scholars.

The first step in such an assessment is development of criteria for good global governance related to SDH, based on the preliminary criteria discussed in this chapter. As an initial product of the larger reform process of global governance, WHO member states could be encouraged to give higher priority to addressing SDH themselves, while allocating more core funding to the WHO. The WHO should reflect that priority by allocating substantial and commensurate core funding, by hiring more social scientists and nurses, and by building the corresponding capacity of its staff.

The WHO further needs to play a lead role in providing scientific and technical support to address SDH, and should focus its own work to give much greater emphasis to SDH. Its conception of health and institutional structure should also move decisively beyond a vertical, disease-specific, and biomedically focused model, towards a more holistic and multidisciplinary model. To play this lead role effectively, the WHO's independence from sectional interests, and the symmetry of its accountability to member states, needs to be more effectively ensured.

There remains a need for stronger consensus and for more concerted coordination of relevant global institutions if SDH are to be tackled effectively. The UN's Economic and Social Council could be strengthened and, with the WHO, formally tasked to oversee such work, with relevant UN organizations, including the WHO, reporting to it. In this work, the human rights–based approach should be used as a key analytical and normative framework and advocacy tool. In addition to the WHO, global institutions whose policies impact significantly on SDH, notably the World Bank, IMF, and WTO, should be required to include health ministries and relevant CSOs in key decision-making bodies and negotiations on issues substantially affecting SDH.

Finally, alternative financing mechanisms, more independent of political interference by individual donors, should be systematically assessed and adopted.

NOTES

1. http://www.codexalimentarius.net/web/index_en.jsp.
2. See http://www.ifitransparencyresource.org/en/index.aspx (accessed October 17, 2006).
3. See www.gppi.net (accessed October 17, 2006).
4. International Tobacco Growers Association. Who we are and what we do. http://www.tobaccoleaf.org/ (accessed October 17, 2006).

REFERENCES

AusAID. (2000). *Good governance: Guiding principles for implementation*. Canberra: AusAID.

Bale, H. (2003). WHO should build partnerships with the pharmaceutical industry to improve public health. *Lancet, 361*, 4.

Banerjee, A., Deaton, A., Lustig, N., Rogoff, K., & Hsu, E. (2006). *An evaluation of World Bank Research, 1998–2005*. Washington, DC: World Bank. Retrieved from: http://siteresources.worldbank.org/DEC/Resources/84797–1109362238001/726454–1164121166494/RESEARCH-EVALUATION-2006-Main-Report.pdf.

Barder, O., & Birdsall, N. (2006). *Payments for progress: A hands-off approach to foreign aid.* CGD Working Papers No. 102. Washington, DC: Center for Global Development.

Barnett, M. (2005). *Power in global governance.* Cambridge: Cambridge University Press.

Biden, J. R. (2001). "Floor statement: Helms-Biden legislation on UN arrears." Statement to the U.S. Senate, Washington, DC, February 7 [online]. Retrieved from: http://biden.senate.gov/newsroom/details.cfm?id=229891&&.

Birdsall, N. (2006). *Stormy days on an open field: Asymmetries in the global economy.* Research Papers No. 2006/31. Helsinki: World Institute for Development Economics Research. Retrieved from: http://www.wider.unu.edu/publications/rps/rps2006/rp2006–31.pdf.

Blagescu, M., de Las Casas, L., & Lloyd, R. (2005). *Pathways to accountability: A short guide to the GAP Framework.* London: One World Trust.

Blagescu, M., & Lloyd, R. (2006). *2006 Global Accountability Report: Holding power to account.* London: One World Trust.

Bloche, M.G. (2002). WTO deference to national health policy: Toward an interpretive principle. *Journal of International Economic Law, 5,* 825–48.

Braithwaithe, J., & Drahos, P. (2004). *Global business regulation.* Cambridge: Cambridge University Press.

Buse, K., & Walt, G. (1997). An unruly mélange? Coordinating external resources to the health sector: A review. *Social Science and Medicine, 45,* 449–63.

———. (2000). Global public-private partnerships: Part I—a new development in health? *Bulletin of the World Health Organization, 78,* 549–61.

Cohen, D., & Laporte, B. (2004). *The evolution of the knowledge bank.* Retrieved from: http://siteresources.worldbank.org/KFDLP/Resources/461197–1148594717965/EvolutionoftheKnowledgeBank.pdf.

Cohen, J. (1999). Philanthropy's rising tide lifts science. *Science, 286,* 214.

Collin, J., Lee, K., & Bissell, K. (2002). The Framework Convention on Tobacco Control: The politics of global health governance. *Third World Quarterly, 23,* 265–82.

Commission on Global Governance. (1995). *Our global neighbourhood: Report of the Commission on Global Governance.* Oxford: Oxford University Press. Retrieved from: http://www-old.itcilo.org/actrav/actrav-english/telearn/global/ilo/globe/gove.htm.

Cornia, G. A., Jolly, R., & Stewart, F. eds. (1987). *Adjustment with a human face. Vol. 1: Protecting the vulnerable and promoting growth.* Oxford: Clarendon Press.

Deacon, B., Ollila, E., Koivusalo, M., & Stubbs, P. (2003). *Global social governance: Themes and prospects.* Helsinki: Ministry of Foreign Affairs for Finland.

Dobriansky, P. (2003). Principles of good governance. U.S. Undersecretary of State for Global Affairs [online]. Retrieved from: http://usinfo.state.gov/journals/ites/0303/ijee/dobriansky.htm

Dodgson, R., Lee, K., & Drager, N. (2002). *Global health governance: A conceptual review* [online]. Discussion paper No. 1. London: London School of Hygiene & Tropical Medicine/WHO Department of Health and Development. Retrieved from: http://www.lshtm.ac.uk/cgch/globalhealthgovernance.pdf.

Falk, R. (1999). *Predatory globalization.* London: Polity Press.

Fidler, D. (2005a). Health, globalization and governance: An introduction to public health's "new world order." In K. Lee & J. Collin (eds.), *Global change and health* (pp. 161–77). Maidenhead, UK: Open University Press.

———. (2005b). From international sanitary conventions to global health security: The new international health regulations. *Chinese Journal of International Law, 4* (2), 1–68.

Grindle, M. S. (2004). Good enough governance: Poverty reduction and reform in developing countries. *Governance, 17,* 525–48.

Hardon, A. (2003). New WHO leader should aim for equity and confront undue commercial influences. *The Lancet, 361,* 6.

Held, D. (1995). *Democracy and the global order.* Stanford, CA: Stanford University Press.

Horton, R. (2003). WHO's mandate: A damaging reinterpretation is taking place. *The Lancet, 360,* 960–61.

———. (2006). The next director-general of WHO. *The Lancet, 368,* 1213–14.

House, R. J. (2004). *Culture, leadership, and organizations: The GLOBE study of 62 societies.* Thousand Oaks, CA: SAGE Publications.

Hunt, P. (2005a). *The right of everyone to the enjoyment of the highest attainable standard of physical and mental health.* A/60/348. UN General Assembly: 60th Session.

———. (2005b). *Economic, social and cultural rights: The right of everyone to the enjoyment of the highest attainable standard of physical and mental health.* Report of the Special Rapporteur—E/CN.4/2005/51. Geneva: United Nations Economic and Social Council. Retrieved from: http://daccessdds.un.org/doc/UNDOC/GEN/G05/108/93/PDF/G0510893.pdf?OpenElement.

Huther, J., & Shah, A. (1998). *Applying a simple measure of good governance to the debate of fiscal decentralization.* World Bank Policy Research Working Paper No. 1894. Washington, DC: World Bank.

International Labour Organization. (2004). *A fair globalization: Creating opportunities for all.* Report of the World Commission on the Social Dimension of Globalization. Geneva: International Labour Organization. Retrieved from: http://www.ilo.org/public/english/wcsdg/docs/report.pdf.

———. (2006). *The end of child labour: Within reach—Global Report under the follow-up to the ILO Declaration on Fundamental Principles and Rights at Work.* Geneva: International Labour Office. Retrieved from: http://www.ilo.org/public/english/standards/relm/ilc/ilc95/pdf/rep-i-b.pdf.

Kickbusch, I. (1997). Think health: What makes the difference? *Health Promotion International, 12,* 265–72.

———. (2003). Global health governance: Some theoretical considerations on the new political space. In K. Lee (ed.), *Health impacts of globalization: Towards global governance* (pp. 192–203). London: Palgrave Macmillan.

Koivusalo, M. (2003). *The impact of WTO agreements on health and development policies.* Global Social Governance. Themes and Prospects. Helsinki: Globalism and Social Policy Programme. Retrieved from: www.gaspp.org.

Koivusalo, M., & Ollila, E. (1997). *Making a healthy world.* London: Zed Books.

Labonté, R., & Schrecker, T. (2007a). Globalization and social determinants of health: Introduction and methodological background (part 1 of 3). *Globalization and Health, 3,* 1–10.

———. (2007b). Globalization and social determinants of health: Promoting health equity in global governance (part 2 of 3). *Globalization and Health, 3,* 1–15.

———. (2007c). Globalization and social determinants of health: The role of the global marketplace (part 3 of 3). *Globalization and Health, 3,* 1–17.

Lee, E., & Vivarelli, M. (2006). *The social impact of globalization in the developing countries.* No. 1925. Bonn: Institute for the Study of Labour. Retrieved from: http://papers.ssrn.com/sol3/papers.cfm?abstract_id=878329.

Lee, K., & Buse, K. (2006). Assuming the mantle: The balancing act facing the new director-general. *Journal of the Royal Society for Medicine, 99,* 494–96.

Lee, K., Collinson, S., Walt, G., & Gilson, L. (1996). Who should be doing what in international health: A confusion of mandates in the United Nations? *British Medical Journal, 312,* 302–07.

314 Kelley Lee et al.

Leftwich, A. (1994). Governance, the state and the politics of development. *Development and Change*, 25, 363–86.

Lucas, A., Mogedal, S., Walt, G., Hodne Steen, S., Kruse, S. E., Lee, K., et al. (1997). *Cooperation for health development: The World Health Organisation's support to programmes at country level*. London: Governments of Australia, Canada, Italy, Norway, Sweden and UK.

Malhotra, K. (2002). *Making global trade work for people*. New York: UNDP/ Rockefeller Brothers Fund.

Martin, G. (2006). The global health governance of antimicrobial effectiveness. *Global Health*, 2, 7.

Martinez, J. (2006). *Implementing a sector wide approach in health: The case of Mozambique*. London: HLSP Institute. Retrieved from: http://www.hlspinstitute.org/files/project/100615/Mozambique_SWAP.pdf.

McGrew, A. (2000). Power shift: From national government to global governance? In D. Held (ed.), *A globalizing world? Culture, economics, politics* (pp. 125–66). London: Routledge.

McGrew, A., & Held, D., eds. (2002). *Governing globalization, power, authority and global governance*. London: Polity Press.

Microcredit Summit Campaign/United Nations Population Fund. (2005). *From microfinance to macro change: Integrating health education and microfinance to empower women and reduce poverty*. New York. Retrieved from: http://www.unfpa.org/upload/lib_pub_file/530_filename_advocacy.pdf.

Must, E. (2001). *International Tobacco Growers' Association, (ITGA). ITGA uncovered: Unravelling the spin—the truth behind the claims*. Ottawa: PATH Canada. Retrieved from: http://www.healthbridge.ca/assets/images/pdf/Tobacco/Publications/itgabr.pdf.

Neidell, S. (1998). Women's empowerment as a public problem: A case study of the 1994 International Conference on Population and Development. *Population Research and Policy Review*, 17, 247–60.

Ng, F., & Yeats, A. (1999). *Good governance and trade policy: Are they the keys to Africa's global integration and growth?* World Bank Policy Research Working Paper No. 2038. Washington, DC: World Bank.

Ollila, E. (2003). *Global health-related public-private partnerships and the United Nations*. Globalisation and Social Policy Programme Policy Brief No. 2. Helsinki: GASPP.

———. (2005). Restructuring global health policy making: The role of global public-private partnerships. In M. McIntosh & M. Koivusalo (eds.), *Commercialization of health care: Global and local dynamics and policy responses* (pp. 187–200). Houndmills, UK: Palgrave.

Organisation for Economic Cooperation and Development. (2003). *Policy coherence: Vital for global development*. Paris: OECD. Retrieved from: http://www.oecd.org/dataoecd/11/35/20202515.pdf.

Pan American Health Organization. (2000). *Revolving fund* [online]. Retrieved from: http://www.paho.org/english/hvp/hvi/revol_fund.htm.

Pangestu, M. (2001). *Social impact of globalisation in Southeast Asia*. No. 187. Paris: OECD. Retrieved from: http://www.eldis.org/cache/DOC8096.pdf.

Ranson, M., Beaglehole, R., Correa, C., Mirza, Z., Buse, K., & Drager, N. (2002). The public health implications of international trade. In K. Lee, K. Buse, & S. Fustukian (eds.), *Health policy in a globalising world* (pp. 18–40). Cambridge: Cambridge University Press.

Reinicke, W., Deng, F., Benner, T., & Witte, J. M. (2000). *Critical choices: The United Nations, networks, and the future of global governance*. Ottawa: IDRC Publishers.

Richter, J. (2002). *Holding corporations accountable: Corporate conduct, international codes, and citizen action*. London: Zed Books.

———. (2004). Public-private partnerships for health: A trend with no alternatives? *Development, 47,* 43–48.

Rosenau, J. N. (1995). Governance in the twenty-first century. *Global Governance,* 1, 13–43.

Shiffman, J. (2006). Donor funding priorities for communicable disease control in the developing world. *Health Policy and Planning,* 21, 411–20.

Smith, R., Beaglehole, R., Woodward, D., & Drager, N., eds. (2003). *Global public goods for health: Health economic and public health perspectives*. Oxford: Oxford University Press.

Solar, O., & Irwin, A. (2006). Social determinants, political contexts, and civil society action: A historical perspective on the Commission on Social Determinants of Health. *Health Promotion Journal of Australia,* 17, 180–85.

Ståhl, T., Wismar, M., Ollila, E., Lahtinen, E., & Leppo, K., eds. (2006). *Health in all policies: Prospects and potentials*. Helsinki: Ministry of Social Affairs and Health. Retrieved from: http://ec.europa.eu/health/ph_information/documents/health_in_all_policies.pdf.

Stiglitz, J., & Charlton, A. (2004). Common values for the Development Round. *World Trade Review,* 3, 495–506.

UN Millennium Project. (2005). *Investing in development: A practical plan to achieve the Millennium Development Goals*. London: Earthscan. Retrieved from: http://www.unmillenniumproject.org/documents/MainReportComplete-lowres.pdf.

UNICEF (2005). *Child poverty in rich countries 2005*. Florence, Italy: UNICEF Innocenti Research Centre. Retrieved from: http://www.unicef.org/brazil/repcard6e.pdf.

United Kingdom Department for International Development. (2001). *Sector-wide approaches (SWAps): Key sheets for sustainable livelihoods*. London: Department for International Development. Retrieved from: http://www.keysheets.org/red_7_swaps_rev.pdf.

———. (2006). Policy coherence for development. Department for International Development [online]. Retrieved from: http://www.dfid.gov.uk/mdg/aid-effectiveness/policy-coherence.asp.

United Nations. (1995). *Report of the World Summit for Social Development*. No. A/RES/55/2. New York: United Nations.

———. (2000). Resolution adopted by the General Assembly: Further initiatives for social development. In *A/RES/S-24/2*. New York: United Nations.

———. (2004). United Nations Millennium Declaration. In *A/RES/55/2*. New York: United Nations.

United Nations Development Program. (1997). Governance for sustainable human development [online]. http://mirror.undp.org/magnet/policy/.

United Nations Economic and Social Commission for Asia and the Pacific. (2007). *What is good governance?* Bangkok, Thailand: United Nations Economic and Social Commission for Asia and the Pacific. Retrieved from: http://www.unescap.org/pdd/prs/ProjectActivities/Ongoing/gg/governance.pdf.

van Diesen, A., & Walker, K. (1999). *The changing face of aid to Ethiopia: Past experience and emerging issues in British and EC aid*. London: Christian Aid. Retrieved from: http://www.christian-aid.org.uk/indepth/9901ethi/ethiopi1.htm.

Vaughan, J. P., Mogedal, S., Kruse, S., Lee, K., Walt, G., & de Wilde, K. (1995). *Cooperation for health development: Extrabudgetary funding in the World Health Organization*. Oslo: Governments of Australia, Norway and UK.

Walt, G., Pavignani, E., Gilson, L., & Buse, K. (1999). Health sector development: From aid coordination to resource management. *Health Policy and Planning,* 14, 207–18.

Ware, G. (2006). Filling the regulatory gap: The emerging transnational regulator. *Global Governance,* 12, 135–39.

Wei, S. J. (2000). *Natural openness and good government.* Policy Research Working Paper No. 2411. Washington, DC: World Bank.

Wolfowitz, P. (2006). *Good governance and development: A time for action (speech).* Jakarta, Indonesia.

Woodward, D. (2005). The GATS and trade in health services: Implications for health care in developing countries. *Review of International Political Economy,* 12, 511–34.

World Bank. (1994). *Governance: The World Bank experience.* Washington, DC: IBRD.

———. (2006). *PRSP sourcebook.* Retrieved from: http://web.worldbank.org/WBSITE/EXTERNAL/TOPICS/EXTPOVERTY/EXTPRS/0,,contentMDK:20175742~pagePK:210058~piPK:210062~theSitePK:384201,00.html.

World Health Organization. (1999). *Management of childhood illness in developing countries: Rationale for an integrated strategy.* Geneva: WHO Department of Child and Adolescent Health and Development. Retrieved from: http://www.who.int/child-adolescent-health/New_Publications/IMCI/WHO_CHS_CAH_98.1/Rev99.A.pdf.

———. (2001). *Strategic alliances: The role of civil society in health.* Geneva: Civil Society Initiative, External Relations and Governing Bodies. Retrieved from: http://www.who.int/civilsociety/documents/en/alliances_en.pdf.

World Social Forum. (2006). World Social Forum India [online]. Retrieved from: http://www.wsfindia.org/.

Zammit, A. (2003). *Development at risk: Rethinking UN-business partnerships.* Geneva: South Centre/United Nations Research Institute for Social Development. Retrieved from: http://www.globalpolicy.org/reform/business/2003/risk.pdf.

13 Rights, Redistribution, and Regulation

Ronald Labonté and Ted Schrecker

INTRODUCTION

The authors of Chapter 5 noted Birdsall's description of globalization as "disequalizing" and her identification of three distinct, although interrelated, kinds of "asymmetries" that characterize its operations. These characteristics must be addressed, at multiple institutional levels, in any serious effort to reduce the toll of millions of readily preventable deaths every year by way of social determinants of health (SDH). In today's world economic order, unprecedented affluence for a minority (Figure 13.1)[1] coexists with continued massive deprivation for literally billions of people, with dramatic effects on health. Consider, as just one example, the fact that the lifetime risk of death from complications of pregnancy and childbirth for Canadian women is one in 11,000. For women in Niger, one of the world's poorest countries, it is one in seven (Say, Inoue, Mills, & Suzuki, 2007). Policy prescriptions that presume the ability of countries outside the industrialized world to grow their way out of poverty and into better health (and reductions in health inequity) for their populations have been tried and found wanting over the past two or three decades.

During that period, neoliberal social and economic policies were actively promoted on pragmatic grounds, as the only ones that "worked." The superficial credibility of that claim relied on systematic amnesia about the recent history that created the context in which social and economic policies were applied, and about how that recent history embodied the asymmetries identified by Birdsall. In extreme cases, those asymmetries included U.S. support for military coups against egalitarian governments, notably that of Salvador Allende in Chile (see Chapter 3, this volume). More often, the promotion of neoliberal policies took the form of conditionalities attached to loans from the international financial institutions (IFIs), and—as noted in Chapter 5, this volume—of the "implicit conditionalities" that technological change and financial deregulation enabled the owners of mobile financial assets to impose on national governments.

As a number of authors have noted, globalization could offer tremendous benefits in terms of reducing health inequity worldwide. However,

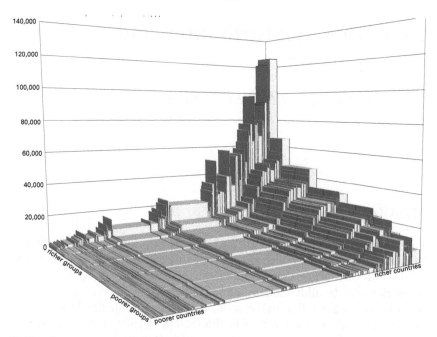

Figure 13.1   Gross annual national income per head by deciles (US$ at purchasing power parity).

© 2007 Bob Sutcliffe. Used with permission.

this would require changes that go far beyond those that are normally described in terms of "managing" globalization, or (less frequently) in terms of ameliorating its negative effects (see, for instance, the discussion of social protection policies in Chapter 6, this volume). Here, we build on the discussion in Chapter 12 but also go beyond it.

FIRST, DO NO HARM

A starting point must be recognition that many neoliberal policies of the past thirty years have failed to produce the results claimed by their proponents. Hence the generic policy recommendation: *First, do no harm.* Specifically, abandon policy measures that demonstrably increase health inequity, such as those limiting the scope for public provision for basic health-related needs, or resulting in their commodification.

Chapter 8 (this volume) described the way in which the World Bank has promoted the reorganization of health services on commercial lines, emphasizing private insurance and cost recovery, thereby increasing both the direct and indirect costs of illness. Since a recent report on chronic poverty noted with particular reference to rural locations that "ill health and the costs of healthcare are overwhelmingly the single most important reason why households enter into poverty" (Addison et al., 2008, p. 14), the implications for health equity are especially disturbing. In addition to general critiques of the effects on incomes, income security, and social protection of structural adjustment conditionalities attached to Bank and International Monetary Fund (IMF) lending (see the discussion in Chapter 1, this volume), recent evidence suggests that wage expenditure ceilings insisted upon by the IMF have restricted the ability of governments—especially in sub-Saharan Africa—to spend on health care and education, thus potentially working against the benefits of debt cancellation and development assistance (see the discussion in Chapter 7, this volume, and, for more extensive analysis, Center for Global Development, 2007; Independent Evaluation Office, 2007; Ooms, Van Damme, Baker, Zeitz, & Schrecker, 2008). It is not entirely fair to criticize the IMF for this stance, given its mandate; it is fair—and in our view essential—to insist on policy coherence around a set of values that emphasizes meeting human needs, and includes global redistribution in support of efforts to meet those needs. We return to this theme in later sections of the chapter.

Because the importance of water and sanitation as determinants of health was underscored in a recent WHO report (World Health Organization/ UNICEF Joint Monitoring Programme for Water Supply and Sanitation, 2008), it is useful briefly to consider these as an additional illustration of how globalization has influenced access and affordability. IMF loan policies systematically promoted privatization of water utilities, the operation of publicly owned utilities on commercial principles of full cost recovery, or both (Grusky, 2001). "In general," according to Grusky, "it [was] African countries, and the smallest, poorest and most debt-ridden countries that [were] being subjected to IMF conditions on water privatisation and full cost recovery." However, abundant evidence exists that privatization has failed to provide higher quality, more affordable and accessible services, and in many cases has increased the cost of access (Loftus & McDonald, 2001; Jaglin, 2002; McDonald, 2002; Budds & McGranahan, 2003; International Consortium of Investigative Journalists, 2003; Freedom from Debt Coalition, 2005; Cashmore, Gleick, Newcomb, Morrison, & Harrington, 2006; Public Services International Research Unit, 2006). An alternative strategy, which is preferable from an equity perspective, starts from the premise that water provision should be "decommodified" because access for certain purposes is a basic health-related human need and arguably, therefore, a human right as recognized by the United Nations Committee on Economic, Social and Cultural Rights (Committee on Economic, Social and Cultural Rights, 2003).[2] Strategies of decommodification demand not only the formal recognition of rights but also their use as a basis for mobilizing of resources, domestically and (at least in low-income countries) from development assistance, sufficient to support provision independently of ability to pay. We expand upon this point about the nature of human rights in the section of the chapter that follows.

RIGHTS AGAINST THE GLOBAL MARKETPLACE

Ten years after the United Nations' 1995 Copenhagen social policy summit, a team from the Finnish National Research and Development Centre for Welfare and Health (STAKES) argued the need to organize economic and social policies organized around the "three Rs" of:

1. systematic resource **redistribution** between countries and within regions and countries to enable poorer countries to meet human needs,
2. effective supranational **regulation** to ensure that there is a social purpose in the global economy, and
3. enforceable social **rights** that enable citizens and residents to seek legal redress (Deacon, Ilva, Koivusalo, Ollila, & Stubbs, 2005).

Their policy brief was explicit in arguing that national governments must do more in terms of implementing the three Rs, and more must be demanded of them in countries rich and poor alike. At the same time, national and subnational governments' options are limited by globalization and the actions of various supranational institutions and processes. Only some of those constraints are embodied in formal institutional arrangements like trade agreements; others arise from the operations of global financial markets, and from a policy environment in which competition for foreign direct investment and outsourced production "mercilessly weeds out those centers with below-par macroeconomic environments, services, and labor-market flexibility" (World Bank, 1999, p. 50). Achieving "a vision of the world where people matter and social justice is paramount," in the words of Commission Chair Sir Michael Marmot (2005, p. 1099), therefore *requires coordinated action on an international scale by national governments and multilateral institutions.*

An important background paper prepared for the Commission on Social Determinants of Health concluded that "The international human rights framework is the appropriate conceptual structure within which to advance towards health equity through action on SDH" (Solar & Irwin, 2007, p. 8). Key texts in international law include the 1948 Universal Declaration of Human Rights (UDHR), which states that "Everyone has the right to a standard of living adequate for the health and well-being of himself and his [*sic*] family" (Article 25); the 1966 International Covenant on Economic, Social and Cultural Rights (ICESCR), which specifies the "right of everyone to the enjoyment of the highest attainable standard of physical and mental health" (Article 12); and General Comment 14 by the UN Committee on Economic, Social and Cultural Rights (2000), which sets out states' specific legal obligations "to *respect, protect* and *fulfill*" the rights cited under

Article 12.[3] Conventional wisdom is that these obligations apply only to the actions of national governments with respect to people living within their borders. Even if one chooses to disregard the 1966 Covenant, which has not been ratified by the United States, it is essential to consider the argument made by Pogge (2002, 2005) that cross-border obligations follow from Article 28 of the UDHR, which specifies that "Everyone is entitled to a social and international order in which the rights and freedoms set forth in this Declaration can be fully realized."

In 2002, the United Nations Commission on Human Rights appointed a special rapporteur on the Article 12 right under ICESCR for a three-year period (an appointment renewed in 2005, and then again with a new rapporteur in 2008). Over the first six years of the term, Special Rapporteur Paul Hunt addressed issues including health worker migration, poverty-reduction strategies, trade agreements, health systems, mental health care, neglected diseases, access to medicines, maternal mortality, and indigenous populations through the prism of the right to health (Labonté et al., 2007, pp. 79–80). Notably, following a 2004 mission to the World Trade Organization he observed that "the progressive realization of the right to health and the immediate obligations to which it is subject, place reasonable conditions on the trade rules and policies that may be chosen" (Hunt, 2004, p. 24), and recommended "that urgent attention be given to the development of a methodology for right to health impact assessments in the context of trade" (Hunt, 2004, p. 74). Subsequently, he provided examples of how the Article 12 obligations had been implemented within individual national jurisdictions (Hunt, 2007). These observations indicate the importance of devising mechanisms to ensure that trade policy outcomes are consistent with human rights norms, including—but not limited to—the right to health. The challenge is perhaps best viewed as part of the larger imperative of ensuring that the commercial objectives of trade agreements do not undermine achievement of social objectives such as poverty elimination (McGill, 2004), and as a response to the need, identified by the UN Special Rapporteurs on globalization and human rights, "to move away from approaches that are ad hoc and contingent" in ensuring that human rights are not compromised by trade liberalization (Oloka-Onyango & Udagama, 2003, p. 25).

The human rights framework represents an important foundation for legally enforceable obligations. For the moment, these remain contingent on implementation by national and subnational governments. National governments are obviously capable of entering into agreements that establish supranational mechanisms of implementation and enforcement, as illustrated by the European Union's Convention for the Protection of Human Rights and Fundamental Freedoms, but this example (which has not been studied further for purposes of this chapter) reflects a distinctive institution that has taken decades to build. Meanwhile, even if countries have not incorporated recognition of a human right in their national legislation, their ratification of the ICESCR may be sufficient for courts to require action by national governments. This has happened at least twice (in Argentina and in Ecuador) with respect to the right to health (Singh, Govender, & Mills, 2007). The human rights framework also, and perhaps more importantly, offers a normative challenge to the priorities of the global marketplace. If what human rights scholar Audrey Chapman, one of the drafters of General Comment 14, describes as the "intrinsic value and worth of all human beings" (Chapman, 1993, p. 21) is to have much meaning, then it cannot be contingent on accidents of birth that mean some people are born in Zambia, where life expectancy at birth is now thirty-eight years, and others in Canada, where life expectancy at birth is eighty years and all but the country's poorest residents can anticipate far better health from the moment of their birth. And when priorities are set for allocating resources among competing options for improving social determinants of health, it must be kept in mind that human rights of any kind lose meaning when their realization must be vindicated with reference to an external criterion such as the right holder's future income earning potential (human capital), or the contribution that improving her health might make to a regional or national economy.

An immediate step toward solidifying the human rights foundations for action to improve SDH would be to establish the post of the UN Special Rapporteur on the Article 12 right as a permanent position within the UN system, supported by a secretariat with the necessary research and advocacy capabilities; this secretariat might have a permanent location or might "float" geographically to follow the rapporteur. Research and advocacy have their limitations, since producing yet another series of critical reports (however authoritative the source) to add to the existing pile is likely to have only limited value. In particular, such reports cannot in themselves directly address the "asymmetry between enforceable economic (market-based) rules and unenforceable social and environmental obligations," which has been described as "arguably the biggest governance challenge of the new millennium"(Labonté, Schrecker, Sanders, & Meeus, 2004, p. 3). Caution is in order about formal linkages between trade policy and human rights, because of the risk (noted in Chapter 4, this volume, with respect to labor standards) that such linkages could be used in a self-interested way as disguises for protectionist policies that injure those they are supposedly intended to protect. However, again as noted in that chapter, this is almost certainly a problem that could be overcome through thoughtful institutional design. In general, institutional innovation to establish effective linkages between human rights standards (including labor standards) and trade is one of the critical challenges for advocacy and multilateral action.

REDISTRIBUTING RESOURCES

As noted at several points in the book, a need exists both to redistribute more resources across national borders and to make existing mechanisms of redistribution work more effectively in support of health equity. Despite fashionable skepticism about the effectiveness of development assistance, in our view the burden of proof has now shifted decisively to those who argue against substantial long-term increases in development assistance—recognizing, at the same time, that this is a necessary rather than a sufficient condition for ameliorating global inequities that threaten health. Chapter 7 (this volume) refers to Sachs's calculations of the gap between the amount needed to provide basic health care in low-income countries and the amount that their governments can realistically expect to raise from domestic revenue sources: Chapter 5 (this volume) points out that in many cases, import liberalization promoted by the industrialized world has substantially *reduced* the tariff revenues available to these same countries.

Here, we provide only two illustrations of the magnitudes involved. First, Ooms et al. (2008) use Sachs's $40/capita cost figure to estimate the amount that would be needed to transform the Global Fund to fight AIDS, Tuberculosis and Malaria into a Global Health Fund that supported comprehensive health system strengthening. Assuming that all countries that received grants from the expanded Fund were to commit 15 percent of their general government budgets to health—which may be an optimistic assumption—such a fund would need to disburse approximately US$28 billion per year. This is a dramatic increase relative to the estimated US$12–14 billion value of all development assistance for health, of which support for the Fund of course represents only a part. However, it is also equivalent to the cost, circa 2007, of the US war in Iraq for roughly one month (Leonhardt, 2007). Second, the long-standing United Nations target of committing 0.7 percent of the rich countries' gross national income (GNI) to development assistance has consistently been met only by a few northern European countries. The G7 countries have never come close. Figure 13.2 shows how much it would have cost the population of each G7 country to have met the target in 2007, stated not as an aggregate figure but rather in terms of the cost to each man, woman, and child in those countries, measured using a ubiquitous gastrocommodity: the Big Mac. The amounts needed, although not large, do not appear to be beyond the realm of possibility when stated in this way, and the result would have been to mobilize an additional US$140 billion per year for development assistance: in other words, more than doubling the G7's spending.

Chapter 7 (this volume) also notes that existing mechanisms for debt cancellation have a number of limitations. These must be addressed in order to eliminate the current process in which "dozens of heavily indebted poor and middle-income countries are forced by creditor governments to spend large parts of their limited tax receipts on debt service, undermining their ability to finance investments in human capital and infrastructure. In a pointless and debilitating churning of resources, the creditors provide development assistance with one hand and then withdraw it in debt servicing with the other" (UN Millennium Project, 2005, p. 35). In

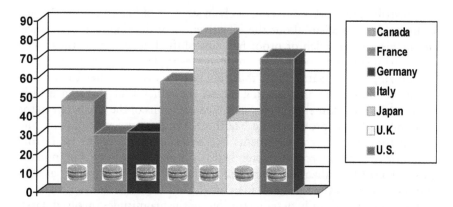

Figure 13.2   Additional cost to the G7 nations in 2007 of spending 0.7 percent of their gross national income on development assistance, in Big Macs per capita.

Source: OECD Development Assistance Committee, 2008; Big Mac prices from Anon., 2007.

this case, one illustration indicates the magnitudes involved: the proposal briefly described in Chapter 7 of this volume to structure debt cancellation around ensuring that debtor countries have available the resources needed to raise the living standard of their poorest residents to an "ethical poverty line" of $3/person/day implies that a total of 136 countries would require either complete or partial debt cancellation with a net present value of between $424 and $589 billion. This represents a fivefold increase relative to the amounts of debt cancellation available under the combined enhanced HIPC and MDRI initiatives, spread over a much larger number of countries (Mandel, 2006) and probably over a number of years. It is possible, of course, that the tremendous opportunity offered by such cancellation would be squandered by debtor governments. Multilateral measures need to be developed both to minimize the chances of such an outcome and to prioritize the cancellation of odious debts. Although the point is not fully explored here, the close connection between foreign debt burdens and domestic capital flight (Rodriguez, 1987; Helleiner, 2001) and the constraint that capital flight can create on domestic social and macroeconomic policy suggest a need to rethink today's widespread opposition to capital controls, and indeed consider measures to facilitate their effective use in certain equity-related contexts.

Then there is trade. Development policy protagonists who disagree about much else agree on the need for high-income countries to open up their markets, although both the magnitude and the distribution of the economic benefits that result is a matter of continued debate. At this writing (July 2008), talks aimed at ending the impasse that has characterized the so-called development round of WTO negotiations, begun in 2001, have just collapsed. This means that at least in the near future, bilateral and regional trade agreements that reflect asymmetries in bargaining power and resources even more glaring than those present within the WTO framework will continue to proliferate. (The existence of "TRIPS-plus" provisions in a number of such agreements, as noted in Chapter 11 (this volume), is just one cause for concern among many about the health consequences of such an outcome.) An interesting proposal by development economist Paul Collier would see the OECD countries periodically offer nonreciprocated access to certain sectors of their markets, essentially as a way of revitalizing the negotiating process by offering low- and middle-income countries something of clear value to them in advance of bargaining over further trade liberalization—in other words, adding an explicitly redistributive component to the WTO process (Collier, 2006). Arithmetically, a logical starting point involves market access concessions that would in short order generate taxable revenues sufficient to compensate for past losses resulting from tariff reductions. As with many of the institutional innovations described in this chapter, the fundamental question here is one of political will: are national governments in general, and those of high-income countries most particularly, willing to exercise leadership in support of policies that are specifically focused on redistributing resources to reduce inequities in health by way of the SDH?

REGULATING FOR HEALTH EQUITY: IMPROVING GLOBAL GOVERNANCE

Many of the policies driving the past three decades of globalization have placed economic growth ahead of health improvements or human development, regarding the latter as positive externalities and the former as their essential prerequisite. The past decade, however, has seen an accumulation of evidence suggesting a more complex relation between growth and health. It is characteristic of that relation that improvements in population health and education ("human capital") often precede growth (Commission on Macroeconomics and Health, 2001); growth does not automatically improve health (Deaton, 2006) and has proved remarkably ineffective in reducing poverty (Woodward & Simms, 2006); and under some circumstances health can be improved dramatically at quite low levels of GDP/capita by universal and relatively generous social protection and provision (Halstead, Walsh, & Warren, 1985). This implies that both national government policies and the policies of supranational institutions that establish the context for those policies, especially in low- and middle-income countries, should be organized more effectively around improving health equity and not only or primarily on increasing economic growth.

While there has been increased nominal recognition of the importance of health globally, reflected in the Millennium Development Goals (MDGs) and increased aid for health, global governance for health remains weak or nonexistent, whereas global governance for economic integration via trade and financial liberalization is strong. As shown in Chapter 5 (this volume), this is weakening some of the policy options national governments can pursue to improve health equity within their own borders. In addition to their more directly observable negative effects, conditionalities associated with loans and grants from the international financial institutions often reproduce this set of priorities. So too, of course, do the priorities of hypermobile capital as they are manifested in financial markets.[4]

Three responses follow from this analysis: first, a reduction in the reach of trade and financial market rules that limit national governments' flexibilities to manage their domestic economies for health and other social purposes (Chapter 5, this volume); second, a reduction in the conditionalities set by the IFIs or donor countries alongside a more profound overhaul of the entire aid and debt relief architecture (Chapter 7, this volume); and third, a strengthening of systems of global governance in order to achieve policy coherence around the explicit objective of health equity via improvements in social determinants of health (Chapter 12, this volume, and, for a more extensive treatment, see Lee et al., 2008). This third response has implications not only for the role of the World Health Organization (WHO) and the priorities of member states, but also (and just as importantly) for the overall structure of multilateral institutions and global governance.

At present, there are few multilateral institutions, apart from WHO, with a mandate to improve global health, and, as Chapter 12 (this volume) noted, none with an explicit or legal obligation to take health into consideration when formulating policies or engaging in international negotiations in their respective sectors (e.g., trade, finance, environment). Moreover, existing global governance structures that affect SDH are weak with respect to most of the conventions of good governance such as transparency, accountability, and participation (Lee et al., 2008), while in health more "public" organizations such as WHO are being overshadowed by private philanthropies and public-private partnerships. Various aspects of the contemporary international environment call for a fundamental review of present systems and institutions. These aspects include: global power dynamics that have changed substantially since the immediate postwar era; persistent poverty and health inequities throughout much of the world; and the uncoordinated manner in which global governance is emerging in the absence of an ethical foundation or a consensus on the purpose of such governance. Ideally, such a review would be in a purpose-specific forum comparable to the Bretton Woods Conference in 1944 that established the key multilateral institutions of the postwar era, but with far greater transparency and inclusiveness. As noted in a background paper for the Globalization Knowledge Network (GKN), "Building global institutional and intergovernmental support for such a large but important governance initiative requires WHO to promote this goal among its member nations, and the global institutions with which it presently actively partners" (Lee et al., 2008, p. 65).

The need for restructuring of this kind in response to globalization's asymmetries has been identified by others, for example, by the International Labour Organization's World Commission on the Social Dimension of Globalization (World Commission on the Social Dimension of Globalization, 2004) and in the Helsinki Process on Globalisation and Democracy (Helsinki Process on Globalisation and Democracy, 2007) hosted jointly by the governments of Finland and Tanzania.[5] In June 2008, the Commonwealth Heads of Government issued an important statement on the need for reform of international institutions (Commonwealth Heads of Government Meeting on Reform of International Institutions, 2008). However, WHO has so far remained peripheral to these and other efforts, and none of them has so far been supported by consistent and decisive leadership on the part of powerful nations like the members of the G8.

CONCLUSION: THE NEED FOR A VALUES-BASED APPROACH TO SDH

As suggested by Marmot's observation quoted earlier in this chapter, the ultimate need is for institutions that embody a global health ethic. Such an ethic must explicitly acknowledge that "Global actors and institutions, whether they act bilaterally (especially direct overseas development assistance, trade agreements) or multilaterally (through, e.g., the United Nations system, World Bank or International Monetary Fund), are obligated to remedy global inequalities that exist in affluence, power, and social, economic and political opportunities" (Ruger, 2006, p. 1001). Multiple arguments can be made in support of such an ethic, but it clearly must (a) explicitly acknowledge the existence of obligations across national borders, and (b) challenge the priorities of the global marketplace by defining the scope of those obligations broadly enough to include redistribution both within and across those borders.

As Sachs (2003, p. 3) has noted, "in a world of trillions of dollars of income every year, the amount of money that you need to address the health crises is easily available in the world." Scarcity of resources, in any absolute sense, is not the issue. Rather, the issue is one of whether and how resources necessary to meet basic health-related needs will be mobilized rapidly and effectively and distributed equitably. Some movement on this has occurred. The UN High-Level Panel on Financing for Development in 2001 (Zedillo et al., 2001) stressed the need for new sources of development financing, and proposed the establishment of an international tax organization as a starting point for limiting tax competition and evasion. Another initiative, focused on a specific set of policy instruments, is the Leading Group on Solidarity Levies to Fund Development, established at the 2006 Paris Conference on Innovative Development Financing Mechanisms. The second plenary meeting of this group, hosted by Norway in February 2007

(Norwegian Ministry of Foreign Affairs, 2007), considered not only taxes on air travel—already implemented by a number of countries (Farley, 2006; Ministries of the Economy, 2006)—but also research commissioned by the Norwegian Foreign Ministry on a currency transaction development levy (CTDL) (Hillman, Sony, & Spratt, 2006) and on policy options to address tax evasion and tax competition (Murphy, Christensen, Kapoor, Spencer, & Pak, 2007). In 2008, a background note for the United Nations' annual high-level meeting on financing for development noted "renewed international interest in a possible currency-transaction 'development levy' of 0.005 per cent" (United Nations Economic and Social Council, 2008, p. 3). If levied and based on the current estimated daily value of foreign exchange transactions of $3.2 trillion (Chapter 5, this volume), this would generate almost $60 billion a year in new development financing. The Helsinki Process and the Leading Group on Solidarity Levies, in particular, reflect the importance of establishing both new governance mechanisms and new sources of financing for redistributing resources; they also illustrate the range of available opportunities to build important multisectoral linkages both with WHO member governments and with civil society organizations worldwide.

Global political discourse is replete with clichéd references to an international or "global community," even though many political scientists regard such a community only as a utopian ideal. If we take health as one of the shared values that might come to define such a community, then addressing the asymmetrical impacts of globalization on health and the underlying distributions of power and resources they reflect assumes special importance. Two well-known economists have written:

> At the very least . . . those who stand to benefit from the process [of globalization] should be expected to agree to provide systematic and substantial assistance to the victims, presumably via government channels, and supported liberally by the wealthier communities. If that is not acceptable politically, there is surely little that can be said convincingly in support of a contention that the suffering of the victims will be justified by the promised future benefits to their descendants. (Gomory & Baumol, 2004, p. 430)

That assistance, and the commitment to shared values that must drive it, will not be mobilized in the absence of decisive leadership and political action.

NOTES

1. The figure updates a multidimensional earlier description (Sutcliffe, 2005) of global economic inequality based on the most recent World Bank data. It shows the distribution of income based on global income deciles (adjusted for purchasing power) both within and among countries. In the graph, countries have been

allotted a number of rows of columns based on their populations. "So each country gets one row of columns for every 10 million population. That means that the big countries come out about right but the very small ones occupy more space in the graph than in the world"—an unavoidable compromise if the graph is not to have 60,000 rather than 6,000 columns" (B. Sutcliffe, personal communication, March 2007). The graph makes it clear that while intracountry income disparities are dramatic even in some countries that are relatively poor as ranked by income per capita, the commanding heights of the worldwide income distribution are occupied by relatively rich people in rich countries. "The top one-tenth of US citizens now receives a total income equal to that of the poorest 2,200,000,000 citizens in the world" (Sutcliffe, 2005, p. 12).

2. For explication and analysis of policy implications, see World Health Organization, 2003; Mehta & Madsen, 2004, 2005; Mehta, 2005.
3. These obligations are explicated by Chapman, 2002; Nygren-Krug, 2002.
4. "The markets" are an abstraction: their judgment of a country's policies is simply the resource-weighted aggregation of choices made by asset owners and managers with broadly similar interests and motivations, including not only those in London, New York, and Geneva but also an increasing number of rich households in many low- and middle-income countries.
5. For illustrations of the perspectives articulated as part of the process, see Helsinki Process Secretariat, 2005.

REFERENCES

Addison, T., Harper, C., Prowse, M., Shepherd, M., Barrientos, A., Braunholtz-Speight, T., et al. (2008). *The Chronic Poverty Report 2008–09*. Manchester: Chronic Poverty Research Centre. Retrieved from: http://www.chronicpoverty.org/pubfiles/CPR2_whole_report.pdf.

Anonymous. (2007, July 7). Sizzling: The Big Mac index. *The Economist*, p. 82.

Budds, J., & McGranahan, G. (2003). Are the debates on water privatization missing the point? Experiences from Africa, Asia and Latin America. *Environment and Urbanization, 15*, 87–114.

Cashmore, N., Gleick, P., Newcomb, J., Morrison, J., & Harrington, T. (2006). *Remaining drops: Fresh water resources a global issue*. Oakland, CA: CLSA Asia-Pacific Markets. Retrieved from: http://www.pacinst.org/reports/remaining_drops/CLSA_U_remaining_drops.pdf.

Center for Global Development. (2007). *Working group on IMF-supported programs and health spending. Center for Global Development* [online]. Retrieved from: http://www.cgdev.org/section/initiatives/_active/ghprn/workinggroups/imf.

Chapman, A. R. (1993). *Exploring a human rights approach to health care reform*. Washington, DC: Science and Human Rights Program, American Association for the Advancement of Science.

———. (2002). Core obligations related to the right to health. In A. Chapman & S. Russell (eds.), *Core obligations: Building a framework for economic, social and cultural rights* (pp. 185–215). Antwerp: Intersentia.

Collier, P. (2006). Why the WTO is deadlocked: And what can be done about it. *The World Economy, 29*, 1423–49.

Committee on Economic, Social and Cultural Rights (2003). *General comment No. 15: The right to water (arts. 11 and 12 of the International Covenant on Economic, Social and Cultural Rights)*. No. E/C.12/2002/11. United Nations High Commission for Human Rights. Retrieved from: http://www.fao.org/righttofood/kc/downloads/vl/docs/AH355.pdf.

Commission on Macroeconomics and Health. (2001). *Macroeconomics and health: Investing in health for economic development.* Geneva: World Health Organization. Retrieved from: http://www.cid.harvard.edu/cidcmh/CMHReport.pdf.

Commonwealth Heads of Government Meeting on Reform of International Institutions. (2008). Marlborough House Statement on Reform of International Institutions. London: Commonwealth Secretariat.

Deacon, B., Ilva, M., Koivusalo, M., Ollila, E., & Stubbs, P. (2005). *Copenhagen Social Summit ten years on: The need for effective social policies nationally, regionally and globally.* GASPP Policy Briefs No. 6. Helsinki: Globalism and Social Policy Programme, STAKES. Retrieved from: http://gaspp.stakes.fi/NR/rdonlyres/4F9C6B91-94FD-4042-B781-3DB7BB9D7496/0/policybrief6.pdf.

Deaton, A. (2006). Global patterns of income and health. *WIDER Angle, 2,* 1–3.

Farley, M. (2006, June 3). 14 nations will adopt airline tax to pay for AIDS drugs. *Los Angeles Times.*

Freedom from Debt Coalition. (2005). Lessons from a failed privitization experience: The case of the Philippines' metropolitan waterworks and sewerage system (MWSS). Manila: Freedom from Debt Coalition.

Gomory, R. E., & Baumol, W. J. (2004). Globalization: Prospects, promise and problems. *Journal of Policy Modeling, 26,* 425–38.

Grusky, S. (2001). *The World Bank, the International Monetary Fund, and the right to water.* Accra, Ghana: National Forum on Water Privatisation.

Halstead, S. B., Walsh, J. A., & Warren, K. S., eds. (1985). *Good health at low cost.* New York: Rockefeller Foundation.

Helleiner, E. (2001). Regulating capital flight. *Challenge, 44,* 19–34.

Helsinki Process on Globalisation and Democracy. (2007). Ministry for Foreign Affairs of Finland [online]. Retrieved from: http://www.helsinkiprocess.fi/.

Helsinki Process Secretariat, ed. (2005). *Helsinki Process papers on global economic agenda.* Helsinki: Foreign Ministry of Finland.

Hillman, D., Sony, K., & Spratt, S. (2006). *Taking the next step: Implementing a currency transaction development levy.* London: Stamp Out Poverty. Retrieved from: http://www.innovativefinance-oslo.no/pop.cfm?FuseAction=Doc&pAction=View&pDocumentId=11626.

Hunt, P. (2004). *Economic, social and cultural rights: The right of everyone to the enjoyment of the highest attainable standard of physical and mental health—Addendum: Mission to the World Trade Organization.* E/CN.4/2004/49/Add.1. Geneva: United Nations Economic and Social Council Commission on Human Rights. Retrieved from: http://www.unhchr.ch/Huridocda/Huridoca.nsf/e06a53 00f90fa0238025668700518ca4/5860d7d863239d82c1256e660056432a/$FILE/G0411390.pdf.

———. (2007). *Implementation of General Assembly Resolution 60/251 of 15 March 2006 entitled "Human Rights Council": Report of the Special Rapporteur on the right of everyone to the enjoyment of the highest attainable standard of physical and mental health.* No. A/HRC/4/28. Geneva: Office of the United Nations High Commissioner for Human Rights. Retrieved from: http://www.ohchr.org/english/bodies/hrcouncil/docs/4session/A.HRC.4.28.pdf.

Independent Evaluation Office, I. M. F. (2007). *The IMF and aid to sub-Saharan Africa.* Washington, DC: IMF. Retrieved from: http://www.imf.org/external/np/ieo/2007/ssa/eng/pdf/report.pdf.

International Consortium of Investigative Journalists. (2003). *The water barons.* Center for Public Integrity [online]. Retrieved from: http://www.icij.org/water/.

Jaglin, S. (2002). The right to water versus cost recovery: Participation, urban water supply and the poor in sub-Saharan Africa . *Environment and Urbanization, 14,* 231–45.

Labonté, R., Blouin, C., Chopra, M., Lee, K., Packer, C., Rowson, M., et al. (2007). *Towards health-equitable globalization: Rights, regulation and redistribution.* Globalization Knowledge Network Final Report to the Commission on Social Determinants of Health. Ottawa: Institute of Population Health, University of Ottawa. Retrieved from: http://www.who.int/social_determinants/resources/gkn_final_report_042008.pdf.

Labonté, R., Schrecker, T., Sanders, D., & Meeus, W. (2004). *Fatal indifference: The G8, Africa and global health.* Cape Town: University of Cape Town Press.

Lee, K., Koivusalo, M., Ollila, E., Labonté, R., Schrecker, T., Schuftan, C., et al. (2008). *Globalization, global governance and the social determinants of health: A review of the linkages and agenda for action.* Globalization Knowledge Network Papers. Ottawa: Institute of Population Health, University of Ottawa. Retrieved from: http://www.globalhealthequity.ca/electronic%20library/Globalization%20Global%20Governance%20and%20SD%20of%20H.pdf.

Leonhardt, D. (2007, January 12). What $1.2 trillion can buy. *New York Times.*

Loftus, A. J., & McDonald, D. A. (2001). Of liquid dreams: A political ecology of water privatization in Buenos Aires. *Environment and Urbanization*, 13, 179–200.

Mandel, S. (2006). *Debt relief as if people mattered: A rights-based approach to debt sustainability.* London: New Economics Foundation. Retrieved from: http://www.neweconomics.org/gen/z_sys_publicationdetail.aspx?pid=223.

Marmot, M. (2005). Social determinants of health inequalities. *Lancet*, 365, 1099–1104.

McDonald, D. (2002). No money, no service: South Africa's poorest citizens lose out under attempts to recover service costs for water and power. *Alternatives Journal*, 28, 16–20.

McGill, E. (2004). Poverty and social analysis of trade agreements: A more coherent approach? *Boston College International and Comparative Law Review*, 27, 371–427.

Mehta, L. (2005). *Unpacking rights and wrongs: Do human rights make a difference? The case of water rights in India and South Africa.* IDS Working Papers No. 260. Brighton, UK: Institute of Development Studies. Retrieved from: http://www.ntd.co.uk/idsbookshop/details.asp?id=904.

Mehta, L., & Madsen, B. (2004). The General Agreement on Trade in Services (GATS) and poor people's right to water. *IDS Bulletin*, 35, 92–102.

Mehta, L., & Madsen, B. L. (2005). Is the WTO after your water? The General Agreement on Trade in Services (GATS) and poor people's right to water. *Natural Resources Forum*, 29, 154–64.

Ministries of the Economy, Finance and Industry and Foreign Affairs, Government of France. (2006). Solidarity and Globalization: Paris Conference on Innovative Development Financing Mechanisms, 28 February – 1 March 2006. Paris: Government of France.

Murphy, R., Christensen, J., Kapoor, S., Spencer, D., & Pak, S. (2007). *Closing the floodgates: Collecting tax to pay for development.* London: Tax Justice Network. Retrieved from: http://www.innovativefinance-oslo.no/pop.cfm?FuseAction=Doc&pAction=View&pDocumentId=11607.

Norwegian Ministry of Foreign Affairs. (2007). *Leading Group on Solidarity Levies to Fund Development.* Norwegian Ministry of Foreign Affairs [online]. Retrieved from: http://www.innovativefinance-oslo.no/

Nygren-Krug, H. (2002). *25 questions and answers about health and human rights.* Geneva: World Health Organization. Retrieved from: http://www.who.int/entity/hhr/NEW37871OMSOK.pdf.

OECD Development Assistance Committee. (2008). Debt relief is down: Other ODA rises slightly. Organization for Economic Cooperation and Development

[online]. Retrieved from: http://www.oecd.org/document/8/0,3343,en_2649_3
4447_40381960_1_1_1_1,00.html.

Oloka-Onyango, J., & Udagama, D. (2003). *Economic, social and cultural rights:
Globalization and its impact on the full enjoyment of human rights—final
report*. No. E/CN.4/Sub.2/2003/14 Fifty-fifth session Item 4 of the provisional
agenda. Geneva: United Nations Economic and Social Council. Retrieved from:
http://www.unhchr.ch/huridocda/huridoca.nsf/AllSymbols/276821C18F7CDF
F0C1256D780028E74B/$File/G0314784.pdf?OpenElement.

Ooms, G., Van Damme, W., Baker, B. K., Zeitz, P., & Schrecker, T. (2008). The
"diagonal" approach to Global Fund financing: A cure for the broader malaise
of health systems? *Globalization and Health, 4.*

Pogge, T. (2002). Human rights and human responsibilities. In P. De Greiff & C.
Cronin (eds.), *Global justice & transnational politics* (pp. 151–95). Cambridge,
MA: MIT Press.

———. (2005). Human rights and global health: A research program. *Metaphi-
losophy, 36*, 182–209.

Public Services International Research Unit. (2006). *Pipe dreams: The failure of the
private sector to invest in developing countries.* Greenwich, UK: World Development Movement.

Rodriguez, M. A. (1987). Consequences of capital flight for Latin American debtor
countries. In D. R. Lessard & J. Williamson (eds.), *Capital flight and third world
debt* (pp. 129–52). Washington, DC: Institute for International Economics.

Ruger, J. P. (2006). Ethics and governance of global health inequalities. *Journal of
Epidemiology and Community Health, 60*, 998–1002.

Sachs, J. (2003). *Achieving the Millennium Development Goals: Health in the
developing world.* Speech at the Second Global Consultation of the Commission on Macroeconomics and Health. Geneva: World Health Organization.
Retrieved from: http://www.earthinstitute.columbia.edu/about/director/pubs/
CMHSpeech102903.pdf.

Say, L., Inoue, M., Mills, S., & Suzuki, E. (2007). *Maternal mortality in 2005: Esti-
mates developed by WHO, UNICEF, UNFPA, and the World Bank.* Geneva:
Department of Reproductive Health and Research, World Health Organization.
Retrieved from: http://www.unfpa.org/publications/detail.cfm?ID=343.

Singh, J. A., Govender, M., & Mills, E. J. (2007). Do human rights matter to
health? *The Lancet, 370*, 521–27.

Solar, O., & Irwin, A. (2007). *A conceptual framework for action on the social
determinants of health.* Geneva: Commission on Social Determinants of Health,
World Health Organization. Retrieved from: http://www.who.int/entity/social_
determinants/resources/csdh_framework_action_05_07.pdf.

Sutcliffe, B. (2005). *A converging or diverging world?* ST/ESA/2005/DWP/2,
DESA Working Paper Series No. 2. New York: United Nations Department of
Economic and Social Affairs.

UN Millennium Project. (2005). *Investing in development: A practical plan to achieve
the Millennium Development Goals.* London: Earthscan. Retrieved from: http://
www.unmillenniumproject.org/documents/MainReportComplete-lowres.pdf.

United Nations Committee on Economic, Social and Cultural Rights. (2000). General Comment 14: The right to the highest attainable standard of health. Geneva:
United Nations High Commission for Human Rights.

United Nations Economic and Social Council. (2008). *Coherence, coordination
and cooperation in the context of the implementation of the Monterrey Consensus, including new challenges and emerging issues (note by the Secretary-
General).* Prepared for special high-level meeting of the Economic and Social
Council with the Bretton Woods Institutions, the World Trade Organization
and the United Nations Conference on Trade and Development, 14 April 2008.

No. E/2008/7. New York: United Nations. Retrieved from: http://daccess-ods. un.org/access.nsf/Get?OpenAgent&DS=E/2008/7&Lang=E.

Woodward, D., & Simms, A. (2006). *Growth isn't working: The unbalanced distribution of benefits and costs from economic growth.* London: New Economics Foundation. Retrieved from: http://www.neweconomics.org/NEF070625/ NEF_Registration070625add.aspx?returnurl=/gen/uploads/hrfu5w555mzd3f-55m2vqwty502022006112929.pdf.

World Bank. (1999). *World Development Report 1999/2000: Entering the 21st century.* New York: Oxford University Press. Retrieved from: http:// go.worldbank.org/YH54DW4WS0.

World Commission on the Social Dimension of Globalization. (2004). *A fair globalization: Creating opportunities for all.* Geneva: International Labour Organization. Retrieved from: http://www.ilo.org/public/english/wcsdg/docs/ report.pdf.

World Health Organization. (2003). *The right to water.* Geneva: WHO. Retrieved from: http://www.who.int/docstore/water_sanitation_health/Documents/right-towater/righttowater.pdf.

World Health Organization/UNICEF Joint Monitoring Programme for Water Supply and Sanitation. (2008). *Progress on drinking water and sanitation: Special focus on sanitation.* New York and Geneva: UNICEF. Retrieved from: http:// www.unicef.org/media/files/Joint_Monitoring_Report_-_17_July_2008.pdf.

Zedillo, E., Al-Hamad, A. Y., Bryer, D., Chinery-Hesse, M., Delors, J., Grynstpan, R., et al. (2001). *Recommendations of the High-Level Panel on Financing for Development.* No. A/55/1000 . New York: United Nations.

14 Globalization, Social Determinants, and the Struggle for Health

David Sanders

Over the past half century the global health situation has significantly improved in aggregate terms, with a continuous rise in life expectancy, albeit at slowing rates in the past two decades and with sharp reversals in the former Soviet Union and sub-Saharan Africa. The change in the pattern of disease from one where premature mortality is at high levels and communicable diseases predominate to one where premature mortality declines and noncommunicable causes account for the great majority of morbidity and mortality is referred to as the "health transition." *Transition*, however, is a somewhat misleading term since, in many low- and middle-income countries (LMICs), a pattern has emerged in which communicable diseases persist as significant contributors to overall disease burden, especially in poor communities, but coexist with high levels of noncommunicable diseases, including violent injury (Frenk, Bobadilla, Sepulveda, & Lopez Cervantes, 1989). Moreover, it is rapidly growing inequalities in health status indicators between and within countries that uniquely characterize the current global situation.

The relatively recent emergence of dual (or triple) burdens of disease can be traced to various determinants associated with processes of globalization analyzed in this volume. Rural environmental degradation and the accompanying pauperization of LMIC rural communities are resulting in accelerating squalid urbanization; these processes underlie the persistence of communicable diseases as prominent causes of morbidity and mortality, especially among young children. Greatly increased and liberalized trade has accelerated the penetration of "obesogenic" (processed, high-fat, high-sugar, high-salt) diets. Increased sedentariness and the spread of global "bads" (e.g., tobacco, alcohol, and habit-forming drugs), together with insecure employment associated with increased labor-market flexibility, largely explain the rise of noncommunicable diseases, including mental ill health, as well as the escalation of injuries, especially in poor communities. Globalization, with increased and accelerated movement of humans and animals (and animal products) and more porous borders, is also facilitating the rapid spread of both old communicable diseases such as cholera and TB and new ones such as HIV, SARS, and avian influenza.

Trade is just one of the dimensions of globalization that has a big impact on (especially poor) countries' abilities to implement healthy public policies. Amongst other important factors undermining equitable economic growth—and health—are unregulated financial flows ("hot money") and corporate and individual tax evasion. Disinvestment by states in social provisioning has been a feature of neoliberal policies, and, with promotion of the private sector and stagnating or "verticalized" development assistance, public sectors have been considerably weakened in many places, often resulting in tiered and fragmented health care systems.

Although they influence health outcomes significantly, the majority of social determinants of health (SDH) are beyond the reach of policy instruments available to health ministries, with responsibility residing in other government departments (e.g., trade, commerce, finance, etc.) or, increasingly, with global bodies such as the World Trade Organization. Policy space for health is further influenced by both real and presumed shifts of power associated with globalization, which constrain the kind of action that can be taken with respect to health and SDH (Chapter 5, this volume). The development of policy and allocation of resources by LMIC health sectors themselves is also significantly constrained by the fact that health care resources are increasingly controlled by remote, often global institutions dominated by the wealthy donor countries, such as the World Bank, the Global Fund, and the U.S. President's Emergency Plan for AIDS Relief (PEPFAR). Thus, the formulation and implementation of public policies that might address SDH are influenced not only by national power arrangements, but are increasingly circumscribed by factors that derive from global economic structures and geopolitical relationships. This is especially the case for poor countries whose health needs are profound and urgent and whose bargaining power in (especially the new) international bodies is relatively weak.

As is noted in the chapter on global governance, this situation—of limitations on countries' ability to implement policies that address SDH—is aggravated by the fact that "efforts to improve coherence and coordination (in health cooperation) have been hindered foremost by the absence of any overarching authority in global governance above sovereign states. Key institutional actors concerned with global governance operate largely independently of one another, formally accountable to certain constituencies such as powerful donor governments, but not to a higher level of authority" (Chapter 12, this volume). Notwithstanding its formal status as the key health governance structure, deriving from its accountability to and representation of its member states, WHO's weakened independence and authority starkly reflect its declining regular budget, over which it has discretionary control, and its simultaneous increasing dependence on donor funding, which now accounts for over two-thirds of its total spending. "Within each type of institution, there is a greater concentration of power in fewer hands at the global level" (Chapter 12, this volume).

The preceding challenges require actions that ameliorate underlying national and global social determinants of (ill) health, ensure greater equity in access to sustainable health systems, and assist in the rebuilding of public health capacity in poor countries.

Considerable historical evidence indicates the importance of power and politics in influencing the emergence of policies that have resulted in health improvement. The health historian Simon Szreter underlines the disruptive influence that the rapid economic change that occurred during the Industrial Revolution in Britain had on population health, in particular affecting those living in the poor, unplanned settlements of the manufacturing and rapidly growing cities. Although his analysis is limited to the situation in British towns in the nineteenth century, important policy lessons can be drawn. Relevant to currently dominant neoliberal policies that prioritize economic growth above all else and reduce the size and role of the state, Szreter notes: "A discriminating evaluation of the historical evidence indicates . . . that without a strongly interventionist role for local government, supported with the resources of the central state, economic growth will seriously compromise population health" (Szreter, 2003, p. 428). He further observes, with reference to the British experience: "[w]hile economic growth may be necessary, it is never a sufficient condition for improved population health. . . . Significant health improvements only began to appear when the increasing political voice and self-organization of the growing urban masses finally made itself heard, increasingly gaining actual voting power from the late 1860s onwards (a process not completed until 1928)." Support from sections of the new urban elite "snowballed into a social movement. Recognizing the need for an extensive program of investment in municipal health amenities and social services, this new generation of civic leaders devised new sources of funding from the massive revenues of local utility monopolies" (Szreter, 2003, p. 424).

More recent evidence for the role of power, politics, and policies—and confirming Szreter's analysis—comes from a number of poor developing countries, the *Good Health at Low Cost* examples (described in a 1985 Rockefeller Foundation report) of Sri Lanka, Costa Rica, and Kerala State in India (Halstead, Walsh, & Warren, 1985). These territories demonstrate that investment by the state in the social sectors, and particularly in women's education, health, and welfare, has a significant positive impact on the health and social indicators of the whole population. These examples provide further evidence that a strong, organized demand for government responsiveness and accountability to social needs is crucial in securing healthy public policies. Recognition of this important dynamic informed the call at the Alma-Ata Conference on Primary Health Care in 1978 for strong community participation. A process of social mobilization involving broad civil society, which may take different forms in different contexts, is essential to achieve and sustain such political will. Analysts have noted that political commitment to greater social equity was achieved in Costa

Rica through a long history of egalitarian principles and democracy, in Kerala through agitation by disadvantaged political groups, and through social revolution in China. "Strong" community participation is important not only in securing greater government responsiveness to social needs but also in providing an active, conscious and organized population so critical to the design, implementation and sustainability of comprehensive health systems (Sanders, 2000).

More recently, significant gains in health system development and health outcomes have been achieved in countries such as Brazil, which has successfully pursued relatively autonomous economic development and implemented national social—including health—policies that differ markedly from those promoted as part of mainstream health sector reform. In Brazil over the past approximately fifteen years there has been sustained and significant investment in the creation of a universal health system, the centerpiece of which is the Family Health Programme (Macinko, de Souza, Guanais, & da Silva Simoes, 2007). While this is mostly directed at providing more accessible and equitable health services, particularly at the primary level, it also engages community health workers who identify in their localities social factors that negatively affect health status and enroll other sectors in addressing them. The political context of Brazil's reforms dates back to the late 1980s, when popular mobilization gained momentum against a conservative government with strong promarket policies. Such popular mobilization has waned somewhat over the past decade, but social engagement in local government remains active and is structured through such bodies as the National Health Council, which plays an ongoing role in democratizing policy development.

The above are examples—historical and current—of the interplay between popular struggle and responsiveness of national governments in developing equitable social policies and securing health gains. There are, however, many instances of struggles of civil society, both within and outside the health sector, which, without necessarily achieving fundamental and coordinated government policy change, have nonetheless catalyzed national and sometimes global health gains by successfully addressing key SDH through securing policy change in specific areas.

One of the best-known recent cases relates to the legal battle around the attempt by South Africa to secure pharmaceuticals for HIV/AIDS at a reduced cost. In 1997 Nelson Mandela's government approved a law aimed at lowering drug prices through "parallel importing"—that is, importing drugs from countries where they are sold at lower prices—and "compulsory licensing," which would allow local companies to manufacture certain patented drugs in exchange for royalties. Both provisions are legal under the TRIPS agreement as all sides agreed that HIV/AIDS is an emergency. This was confirmed during the WTO meeting in Doha in 2001. The US administration did not bring its case to the WTO but instead, acting in concert with the multinational pharmaceutical corporations, brought a number of pressures (e.g., threats of trade sanctions and legal action) to bear on the South African government to rescind the legislation. This followed similar successful threats against Thailand and Bangladesh. However, a vigorous campaign mounted by local and international AIDS activists and progressive health NGOs and an uncompromising South African government forced a climbdown by both the US government and the multinational pharmaceutical companies (Bond, 1999).

Another important recent example of civil society activism that catalyzed far-reaching policy change that indirectly impacts on health equity is the campaign against the Multilateral Agreement on Investment (MAI). The Association for the Taxation of Financial Transaction for the Aid of Citizens (ATTAC) was founded in France in 1998 to mobilize support for the Tobin tax on currency transactions as part of a broader movement against inequitable globalization. ATTAC, which has now established itself in many countries, played a leading role in France's decision to withdraw from OECD talks on the MAI, resulting in the failure of the talks, and later to rejection by the French electorate of the proposed EU Constitution in a 2005 referendum (Waters, 2004).

While actions explicitly aimed at securing policy change are often viewed as "political" and somehow the province only of "activists," it can be argued that they fall squarely within the domain of public health practice. Public health is defined by Satcher and Higginbotham as ". . . what we as a society do collectively, to assure the conditions for people to be healthy" (Satcher & Higginbotham, 2008). These authors note the integral location of social determinants of health at the heart of achieving such conditions, but emphasize the related imperative to remove disparities in health (by which they presumably mean health care) provision. The potential roles of those who identify themselves as operating within this broad remit of public health will vary with different contexts, but will consist mainly of a combination of research and advocacy: the likelihood of these activities securing policy advances depends on a number of factors, but ultimately on the extent to which broad social forces are mobilized around the issues of concern.

Given the current health situation and its context, research should give priority to a focus on underlying determinants of health at both local and global levels (Sanders, Labonté, Baum, & Chopra, 2004). Labonté and Spiegel argue that such research should attempt to link local phenomena to globalization processes that influence local possibilities (Labonté & Spiegel, 2003). The constituencies affected should, wherever possible, be involved in such research, and the findings used in increasing their awareness of the need for and necessary content of policy change. The Global Equity Gauge Alliance (GEGA), initiated in 2002, was conceived as an active approach of research to action to bring about sustained reductions in inequities in health and health care. The approach involves three interrelated processes: assessment and monitoring, advocacy, and community empowerment. It has been successfully adopted in different countries by several GEGA initiatives which have identified key local SDH and, in some cases, demonstrated the links to policies and relationships operating at a national or supranational level (Scott, Stern, Sanders, Reagon, & Matthews, 2008).

In response to growing global inequalities, the past decade has seen the emergence of a growing "antiglobalization" movement, epitomized by the World Social Forum, which draws large numbers of organizations and individuals to its annual gatherings. As part of this global social movement, the People's Health Movement (PHM) was formed in late 2000 to combat the economic and political causes of deepening inequalities in health worldwide. The PHM (www.phmovement.org), now present in about eighty countries, is a large global civil society network of grassroots health workers, activist academics and researchers, and concerned citizens supportive of the WHO policy of Health for All. It organizes to combat the economic and political causes of deepening inequalities in health worldwide and calls for a return to the principles of Primary Health Care (PHC) launched as global health policy at the Alma-Ata conference in 1978. The PHM recognizes that inequality, poverty, exploitation, violence, and injustice are at the root of ill health and the premature deaths of poor and marginalized people. Its vision is expressed in the People's Charter for Health, now published in approximately forty languages. At its second People's Health Assembly in Ecuador in 2005, attended by over 1,400 people, PHM committed to a global Right to Health and Healthcare campaign (RTHHC). This campaign involves coordinated national and international level action for time-bound, progressive implementation of the right to health, a key focus being on the local and global SDH.

PHM, together with Medact and the Global Equity Gauge Alliance, coordinates the production of Global Health Watch (GHW), a critical report on global health. Its primary aim is to report critically on the state of global health and initiatives to address it. GHW provides an analysis that stresses the social, economic, and political determinants of ill health. It attempts to ensure that the health professional and policy community as well as civil society are better informed about these issues. GHW offers itself as a tool for strengthening public accountability and public health institutions in an attempt to ensure that, at both the national and global level, they are governed in ways that are fair and transparent, and adequately capacitated to promote and protect health.

This volume has assembled compelling evidence of the fundamental—and growing—influence of globalization as a social determinant of health outcomes and health equity. Hopefully, it has enhanced the reader's understanding of the global health situation and its increasingly complex set of determinants. This brief reflective chapter has attempted to convey the understanding that challenging current power imbalances is fundamental to ameliorating social determinants of health inequity. To paraphrase Marx: public health researchers and policymakers now have a better understanding of social determinants of health; the point, however, is to change them.

REFERENCES

Bond, P. (1999). Globalization, pharmaceutical pricing, and South African health policy: Managing confrontation with U.S. firms and politicians. *International Journal of Health Services, 29*, 765–92.
Frenk, J., Bobadilla, J. L., Sepulveda, J., & Lopez Cervantes, M. (1989). Health transition in middle-income countries: New challenges for health care. *Health Policy and Planning, 4*, 29–39.
Halstead, S. B., Walsh, J. A., & Warren, K. S., eds. (1985). *Good health at low cost.* New York: Rockefeller Foundation.
Labonté, R., & Spiegel, J. (2003). Setting global health research priorities. *British Medical Journal, 326*, 722–23.
Macinko, J., de Souza, M., Guanais, F., & da Silva Simoes, C. (2007). Going to scale with community-based primary care: An analysis of the family health program and infant mortality in Brazil, 1999–2004. *Social Science and Medicine, 65*, 2070–80.
Sanders, D. (2000). *PHC 21—Everybody's Business.* Main background paper for the Meeting: PHC 21—Everybody's Business, an international meeting to celebrate 20 years after Alma-Ata, Almaty, Kazakhstan, 27–28 November 1998, WHO/EIP/OSD/00.7. Geneva: World Health Organization.
Sanders, D., Labonté, R., Baum, F., & Chopra, M. (2004). Making research matter: A civil society perspective on health research. *Bulletin of the World Health Organization, 82*, 757–63.
Satcher, D., & Higginbotham, E. H. (2008). The public health approach to eliminating disparities in health. *American Journal of Public Health, 98*, 400–3.
Scott, V., Stern, R., Sanders, D., Reagon, G., & Matthews, V. (2008). Research to action to address inequities: The experience of the Cape Town Equity Gauge. *International Journal for Equity in Health, 7*.
Szreter, S. (2003). The population health approach in historical perspective. *American Journal of Public Health, 93*, 421–31.
Waters, S. (2004). Mobilising against globalisation: ATTAC and the French Intellectuals. *West European Politics, 27*, 854–74.

Contributors

Aniket Bhushan is a researcher at the North-South Institute. His work focuses on international trade and includes a primer on international trade commitments and human rights obligations; trade liberalisation and social protections strategies in developing countries and an assessment of the impact of the end of the multifiber agreement. He holds an MA in political science from Carleton University, Ottawa.

Chantal Blouin is Senior Research Associate at the Centre for Trade Policy and Law, the Norman Paterson School of International Affairs, Carleton University, Ottawa. She is also one of the Canadian International Council's Inaugural Senior Fellowship recipients. Her recent publications include *International Trade in Health Services and the GATS* (World Bank, 2006) and *Trade and Health: Seeking Common Ground* (McGill-Queen's University Press, 2008). She holds a PhD in political science from the University of Toronto.

Patrick Bond is Director of the Centre for Civil Society, University of Kwa-Zulu-Natal (UKZN). His many books for UKZN Press and Zed Books include several that deal with globalization, environment and health. He received his PhD in 1993 from the Johns Hopkins University Department of Geography and Environmental Engineering.

Mickey Chopra is Director, Health Systems Research Unit, Medical Research Council, South Africa. He is a medical doctor with postgraduate qualifications in public health and child health. He has worked for fifteen years in South Africa, first as a district medical officer, where he established an innovative child health and nutrition program. He then taught and conducted research at the School of Public Health, University of the Western Cape, with a particular focus upon primary health care approaches towards maternal and child health. More recently he has taken over a research unit that specializes in broader health systems improvements working from the policy level down to implementation in communities. He has published over sixty international peer-reviewed papers and contributed to numerous book chapters concerned with international child health and nutrition.

Giovanni Andrea Cornia is Professor of Economics at the University of Florence since 2001. Prior to this position, he was the director of UNU-WIDER based in Helsinki and held several research position in the UN and the private sector. His research has mainly focused on macroeconomics, inequality, poverty, health and well-being, and the transition to the market economy.

Carlos M. Correa is Director of the Center for Interdisciplinary Studies on Industrial Property and Economics and of the Post-graduate Course on Intellectual Property at the Law Faculty, University of Buenos Aires. He has been a visiting professor in postgraduate courses of several universities and consultant to UNCTAD, UNIDO, UNDP, WHO, FAO, IDB, INTAL, World Bank, SELA, ECLA, UNDP, South Centre, and other regional and international organizations. He has advised several governments on intellectual property and innovation policy. He was a member of the UK Commission on Intellectual Property and of the Commission on Intellectual Property, Innovation and Public Health established by the World Health Assembly. He is the author of several books and numerous articles.

Sharon Friel is a social and nutritional epidemiologist and has worked in the area of public health nutrition and inequalities in health since 1992. She is Principal Research Fellow for the global Commission on Social Determinants of Health, International Institute for Society and Health, University College London, and a Fellow at the National Centre for Epidemiology and Population Health at the Australian National University, Canberra.

Corinna Hawkes is a freelance consultant and visiting research fellow, Centre for Food Policy, City University, London. Her research interests lie in developing policies to address the global shift towards unhealthy diets, overweight/obesity, and diet-related chronic diseases, with a specific focus on actions that can be taken throughout the food supply chain in the context of globalization. She is author of numerous articles and reports on food policy issues.

Meri Koivusalo is a medical doctor by training with a PhD in public health epidemiology, appointed to the National Research and Development Centre for Welfare and Health, Helsinki, Finland. She has during the last ten years worked in particular on global social and health policy issues, including globalization, commercialization, trade, and health policies. She has published broadly in the area and also provided policy advice for local and national governments, international agencies (WHO, EU, UN/DESA), and nongovernmental organizations. She is an editor of the scientific journal *Global Social Policy*.

Ronald Labonté is Canada Research Chair, Globalization and Health Equity (Institute of Population Health) and Professor, Faculty of Medicine, University of Ottawa. He chaired the GKN for the WHO Commission on Social Determinants of Health. Professor Labonté has written extensively on issues of health promotion, public health, community development, quality of life, and all aspects of globalization and health. He has authored or edited fourteen books, over 125 scientific articles, forty book chapters and two hundred monographs, technical reports, and non-peer-reviewed articles.

Kelley Lee is Reader in global health and co-director of the WHO Collaborating Centre on Global Change and Health at the London School of Hygiene and Tropical Medicine. She is a Fellow through Distinction of the Faculty of Public Health of the Royal Colleges of Physicians of the United Kingdom. Her research focuses on the impacts of globalization on communicable and noncommunicable diseases, and the implications for global governance. She is the author and coauthor of over sixty articles, thirty book chapters, and seven books on global health.

John Lister is a journalist who has been Principal Policy Researcher for London Health Emergency for twenty-four years, working with health unions and campaigners at national and local levels and writing for many publications on a wide variety of policy issues, including mental health, care of older people, various forms of privatization, and the Private Finance Initiative, as well as two books on the history of the British National Health Service. Building on analysis of the ongoing market style "reforms" in Britain, he completed his doctoral thesis on global health policy reform in 2004, which was subsequently published as a book, now in its second edition. As an Associate Senior Lecturer, he leads an MA module on Health Policy, and also teaches journalism (including health journalism) at Coventry University, UK.

Eeva Ollila is a medical doctor specializing in public health medicine and an adjunct professor. She is also Senior Researcher at the National Research and Development Centre for Welfare and Health in Finland. Combining practical experience and research, she currently works as ministerial advisor in the Ministry of Social Affairs and Health in Finland, holding responsibility for international health policies. She has previously worked for the WHO and the European Commission. Her main research areas are global health policy and the implications of globalization on national health policy.

Corinne Packer is Research Associate, Institute of Population Health, University of Ottawa. She has authored two books on reproductive health and international human rights law and was associate editor of a volume on humanitarian assistance. She has written numerous articles and book chapters on diverse subjects such as on the migration of health professionals, the African Union, Roma women and public health care, and national policies in the field of equality between women and men.

Stefano Rosignoli earned his degree in statistics from the University of Florence. He is currently a researcher at IRPET (Istituto Regionale Programmagione Economica della Toscana) where he works on databases and econometric estimates.

Michael Rowson is a freelance writer on international health issues, former executive director of Medact, a teaching fellow at the Centre for International Health and Development at University College London, and one of the editors of the first "Alternative World Health Report," *Global Health Watch 2006–2007* (Zed Books).

Vivien Runnels is a PhD student in population health at the University of Ottawa in Ontario, Canada, and one of the research associates involved with the Globalization Knowledge Network. Her previous employment has included research coordination and rehabilitation counseling. She has contributed a number of articles to professional journals in disability-related issues and vocational rehabilitation. Her research interests include: social exclusion issues such as homelessness, food insecurity, and disability; rehabilitation and work; breastfeeding; governance of community-based research, and knowledge translation.

David Sanders is founding professor and Director of the School of Public Health at the University of the Western Cape, South Africa. He is a pediatrician qualified also in public health. He has over twenty-five years' experience in health policy development in Zimbabwe and South Africa, having advised governments and UN agencies in primary health care, child health and nutrition, and health human resources. He has published extensively in these fields and on the politics of health, including three books. In 2004–2005 he was Heath Clark Lecturer at the London School of Hygiene and Tropical Medicine. He is on the Global Steering Council of the People's Health Movement and a managing editor of Global Health Watch.

Ted Schrecker is Principal Scientist, Institute of Population Health, and associate professor, Faculty of Medicine, University of Ottawa. A political scientist by background, he coordinated the GKN for the WHO Commission on Social Determinants of Health and has written extensively on issues of environmental health, health ethics, urban health, and all aspects of globalisation and health.

Claudio Schuftan is a medical doctor currently based in Ho Chi Minh City, Viet Nam, where he works as a freelance consultant in public health and nutrition. Dr. Schuftan is the author of two books, several book chapters, over fifty scholarly articles published in refereed journals plus over two hundred other assorted publications. Since 1976, he has carried out over one hundred consulting assignments in fifty countries. He is currently an active member of the Steering Group of the People's Health Movement (PHM) and coordinates PHM's global Right to Health Campaign.

Sebastian Taylor is Senior Research Fellow in the Department of Epidemiology and Public Health at University College London. His academic work is in development economics and in the ethnography of international development institutions. For over fifteen years, he has managed and consulted on aid programs, primarily in rural development and health, in East, Southeast and South Asia, the Middle East, and East and West Africa.

Luca Tiberti is completing doctoral studies in development economics at the University of Florence. His PhD thesis examines the poverty alleviation impact of income transfers to AIDS-affected orphans in South Africa.

David Woodward is an independent consultant on development, author of *Debt, Adjustment and Poverty in Developing Countries* (Pinter, 1992) and *The Next Crisis?* (Zed, 2001), and coeditor of *Global Public Goods for Health* (OUP, 2003). He has previously worked as an economist for WHO and the Foreign and Commonwealth Office, among others.

Index

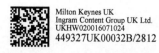
Milton Keynes UK
Ingram Content Group UK Ltd.
UKHW020016071024
449327UK00032B/2812